Healing Relational
Trauma Workbook

ADVANCE PRAISE

"Hughes and Golding's *Healing Relational Trauma Workbook* is a brilliant and essential guide that caters to both seasoned clinicians and novices, presenting a pragmatic and meticulous manual on how to bring the latest in neuroscience and attachment into the therapy room with children and families. Packed with scripts, case examples, and reflective exercises, this masterful resource revolutionizes DDP by embracing diverse cultural perspectives and intersectionality. Unprecedented in its integrative approach, this book is the ultimate compendium to fostering profound and healing connections for traumatized children."

—LETICIA GRACIA, MSW, founding director, Institute of Childhood Trauma and Attachment

"This workbook offers a valuable experience. Along with the helpful review of DDP, instructive dialogue examples, and grounded cultural integration and discussion, practitioners will feel safe as they are invited to reflect on and learn from their experience as a person and practitioner. The reflections and worksheets create a synchronous experience for the practitioner as DDP intends for children and carers; mentalizing abilities and confidence in working with families will grow as a result."

—ALLEN SABEY, PhD, clinical assistant professor and licensed marriage and family therapist, The Family Institute at Northwestern University

"Kim Golding and Dan Hughes risked personal vulnerability by looking inward to sensitive truths while reaching out to find voices unlike theirs. As I read, the same journey was asked of me. I think this is really what DDP is. This is an important step in making intersectionality, community, and uniqueness a way of learning DDP."

—BENJAMIN HARGRAVE, independent therapeutic social worker, practitioner in DDP, EFT, and systemic practice, member of the DDPI Global Development Committee, and cochair of the DDPI Worldwide Board of Directors

Healing Relational Trauma Workbook

DYADIC DEVELOPMENTAL PSYCHOTHERAPY IN PRACTICE

Daniel A. Hughes | Kim S. Golding

Norton Professional Books

An Imprint of W. W. Norton & Company
Independent Publishers Since 1923

This book is intended as a general information resource for professionals practicing in the field of psychotherapy and mental health. It is not a substitute for appropriate training or clinical supervision. Standards of clinical practice and protocol vary in different practice settings and change over time. No technique or recommendation is guaranteed to be safe or effective in all circumstances, and neither the publisher nor the authors can guarantee the complete accuracy, efficacy, or appropriateness of any particular recommendation in every respect or in all settings or circumstances. All case subjects and dialogues described in this book are composites.

The patients and their courses of treatment described in this book are either composites or entirely fictional. Some names of participating therapists have been changed. Any URLs displayed in this book link or refer to websites that existed as of press time. The publisher is not responsible for, and should not be deemed to endorse or recommend, any website, app, or other content that it did not create. The authors, also, are not responsible for any third-party material.

For information about permission to reproduce selections from this book, write to Permissions, W. W. Norton & Company, Inc., 500 Fifth Avenue, New York, NY 10110

For information about special discounts for bulk purchases, please contact W. W. Norton Special Sales at specialsales@wwnorton.com or 800-233-4830

Manufacturing by Versa Press
Book design by Jen Montgomery
Production manager: Gwen Cullen

ISBN: 978-1-324-03058-4 (pbk)

W. W. Norton & Company, Inc., 500 Fifth Avenue, New York, NY 10110
www.wwnorton.com

W. W. Norton & Company Ltd., 15 Carlisle Street, London W1D 3BS

1 2 3 4 5 6 7 8 9 0

Dan and Kim dedicate this book to the global DDP community, past, present, and future.

CONTENTS

ACKNOWLEDGMENTS

This workbook is a companion to *Healing Relational Trauma With Attachment-Focused Interventions*, written with Julie Hudson. Our aim in both books is to help dyadic developmental psychotherapy (DDP) practitioners to develop the skills they use in their DDP practice with families touched by developmental trauma. DDP includes providing psychotherapy, parenting support, and practice support for schools, social workers and networks. We have learned much through our supervision, training, and support of DDP practitioners and wish to acknowledge that our wisdom is enhanced by what DDP practitioners have shared with us.

In writing this book, we, Dan and Kim, have listened to the many colleagues who are asking us to make DDP more relevant to clients and practitioners who live with marginalization and oppression. We have endeavored to go further in our exploration of intersectionality than we have gone before. While this has involved us in our own work through reading, training, and self-reflection, we could not have done this without the inspiration and support of others. We acknowledge the generous time given to us by Georgia Cooper, Nneamaka Edebuisi, Julie Hudson, Ben Hargrave, Delroy Madden, Randy Maldonado, Gill Maxwell, Shani Sephton, Elizabeth Studwell, Hannah Sun-Reid, and Cambell Plant. We hope we have come close to doing justice to the wisdom they have offered to us. Mistakes and omissions are, of course, our own. We will keep listening and learning.

We would also like to thank those who took part in our "In Conversation" features, contributing their lived-experience to our reflections. These conversations are interspersed throughout this workbook, and the contributors are named. We also thank Amber Elliott, Sally Moffatt, Mikenda Plant, and Hannah Sun-Reid for putting us in touch with some of these people.

We have always appreciated the support of colleagues from across the DDP community, and especially those who give time and energy to the development of DDP. Naming some of these people risks omitting many, but we wish to mention Betty Brouwer, Anna Binnie-Dawson, Leila Caston, Joy Gamble, Edwina Grant, Alison Keith, Marie Kershaw, Dafna Lender, Mervin Maier, Philip McAleese, Grey McKellar, Brandon Mock, Sez Morse, Sian Phillips, Courtney Rennicke, Ben Gurney-Smith, Billy Smythe Vicky Sutton, George Thompson, and Liz Tower.

We would also like to acknowledge the great work going into the development of DDP globally, with special mention to our colleagues in Australia, China, Czech Republic, Cayman Islands, Estonia, Finland, Lithuania, Netherlands, New Zealand, and Singapore.

Finally, thanks to those at Norton who have supported this book and offered advice when needed.

Dan Hughes and Kim Golding
January 2023

Healing Relational Trauma Workbook

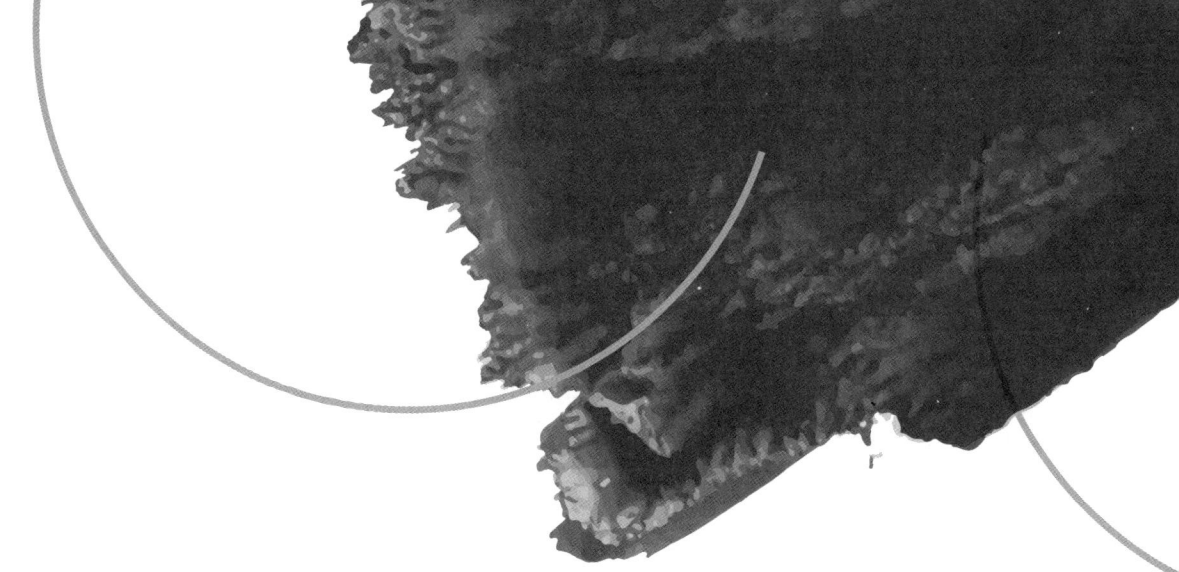

Chapter 1:
Introduction: From Traumatic to Developmental Relationships

DDP is about creating new stories. Traumatic events strike against our minds and hearts and create a story that is fragmented by gaps and is distorted by strong emotions from which the child shrinks and hides. These stories are rigid, with meanings given to the child by the one abusing [them] From these jagged stories of shame and terror that arose from relational trauma, DDP [creates] stories of connection, strength, and resilience. (Hughes et al., 2019, p. 7)

REFRESHER

Relationships are at the heart of DDP.

Relationships are embedded in infants' development, from the moments of conception and birth through the countless challenges and opportunities that they encounter and long into adulthood and old age. Just as relationships are crucial for the child's development, similarly they are crucial to the value of DDP.

In daily life, the shared experience of child and parent become synchronized and leave an impact on both. The same is true in DDP. The intersubjective stance of the DDP practitioner enables the child to integrate the practitioner's regulated, affective presence and remain regulated themselves as they explore stressful themes. The practitioner's discoveries of the child's challenges and strengths allow these experiences to become vital, emerging, aspects of the child's developing sense of self.

When the child meets the DDP practitioner, the child brings to the interaction a sense of self and a life story that is often disorganized and full of shame, doubt, hopelessness, and mistrust. With the practitioner's discoveries of other aspects of the child, a new story begins to unfold. This is a story of trust, resilience, and hope.

DDP practitioners have a complex task. They need to attend to their immediate experience of the child, caregivers, and themself while also synchronizing interactions occurring between themself and the child's emerging story. At the same time, the practitioner needs to be aware of their own past relational experiences and their influence on the present experiences with the child. All the while, the practitioner must stay regulated and ensure that the child is able to remain or to regain their own regulation.

How is the practitioner able to do all this at once?

- By ensuring that their own attachment history is resolved
- By discovering qualities in the child that they can resonate with
- By cocreating the child's emerging story, and allowing it to guide the practitioner's mind and heart

The DDP practitioner uses affective and reflective functioning throughout their engagement with the child. The practitioner's affective functioning is consistently regulated in the child's presence and is sensitively responsive to the child's affective regulation. With the first awareness of any dysregulation in the child, the practitioner focuses on coregulating the child's affective state.

Only when the child is able to remain regulated can the practitioner explore with them the experiences that they are attending to. The practitioner joins with the child in a process of discovering the meaning of the events being explored. Through their joint exploration they are cocreating a new story. This is the heart

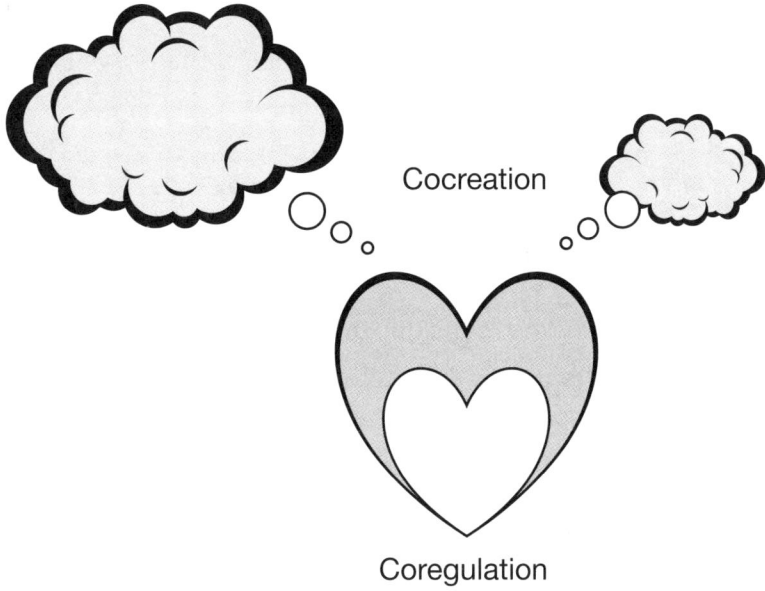

Figure 1.1 Intersubjective Experience

of the intersubjective experiences occurring between the child and the DDP practitioner. While their affective states are being coregulated when needed, the practitioner and child are cocreating a new story—a story that is healing, integrative, and transforming.

THERE IS MORE TO TRAUMA THAN TRAUMA

Traumatic events are a reality in a person's life. The same objective event, experienced by two individuals, may elicit different, equally valid subjective realities. This goes far beyond the specific event.

- One individual may describe an event as traumatic.
- Another individual considers the event as stressful, but not traumatic.
- A third individual finds the event confusing and challenging, but not stressful.

These varying experiences of the event are influenced by the person's complex history, which extends from the past through the present and into the anticipated future.

TIME FOR REFLECTION

Holding a client in mind, consider their life prior to the occurrence of the trauma. Note possible factors that were important in determining the severity of the trauma:

- health and mental health of members of the family
- unique cognitive, emotional, physical, spiritual abilities and disabilities of the individual
- protective and risk factors in the individual's life
- race, religion, class, gender, sexual orientation, and the impact of these aspects of their identity within the context of the larger society

Consider the life of your client at the time of the traumatic event:

- immediate stressors and supports within daily activities, family, and community
- immediate response of family and friends
- impact of the event on the ability to maintain strengths and skills

Consider the life of your client after the traumatic event:

- Has the event undermined their sense of trust and willingness to seek and accept support from family and friends?
- Has the event disrupted their emotional regulation, stability, reflective functioning, and ability to engage in relationship repair with others?

- Are experiences of terror, despair, rage, or withdrawal making it hard for your client to engage in relationships and activities needed for healing and resolution?

A traumatic event happens at a point in time in an individual's life. If we want to understand the impact it is having on a person, we need to explore the complex circumstances that affected the person prior to, at the same time as, and after the event.

TIME FOR REFLECTION

Consider your own life. Have you experienced a traumatic event? If so:

- What were the protective and risk factors that you experienced before, during, and after the event?
- How does this experience affect your ability to stay engaged with your client when they are recalling their trauma?

Reflect on whether this similar experience causes you to:

- minimize the impact of the event on your client
- exaggerate the impact of the event on your client
- focus on rescuing the client from the impact of the event
- recommend a way to deal with the event based on your experience

TRAUMATIC RELATIONSHIPS

When a child or young person is traumatized within their own family, we describe this as developmental trauma (we will be exploring this in Chapter 2). The effects are pervasive and persistent. The child can be described as leading a traumatic life.

The person leading a traumatic life experiences pervasive effects:

- They have trouble with the identification, regulation, and integration of core biological states involving temperature, bodily functions, and identifying and regulating pain.
- They have emotions that often are extreme, unpredictable, dysregulated, and slow to resolve.
- Their cognitive skills are impacted. Their reflective functioning is sparse, as few people have talked to the child about their inner life. The ability to accurately read the thoughts, feelings, and intentions of others is, consequently, mostly lacking.
- The child finds it hard to remain present in the face of stressful circumstances and may rapidly fall into dissociative states.
- Often the child's sense of self is fragmented, and they struggle to remain organized in varying situations. The sense of self that does emerge tends to be laden with shame.
- Their social functioning is impacted. Relationships and events are habitually evaluated as to whether they are safe or threatening, with mistrust predominating. They do not approach relationships or events with an open, curious stance based on acceptance.
- They seek interpersonal safety through attempting to control or avoid most social situations. A child is likely to be persistently dominant or submissive in relationships, depending on which stance feels safer.

All in all, these children are habitually defensive and vigilant to sources of threat. We do not often see what lies beneath their self-protective armor. If we did, what would we see?

- endless anxiety caused by living in a world that is both frightening and confusing
- chronic sadness over the state of it all and a sense that things will never change
- awareness that trying and failing again will only create more pain, so better not to try
- loneliness, wanting to be seen while also wanting to be invisible
- shame that strongly motivates them to remain invisible: being seen might lead to disgust, contempt, rejection, and/or pity from others

TIME FOR REFLECTION

We invite you to think of a child who has experienced developmental trauma.

- While holding in mind their history and symptoms, begin to consider who the child underneath the symptoms is.
- Wonder what it would take to enable this child to reveal the self underneath their defenses.
- How might you respond if you were able to experience their inner life?

Are you aware of liking and/or not liking this child?

- What is the source of your reaction?
- Is your own history contributing to your reaction?

Are you able to perceive this child's defenses as being survival skills that they needed to get through life? Does that evoke compassion? Is your compassion able to evoke a bit of vulnerability within him? Does that awaken the experience of empathy in the child?

DEVELOPMENTAL RELATIONSHIPS

Developmental relationships nurture, guide, lead to discoveries, and comfort. Without such relationships, the developing self will weaken, disorganize, and, in instances of severe neglect, fail to develop at all. In Chapter 2 we will discuss attachment, intersubjectivity, and interpersonal neurobiology—three very comprehensive areas of research that demonstrate the interwoven realities of self and other.

In DDP the practitioner facilitates both the resolution of trauma and the active development and integration of the self of the child. They also indirectly facilitate the same process by encouraging the child's parents, caregivers, teachers, social workers, and mentors to create and maintain similar developmental relationships with the child. It is within this network of relationships that the child can develop a narrative that is coherent and comprehensive, providing opportunities to discover and thrive.

TIME FOR REFLECTION

We invite you to reflect on the developmental relationships in your own life, past and present.

- Think of individuals who have had a positive influence on your development.
- Think of various aspects of these relationships that inspired you,

that deepened your sense of courage and confidence, and that led you to believe that, no matter what, you are lovable and a person of worth.

- See if you can discover links between specific strengths that you have and individuals who helped you to be aware of and develop these strengths.

Now direct your attention toward children with whom you have had a therapeutic relationship.

- What qualities in your relationships had positive influences on the children's development?
- Are you comfortable communicating your experience of a child in therapy with smiles and laughter, excitement and joy, sadness and tears?
- Have there been times when you expressed annoyance toward a child in a way that was therapeutic? (For example, a child spits at you, you convey annoyance at the behavior while accepting their inner life of anger and fear—not simply a cognitive expression of annoyance: Your voice conveys the emotion of your experience of being spat at.) And then with PACE, you used your voice to demonstrate becoming open and engaged again as you repair the relationship that was threatened by your annoyance?
- Have there been times when you expressed annoyance that was hurtful rather than therapeutic? What evoked your strong reaction? Were there connections with your past?
- Do you recall times when you initiated interactive repair? Do you remember how the repair affected the development of the relationship?
- Do you recall times when qualities within you made it difficult to

develop a therapeutic relationship with a child? What were those qualities, what are their origins, and what was the subsequent course of the relationship?

Finally, when you reflect on the developmental relationships in your life, are you able to create in your mind aspects of your life story?

- Are there gaps?
- Are there bits of your story that are difficult to accept?
- What makes it difficult to accept them?
- How might you develop your story further so that it is comprehensive and fully accepted?

Dan read this phrase once: "The greatest gift you have to give your client is yourself."

- Do you experience this in your relationships with your clients?
- Do you experience this gift aiding your client's development?
- How would you describe the gift you are or might be?
- What might stop you from giving this gift?

AN EXAMPLE OF DDP IN ACTION

Throughout this workbook, we will be presenting many relational experiences between children who were traumatized and their caregivers, practitioners, teachers, and social workers as well as other important individuals in the child's life.

As we will explore throughout this book, especially in Chapter 8, the principles of DDP are not restricted to the interactions that occur within the therapy session. Developmental relationships occur in a great variety of situations and involve individuals who assume many roles in the child's development.

Chapters Four and Five discuss the experience of DDP interventions, what we call the "nuts and bolts" of DDP. Throughout the book, we present examples that explore the relationship between a DDP practitioner, a traumatized child, and caregivers. During each exploration, we will reflect on the relational processes that are occurring and how they are impacting both the child and the significant individuals in the child's life. Through such reflections we can also explore connections with our own lives. These examples will help us keep in mind that each child, and each relationship, is unique, and the examples will highlight the individual gifts that are brought to the various encounters.

BACKGROUND INFORMATION

Eleven-year-old Nathan entered foster care at age six, following life with marginal care from parents who were misusing drugs. His father, Lewis, became increasingly violent toward Nathan and his mother, Beth. Nathan now lives in his fourth foster home, with Thad and Jen, who are committed to providing him with long-term care. His DDP practitioner is Tiffany, who has been certified as a DDP practitioner for about one year.

Nathan is frequently oppositional both at home and at school. He relies on himself, seldom expressing his thoughts or feelings to others. His foster parents state that they have no trouble knowing when he is angry, but they are not able to tell if he is experiencing any vulnerable emotions.

Nathan is an above average athlete and functions adequately in academics. He spends little time with his peers, preferring to spend time on screens when he is allowed. After caring for him for two years, Jen and Thad are increasingly frustrated that Nathan expresses such a habitually negative view of his life. He rarely tries to accomplish anything that they believe is important to have a happy and successful life. They don't feel confident that they are making a difference in his life, and they worry that he will be more challenging to care for as he becomes an adolescent. They are worried that his birth parents' chronic use of drugs, as well as the violence his birth parents exposed him to, are having a negative influence on Nathan's development and behavior.

Jen and Thad have low expectations that therapy will be helpful, but they are willing to participate. They can't understand why Nathan does not take advantage of the good life they are providing him. He becomes annoyed and withdraws when they try to reason with him about not taking advantage of opportunities. Both acknowledge that they are increasingly impatient with him. They have two biological children, Jill, age 17, and Russell, age 15, who are functioning well in their daily lives.

INITIAL MEETING

Tiffany asks to meet with Jen and Thad before scheduling a meeting including Nathan. It's a difficult session for all three of them. After hearing their concerns about Nathan's challenging behaviors, Tiffany asks them why they think he acts that way. Jen quickly replies that Nathan knows what he is supposed to do but will deliberately do something else. Thad adds, "Asking why is just excusing him. He just does what he wants."

Tiffany explains that if she doesn't know why he is acting in a certain way, it will be difficult for her to give them suggestions about how to manage his behaviors. She adds that knowing what he feels and wants is often more important than knowing what he does. Both Jen and Thad strongly disagree. They think that what he does is more important than why he does it. They believe they are responsible for ensuring that he behaves appropriately, not for how he feels about it.

Tiffany tries to find another way to explain how important it is to understand Nathan's inner life. Thad forcefully protests because he experiences Tiffany's explanation as her blaming them for the problems with Nathan. When Tiffany says that she is not blaming them, Jen is not persuaded and agrees with Thad's interpretation.

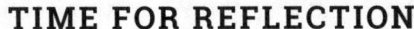

TIME FOR REFLECTION

Recall in your work with parents a time when you became frustrated, similar to Tiffany.

- How did you manage that frustration?
- What did you consider when deciding what to say next?
- Was your response helpful? How did the parents respond?

The more Tiffany tries to explain, the more defensive Jen and Thad become and the more blamed they feel. If she tried to defend herself by insisting that she is not blaming them but rather teaching them another approach to deal with Nathan's behavior, most likely they would become more defensive. And they would also experience Tiffany's defense as invalidating their experience of being blamed!

TIME FOR REFLECTION

- What have you done to reduce a parent's sense of being blamed?
- If that was not helpful, what else could you have done?
- How do you think you can evaluate a parent's behavior without them feeling blamed?

At the first hint that they disagree with her, Tiffany could respond with an attitude similar to the one she wants them to take with Nathan. Central to this attitude is PACE, which we explore in Chapter 3. Without judging them, Tiffany might ask herself why they are resisting her ideas. Rather than giving more information about DDP interventions, she might acknowledge and accept their doubts. She might wonder what it is about her approach that they find uncomfortable, and then express empathy for their discomfort. She might reflect that if they feel she is blaming them, they won't be feeling safe and thus they won't experience her as helpful.

If Tiffany were to ask why—with acceptance, not evaluation—they might have openly responded that they fear they would lose their authority if they took her recommendation. They might express their worry that Nathan would begin to search for excuses whenever they corrected him or that Tiffany's approach would lead to chaos!

Once she has imagined or elicited the parents' whys, Tiffany could respond with understanding about their concerns. She could empathize with their belief that without firm parenting to teach discipline, they would be seen as being weak and permissive and that this would lead to chaos. After affirming their fears that her approach would undermine their authority, she might wonder about the source of their fears. Did their parents raise them to follow behavioral expectations without giving thought to what they felt about it? How were emotions and disagreements handled in their families when they were children? If her ideas were going to create chaos, then she would agree with them that they should not do them!

This is an example, similar to how you would also work with a child, of the need for the practitioner to coregulate the parents' affective state before continuing to explore another way to understand or approach a situation.

CONTINUING WORK WITH THE FOSTER PARENTS

Tiffany continues to meet with Jen and Thad to develop an alliance with them. We explore the development of this alliance in Chapter 6. Tiffany wants to reach the point where she feels confident that they can provide safety for Nathan when he joins the sessions. It is now their fifth session together and Tiffany and the parents are still struggling to feel safe with one another and to develop a joint way forward.

While Jen and Thad are now able to see the value of understanding the meaning of Nathan's behaviors, they often leap to negative assumptions and become critical. Nathan continues to be defensive in response. When Nathan expresses his experience that living with them is hard, they find it hard to respond with empathy and instead react with "If you would just . . . !"

Tiffany often becomes frustrated with Jen and Thad's resistance to her ideas. They seem to agree with her and then to retract their understanding by the next session. She begins to wonder if they are experiencing "blocked care." This is not uncommon when foster parents are caring for a child who does not respond to their guidance and support for weeks or months. Or maybe they are not committed enough to Nathan to do the hard work needed to relate with him differently. Tiffany decides to explore her increasing impatience with her supervisor, Margot.

TIME FOR REFLECTION

Have there been times when you find yourself becoming annoyed with a parent who does not respond to your suggestions or to your PACEful attitude? And then you become more frustrated?

- If a parent does not respond consistently to PACE, how might you make sense of this?
- What could you do that might help in such a situation?

Such negative cycles suggest the need for supervision to regain a state of regulation and to ensure that PACE is a way of being, not something you "do" to a parent to get a desired result. As your regulation increases, you will likely be able to become reflective again.

In Chapter 11 we explore DDP informed supervision. This element is crucial to helping a therapist remain consistently open and engaged with their client. In supervision, the therapist needs to feel safe and confident that the supervisor is not judging the worth of the therapist while exploring the therapist's interventions. The supervisor is standing alongside the therapist, not above them. When the therapist feels safe with the supervisor, the therapist is in a better position to reflect on the process and content of the therapy sessions; the therapist is able to detach from the immediacy of the sessions and experience them from a greater distance while allowing the supervisor's perspective to influence theirs.

SUPERVISION

Here is an example of an effective supervisory process: Margot, the supervisor, creates safety by relating to Tiffany with PACE.

Margot:	Your intention with Jen and Thad seems very clear to me. You want them to understand and use the DDP stance of PACE with Nathan. Yet often they don't do so, or if they do, it doesn't last. And that seems to be very hard for you.
Tiffany:	Yes, I don't know how I could have been clearer about the ways that they might engage their son differently. I also thought that I had made it obvious how important this is.
Margot:	And they didn't do what you were asking?
Tiffany:	Was I approaching it wrong?
Margot:	How does it seem to you? What made it so hard?
Tiffany:	It seemed like they were deliberately defying me. Like they didn't want to acknowledge that I was right . . . and that what they were doing was not very helpful.

Margot:	Your request seemed to be so reasonable to you. Why wouldn't they just do it?
Tiffany:	I don't know!
Margot:	And it seems so painful when they don't follow your lead. Why so painful? Why?
Tiffany:	(*following a long reflective pause*) It just seems to me that Nathan has had so many bad experiences in his life when he was being maltreated that he deserves something better. And I know that what I'm saying will give him something better! I don't understand why they don't see that my ideas will help him with the trauma he has had to live with for so long! I know that they want to help him. I want to help him, but I can't help them to help him! And I want to, so badly! (*another pause, as she experiences both her sense of helplessness and her sadness*) What this reminds me of most are the times with my father when we would go round and round and never get anywhere. And he was always so reasonable! Sometimes I wished he would just get angry with me. I knew he was being reasonable, but I just couldn't make myself do what he wanted.
Margot:	What made it so hard for you to do what he wanted?
Tiffany:	I think it was because he didn't seem to care how hard it was for me. It seemed that it didn't matter what I felt about it—if it was reasonable, I should do it, like it or not. What I felt didn't seem important to him.
Margot:	Oh, Tiffany, I think we're getting close to something that

was very important to you. It seemed to you that what you felt was not important to your father.

Tiffany: I know it was, but I didn't feel it. The only important thing was what he thought was reasonable. If I experienced it differently, it either didn't matter or I was just being selfish . . . and defiant.

Margot: And now . . . with Jen and Thad?

Tiffany: I see two connections between my dad and Jen and Thad. First, I'm frustrated with them, just like my dad was with me! Why won't they just be more reasonable! Why are they defying me and disregarding my ideas. Second, it seems to me . . . when I think about what it's like when we get stuck, it seems that what they feel is not important to me. I'm not willing to step back and really get what makes it hard for them to join me in my ideas regarding Nathan. I don't have empathy for their experience, I just want it to change.

Margot: Any sense why now? I know that you've often come across parents who were challenging you. What seems so hard about Jen and Thad being that way?

Tiffany: (*following a long pause*) That's it! I don't think it's about Jen and Thad. I think it's mostly about Thad. Something about his attitude reminds me of my father . . . and I get locked in a space where I will not allow him to disregard my thoughts and feelings, like my father seemed to do. With Thad it's like I'm thinking, "It's not going to happen!"

Margot:	Leaving you feeling frustrated . . . with him . . . and maybe with yourself too? Like when you were with your father.

Tiffany:	With myself mostly.

Margot:	*(with empathy)* And maybe this is how it felt after the conflicts with your father.

Tiffany:	*(with both a smile and a few tears)* Maybe.

After this supervision session with Margot, Tiffany is able to engage with Jen and Thad again. She is more open to their experiences, including what is hard for them about her suggestions. As she experiences empathy for Thad's stance, defending himself against both her and Nathan, Thad is able to be more vulnerable about his self-doubts. Could he be the father that he wants to be for Nathan? Could Tiffany see his worth? He begins to express his own pain over his sense of failing, which has been made stronger by his perception that both Nathan and Tiffany find him lacking.

WORK WITH PARENTS AND CHILD

After nine sessions during which Tiffany sees the foster parents without Nathan, she begins joint sessions. Fairly quickly, Nathan begins to insist that he does not need any help and that if Jen and Thad don't like his behavior, they should tell him to move. Tiffany responds with PACE, and Jen and Thad, following her lead as she has asked them to do, listen to Nathan's experience as he becomes engaged with Tiffany.

Tiffany:	So, it seems to you that Jen and Thad are blaming you for every problem you guys have at home! No wonder you don't want to see me. Maybe I need to be clear for all three

of you. My goal is to help the whole family with struggles that you all are having. I'm not planning to try to fix any of you. Just help you to understand each other better, and maybe explore how you all might approach things a bit differently.

Nathan: That'll be a surprise. They never seem satisfied with me.

Tiffany: Oh, Nathan, if that's how it seems to you that would be difficult. No wonder you said that if they don't like what you do, they should just tell you to leave.

Nathan: Like, I said, they're never satisfied.

Tiffany: If that's right, Nathan, what would that be about? Why would they not be satisfied with what you do?

Nathan: They just want some perfect kid who always does what he's told. I'm not good enough for them!

Tiffany: That is so hard, to feel that you're not good enough. Seems like you feel that they're disappointed in who you are?

Nathan: They make that pretty obvious. They yell at me all the time. Well, if they don't like me, why should I like them?

Tiffany: Nathan, you're describing a hard life with Jen and Thad, for all three of you! It's hard living as a family when you don't feel close to one another and you feel that they don't like you and you don't like them.

Nathan: They don't care. They're disappointed in me anyway. They wouldn't miss me if I left tomorrow.

Tiffany: If that's right, Nathan . . . that they wouldn't miss you, you must feel so alone living with them. You feel that you don't matter to them. You must feel all alone.

Nathan: I'm used to it!

Tiffany: I think you are, Nathan, and I'm sad about that. I think you must have felt so alone when you were living with your parents, when you were little. They did drugs so much and seemed angry all the time. You probably often felt that they weren't interested in spending time with you. And your other foster homes—they didn't work out. And now it seems to be the same with Jen and Thad.

Nathan: Nothing's ever going to change!

Tiffany: I wonder, Nathan, what Jen and Thad are thinking about what you've told us, that you don't think it would matter to them if you left tomorrow, that they wouldn't care. Can I tell them that you feel that way and see what they say?

Nathan: Go for it.

Tiffany: Jen and Thad, Nathan has given me permission to talk for him a bit. I'd like to hear what you want to say about that. Would you answer with empathy as we've spoken about and be sure to answer honestly (*they nod*).

Tiffany: (*speaking for Nathan*) I meant it! I don't think you care! I think I'm not good enough for you and you'd be better off without me. (*Tiffany makes her voice quieter and more vulnerable*) I thought this time it would be different, but I don't think it is. I don't think anyone will ever think I'm good enough. I don't think I'll ever be special to anyone.

Jen: Oh, Nathan, I'm sorry that you think that. That you think we wouldn't miss you and we don't think you're good enough. If that's how it seems to you, you must feel so alone living with us. I'm sorry.

Thad: I am too, Nathan. If it seems to you that I think that you're more of a bother than you're worth, that would be very hard. No wonder you'd be angry about living with us, if that's how it seems to you.

Tiffany: (*still speaking for Nathan*) Then why do you yell so much if you do want me around?

Jen: Sometimes, when we keep arguing, I guess I get discouraged and worry that I'm doing something wrong. I think I'm angry with you for not being happier with us.

Thad: I agree with Jen, Nathan. Sometimes I don't know what to do to help us get along better. Then I think I take it out on you. I sometimes say that you should be more grateful, and that's not right. I have to get better at handling our conflicts. After all you've been through, you deserve better. I know you're trying, and we're trying too. I'm sorry it doesn't feel like that to you sometimes. I have to do a better job showing you how much I care about you.

Tiffany: Well, Nathan, what do you think? Do you believe them?

Nathan: I don't know.

Tiffany: I can see why you'd have doubts. I imagine experiencing arguments, anger, is hard after all you've been through. Why trust them? Why would they be any different? They're just going to give up, so maybe you should give up too.

Nathan: I guess.

Tiffany: All three of you are being so honest. I think it's hard for all of you not to feel close just now. I sense you all want it to change. You all want to trust that it might change. I want to help if you'll let me. Jen and Thad, am I right? And will you work at this with Nathan and me?

Jen and Thad: (*loudly and together*) Yes, we want this to work!

Tiffany: Nathan?

Nathan: Yeah.

TIME FOR REFLECTION

Sequences, such as the example above, need to occur repeatedly if any changes are to become integrated. Trust, reciprocal trust, needs time to deepen.

- Do you find yourself at times becoming disappointed that the progress evident in one session seems to fade before the next session?
- Do you find yourself becoming discouraged, especially if the parents or child seem quick to give up, making comments such as: "They really didn't mean what they said last time. They haven't changed at all"?
- What will help you to reflect on the wobble in relationships, especially when efforts are being made to make the relationship stronger?
- How can you keep yourself from expecting too much, from placing too many demands on yourself, on the parents, and on the child?

There are no easy answers, but what might come close is to maintain PACE with patience. This also means trusting the process of DDP.

THE CYCLICAL PROCESS OF DDP

Developing relationships and more coherent stories has a healing and transforming power, but the process is not easy. There may be many times when it seems like you are starting over again and again. Relational changes are often hard. If you are patient with the process, the parents are more likely to be patient too. If the parents are more able to be patient, the child will follow.

As DDP has evolved over the years, there is increasing awareness of how important it is to have the initial sessions with the caregivers before beginning the joint sessions with the child. When the caregivers begin to feel safe with the practitioner, they become more open and engaged with the ideas being presented and with their central role in the development of their child. When they feel safe, their child will more readily feel safe. When traumatized children begin to feel safe, both in the session and at home, their defenses are likely to soften. They will be more willing and able to rely on their caregivers.

TIME FOR REFLECTION

Have you been tempted to meet with a child and caregivers together before they are ready because the caregivers, and possibly others, have wanted you to do so? Or because the child's behaviors were becoming more intense and you felt that the joint sessions just could not wait?

- Reflect on times when you have given in to this temptation.
- If it went well, notice what helped you to be successful.
- If it went less well, notice what prevented you from getting the outcome you or others hoped for.

At times like this remember PACE—for the caregivers and for yourself! Of course they are likely to feel desperate! Of course you would have the joint sessions today if they would be of value! While you are building the foundation of safety and trust, you do not know for sure if or when the foundation will be strong enough to support the hard work of change and healing. Remember that without this foundation, healing most likely will NOT occur.

THE PURPOSE OF THE WORKBOOK

The aim of this workbook is to provide a practical book to help practitioners provide DDP interventions via therapy, parenting, and/or practice. It parallels *Healing Relational Trauma* (Hughes et al., 2019) while attempting to add value to that text by presenting the material in a more reflective and experiential manner. Each chapter in *Healing Relational Trauma* is complemented by a chapter in this workbook.

We invite you to reflect on your experience of DDP through the "Time for Reflection" moments and "Reflective Exercises" indicated within the text. These will guide you, through discussion, examples, and reflections, to embed the DDP model further into your practice. Our aim is to facilitate DDP becoming a lived model of practice for each unique practitioner working with each unique child and family.

We consider working therapeutically with children, supported by their families; working with parents (in whichever way they come to this role) to help them to become secure attachment figures providing DDP-informed parenting for their children; and supporting professionals from social care, health, and education to be DDP-informed in their interactions with families.

An important related aim of this workbook is to spur reflection on the diversity of both practitioners and those receiving interventions to promote thinking about how each unique individual's identity can be embraced within the application of DDP interventions. We urge readers to consider DDP from the unique perspective of their own context, identity, culture, and experience.

Our aim is for all those reading this book to feel recognized and welcomed and to experience DDP as having relevance for them. We look forward to the innovation and creativity we hope this workbook sparks as practitioners bring their own unique lived and professional experience to their practice of DDP. In this way DDP will continue to grow and develop, influenced by our global understanding of what it is to be human and our global knowledge about how to increase emotional well-being and heal trauma.

DDP developed because of a perceived need to address trauma occurring within the family, and especially when the child's attachment figures are the source of the trauma. DDP focuses on the various forms of abuse (physical, sexual, verbal, emotional) and neglect (physical and emotional) that some caregivers impose on the children who depend on them for safety and care. DDP also recognizes the additional trauma for children experiencing separation and loss from birth parents and caregivers.

We are also aware that developmental trauma can intersect with trauma that occurs outside of the family, such as through physical, emotional, and verbal assaults because of race, religion, gender, class, sexual orientation, disability, and/or neurodiversity. In these assaults, an "other" is seen as an inferior object, not as a separate individual of equal worth with equal rights and opportunities. We wish for intersections with these sources of trauma to be acknowledged and addressed within DDP interventions. Hopefully, the following is a step in that direction.

RACIAL EQUITY AND SOCIAL JUSTICE

The DDP community is actively embracing a program of racial equity and social justice (RESJ) work. DDP is predominantly Western, white, and heterosexual centered. It has also paid insufficient attention to differences of class, religion, ability or disability and neurodiversity. This has been reflected in our literature and training. Work is happening to change this, starting with the DDP diversity statement:

> Inherent in the values of DDP, embedded in the PACE (Playfulness, Acceptance, Curiosity, and Empathy) stance is our core belief that all people must be treated with dignity, compassion, and respect.
>
> DDPI has made a firm commitment to embrace diversity and inclusion with the aim of making it an integral part of everything that we do. We understand that we are at the beginning of our diversity journey which is one of understanding and learning new ways of engaging with the diverse communities that we work with across the globe where differences of opinion, belief, or culture exist.
>
> We recognize that the development of DDP has been influenced by a dominant Western culture, including the psychological theory and models underlying it. We commit to learning from the global majority to influence its further development.
>
> It is important in cases where we come across diverse ways of being that exist outside of the dominant Western culture we choose to adopt an

attitude of curiosity, acceptance, and empathy. To better understand these differences and perspectives which have been shaped by the lived experiences of people before we collaboratively move forward.

We promote that all those we work with will be treated without discrimination regardless of race, age, religion, sex, national origin, socioeconomic status, sexual orientation, gender identity or expression, disability, veteran status, or source of payment.

To aid us in better understanding the needs of underrepresented groups within DDPI and global societies we have formed the Racial Equity Social Justice (RESJ) Committee. This will help us to embed the principles of equality, diversity, and inclusion into all areas of DDPI.

However, this is not their work alone. This is a task for all of the DDPI community. For some this will mean stepping out of our comfort zones, experiencing discomfort and being courageous in speaking out for social justice and amplifying the voices of those that are underrepresented.

We will find new ways of working and connecting with different communities. In line with our core value of embracing difference, we aspire to make DDPI a place where people can bring their authentic selves into DDP spaces and not feel a need to compartmentalize any of their identities or cultural patterns of behaviors.

Further, we at DDPI pledge to stay actively committed to making our community, training experiences, consultation services, parenting support, and therapy a more diverse culture that reflects the remarkable heterogeneity of the children, families, carers, educators, and therapists we work with.

We commit ourselves to actively integrate the ethos of diversity in our work and will continue to explore this issue with a vigorous action plan for the future. [1]

---

1   DDPI Diversity Statement (ddpnetwork.org/community/diversity-statement/), July 2023

This workbook is about the practice of DDP, holding racial equity and social justice in mind. It is not a book about racial equity and social justice within DDP. That is a book which still needs to be written. However, the DDP community needs to do more of their own work before this can happen. That book also needs to be written by people more expert in racial equity and social justice than we are.

While working through this book, alongside reflecting on your DDP practice, we invite you to reflect on your heritage and identity and its influence on your work. Here are some reflections from Dan and Kim to start us off.

REFLECTIONS FROM DAN

I live and work in the United States. My heritage is Irish, Welsh, and German. I am a white, heterosexual man raised as a Roman Catholic in a section of Pittsburgh, Pennsylvania, that was almost entirely Irish-Catholic, working class. The primary leaders of my community were priests; therefore, it is not surprising that when I was 17 years old, I left home and entered a seminary. I did not want to work in a factory, and I could not imagine any career possibilities other than being a priest.

I was not aware of being poor and working class because everyone was and had been in all of my family stories. My great-great-grandmother, newly arrived from Ireland, worked as a maid for a wealthy family in another section of the city. One day, she broke some expensive China. She was not fired because the family was in turmoil, as President Abraham Lincoln had been killed that day.

My father became a tradesman, like every other man in our family and neighborhood who could manage to avoid repetitive factory work. It was only when I finally went to university (the first in my family to do so) that I became aware of how limited and narrow my experiences had been compared to those from the middle class, whom I was now meeting. Some thought less of me for that reason. I became comfortable making friends with peers from similar working-class backgrounds but did not feel at ease when associating with those from the middle class, even when they showed no signs of class bias.

I thought little about the lives of individuals from other races or religions. Nor did I give much thought to individuals who did not identify as heterosexual. While I certainly had experience living among girls and women, I don't recall thinking that their lives were being limited by the religion and culture in which we were being raised. I do recall believing stereotypes that girls did not have some of the abilities that boys had. Similarly, as I got older and met more individuals from other religions, races, sexual orientations, I was often surprised to discover that the stereotypes that I held about them were prejudicial and unfair. I have a strong commitment to being nonjudgmental and fair and to treating every individual in an open and engaged manner. At times it was hard to grasp that my mind and actions did not coincide with my stated values. I learned an important lesson from a Black friend in university: that positive stereotypes were also hurtful. He was disappointed and annoyed when I commented that Black individuals tended to be superior to white people in athletic and musical skills. I came to realize, more slowly than I now wish, that I needed to challenge the assumptions that I applied to people from races, classes, and religions different from my own and to get to know each individual person with their unique life experiences. I have found that when I am able to set aside such biased assumptions, it is partly due to what I have learned about unconditional acceptance, nonjudgmental, not-knowing curiosity, and empathy through PACE and DDP.

REFLECTIONS FROM KIM

I am white and British, with some Eastern European heritage. I am heterosexual and cisgender. My preferred pronouns are she/her. I am able-bodied and my neurodiversity centers around motor skills and weak proprioception.

Earlier this year I visited a cemetery on the outskirts of London. It was a dark, overcast day with rain threatening. The cemetery was quiet as I made my way through the large number of graves, all crowded together, and then suddenly I was there. I was standing in front of the final resting place of Alec and Sarah Golding, my great-grandparents. In my more than 60 years, I had not before visited this place.

Following my participation in workshops provided by racial equity consultant Dr Nikkia Young during 2021, this is where my RESJ journey had brought me. When I was asked about the impact of the workshops, I was at first embarrassed to say that they had led me inward to self-reflection. It felt a bit self-indulgent, and yet I don't think it was. I had learned that I lacked curiosity about difference and diversity. This got in the way of my understanding racial equity and social justice and my role in achieving these. I was too focused on ignoring difference to truly listen to those whose heritages and identities are different from mine. I needed to understand why.

I started to explore intergenerational trauma and my own ancestors. I wanted to understand some of the trauma that they experienced as they fled from Russia, part of a wave of emigration to London. I needed to discover an ancestry that is about assimilation, fitting in, and achieving wealth. An ancestry that has unconsciously taught me to distance myself from "others" in order to feel secure within the "in group," to ward off the fear of having to leave again. To discover through my own therapy that I hold their trauma in my body still and how this has influenced my own racism, homophobia, and ableism. As I visit the grave of my great-grandparents, I can let this trauma go.

I lift my head and look around and now I see you. I see your oppression caused by race, sexuality, gender, disability, neurodiversity, class, and/or religion. I will be clumsy and make mistakes. I will experience anxiety and discomfort, but I will not look away again. I believe this will strengthen my DDP practice as I hold acceptance, curiosity, and empathy more deeply.

MULTIPLE VOICES

We, Dan and Kim, have written this book together. We are aware that we are just two voices, constrained by our own life experiences, and yet we are writing on behalf of the many families and practitioners who are, or who will become, part of the DDP community. In recognition of this, we have invited other voices to join us in this book. You will find these voices within the conversations interspersed between the chapters.

Many other people have contributed their voices to this book through their advice and guidance. We have been informed by their wisdom; any mistakes herein are our own.

Further, some voices come from the inspiration of other published works. Where these occur, we have attributed them to their original sources.

CONCLUSION

DDP is a complex therapeutic activity. It involves interventions common to both individual and systemic therapies. It focuses on past trauma and current experiences of shame and conflict, while trying to build connections between the past and present. It seeks to develop the child's attachment security with their primary caregivers while ensuring that these caregivers can indeed provide safety for their child. When successful, DDP can blend affective states with reflective functioning to enable therapeutic stories to evolve. These will assist the resolution of the trauma and create opportunities for all members of the family to thrive.

Within this workbook, we focus on therapists, practitioners, children, and families. We explore how they become engaged with one another and maintain these relationships through repair at times of rupture. We demonstrate that DDP is a joint, lived process rather than a series of techniques that a practitioner employs to effect change in a particular child and family.

We also focus on the need for all adults who relate with traumatized children to do so with PACE and to realize that the gift that they have to offer the children, themselves in the context of the relationship, may also be crucial in helping them to develop in a healthy and coherent manner.

We hope that within this exploration we can also increase our awareness of the trauma that people experience and the challenges to healthy relationships that can arise from experiencing discrimination and marginalization based on race, religion, class, gender, sexual orientation, disability, and/or neurodiversity.

We sincerely hope that DDP will contribute to the process of healthy development for all of us who have been traumatized in one or more of the many ways in which trauma occurs.

We hope that this workbook will assist DDP practitioners in maintaining and enriching their relationships with caregivers, children, and the practitioners that support them along the therapeutic journey that addresses trauma through healing relationships.

NOTES

1. DDP is a dyadic, developmental model for psychotherapy, parenting, and practice. Throughout this workbook, the term DDP is used for all three modalities. When referring specifically to one of these areas of intervention, we will indicate this.

2. In recognition of the nonbinary nature of gender, we have chosen to use the terms they and their rather than he or she, except where the gender is known.

3. When we use the term *parents*, we are referring to all those who have a parenting role in the lives of the children in their care, whether they be biological, step, adoptive, foster, kinship, or residential parents. We have used the terms *parents*, *carers*, and *caregivers* interchangeably throughout.

4. DDP is a model practiced by therapists and other practitioners who are embedding the DDP principles into the work they are qualified to engage in. We therefore refer to both DDP therapists and DDP practitioners.

5. We have written a range of case examples and dialogues for readers to reflect upon. Unless indicated, these are fictional examples inspired by the many families and practitioners we have worked with.

6. Within this workbook we provide a range of reflections and reflective exercises. We include worksheets for some of the reflective exercises at the end of the chapters as well as some thoughts from us about possible responses. These are not definitive answers, and we expect that you will have your own creative responses.

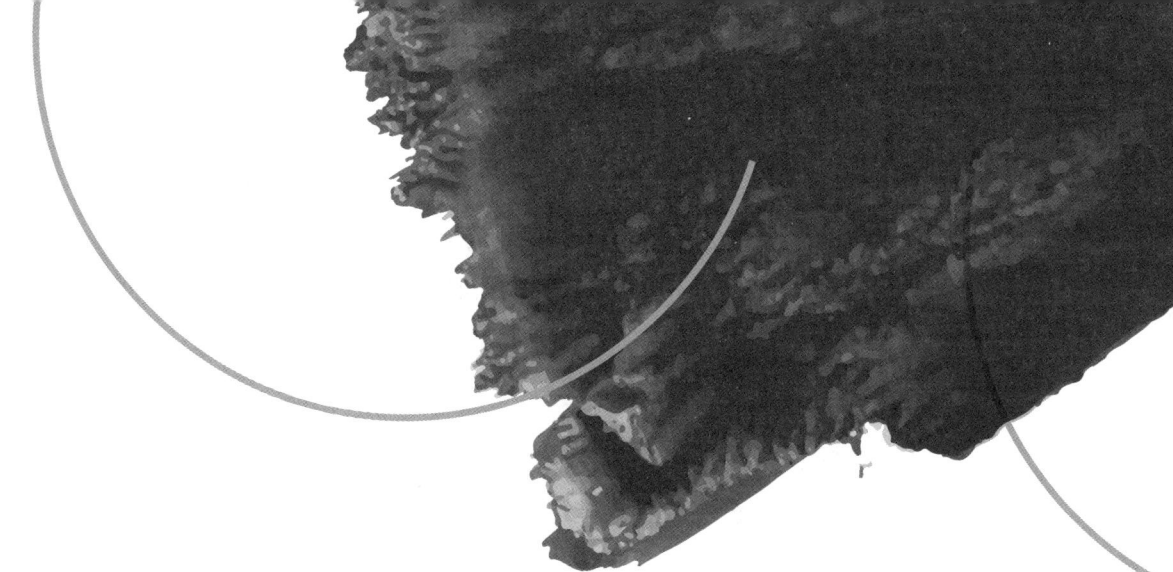

Chapter 2:
Guiding Principles from Trauma, Attachment, Intersubjectivity, and Interpersonal Neurobiology

A child needs new attachment relationships in order to resolve and integrate traumatic experiences that result from violations of trust in attachment relationships, the absence of safety, and stories based on shame and fear. Within these new relationships, the child needs intersubjective conversations that develop into new stories that are embedded in love, compassion, care, and commitment—because of qualities within him. These intersubjective experiences reflect who he is. (Hughes et al., 2019, p. 24)

REFRESHER

In developing DDP as a therapeutic intervention, we relied on the theories and research of attachment, intersubjectivity, interpersonal neurobiology, and trauma. These areas of knowledge describe interwoven features of development and the pervasive developmental impact of relational trauma.

As we explore how these four guiding principles of DDP are important for our complex therapeutic efforts, we keep in mind the foundation upon which they all rest, namely the presence or absence of safety. The comprehensive theory and research that underlie these principles have safety at their core. No matter where we begin in our efforts to understand both the challenges facing traumatized children and ways to assist them in healing and integration, we come back to safety—its absence or its presence.

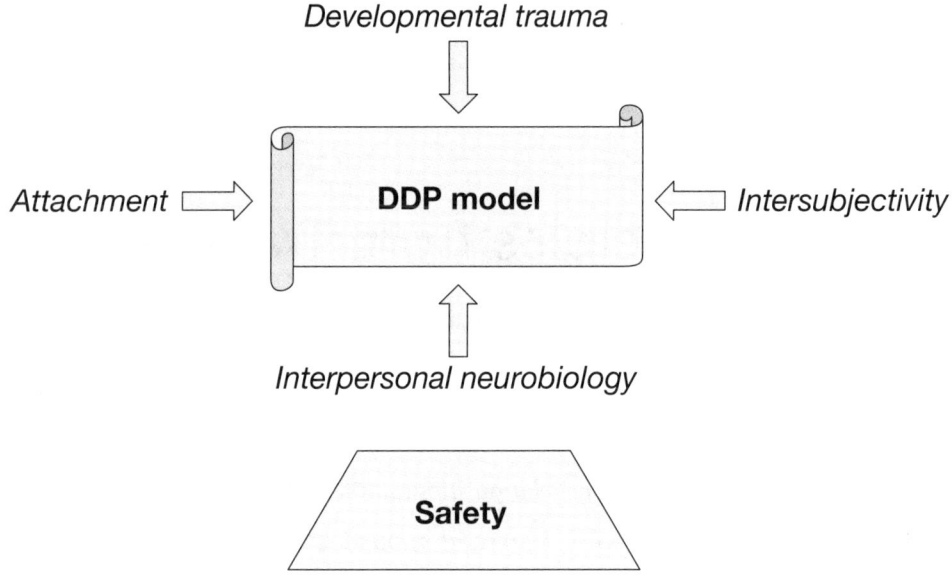

Figure 2.1 Defining Principles

DEVELOPMENTAL TRAUMA

Possibly the most devastating assault against a child's sense of safety is when they experience trauma within their own home, through the eyes, voice, and hands of their parents and/or close family members. This particular form of trauma has persistent and pervasive effects on all aspects of a child's development (Figure 2.2). This is recognized in the term *developmental* trauma (van der Kolk, 2005).

The challenges of trying to engage and assist children who manifest such

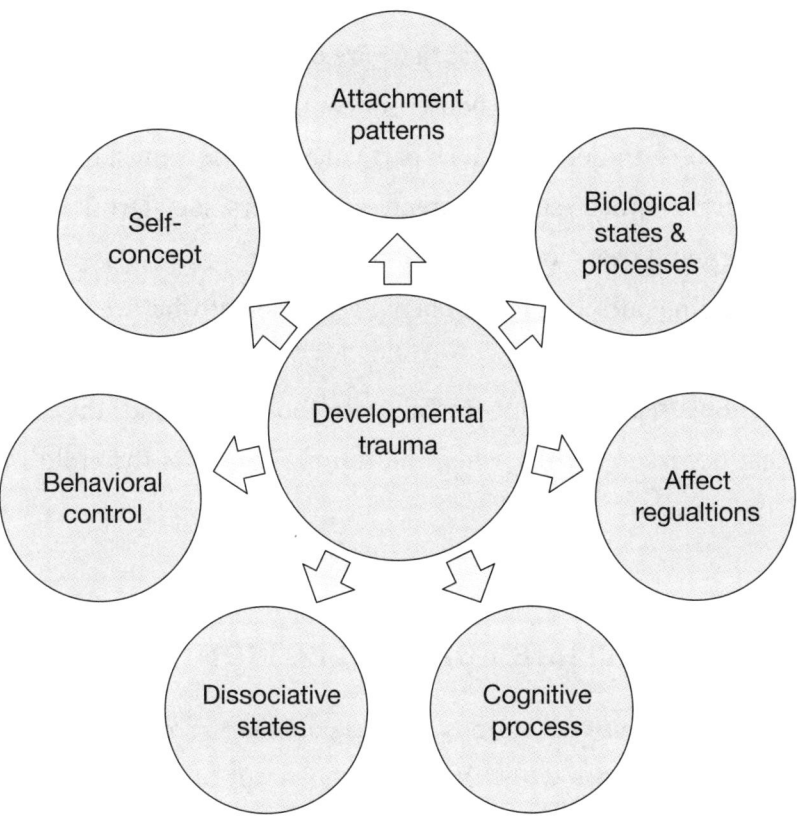

Figure 2.2 Impact of Developmental Trauma
on Development

severe and comprehensive difficulties are profound. Our potential reactions to these children can interfere with the very interventions that we are trying to use. These reactions include:

1. becoming consistently annoyed and impatient with the repetitive quality of the child's behavioral challenges and/or their struggle to connect with us
2. giving up hope that the child will respond to our interventions

3. becoming defensive and trying to control the healing process, which can lead us to believe that there are only two possible solutions: the child must simply "try harder" or comprehensive consequences that reinforce and/or extinguish particular behaviors must be imposed

4. blaming others, such as caregivers, teachers, social workers, neighbors, and peers for the lack of progress

5. blaming ourselves for not being very good at what we do

These reactions represent our inability to hold in mind the severity of trauma that occurs to a child when the trauma source is the child's primary attachment figure.

TIME FOR REFLECTION

Here are a range of reflections to help you keep in mind how hard it is for a child you are working with to move out of consistent states of fear and shame. This involves imagining ways that your life might approximate the child's world. If any of these are your lived experience, reflect on how they impacted your sense of safety.

1. Imagine the effects on your sense of safety and your ability to function if you:
   - were continuously exposed to unpredictable, frightening people and events
   - were hurt and rejected because of your skin color, your religion, your gender, your sexuality, your disability, or other differences
   - once trusted someone but were then betrayed. Would you believe the next person who asks you to trust will be different?

2. Imagine that there is no end in sight to your experience of

> trauma; you cannot recall a time when you felt safe, and you
> don't expect things will ever change.
>
> 3. Imagine that you believe that the trauma is all your fault, but
>   at the same time you're not sure what you've done wrong.
>
> Now think about how these reflections have impacted how you feel
> toward the child.
>
> Do you notice any increase in compassion for the child?

Creating trust and helping children who have experienced developmental trauma is quite a balancing act. What seems to be a matter of children not wanting to do something is more often a sign that they are not able to do something. What seems to be deliberate defiance may be a desperate compulsion to avoid engagement with someone that, though they offer help, seems terrifying. Yes, comfort, support, and care may actually be terrifying.

We know that the traumatized child needs someone who is open and engaged with them even though they are likely to deny it. Yet, in spite of this knowledge, staying open and engaged with a traumatized child who is openly rejecting us, who withdraws from us, or who seems to dissociate in our presence is hard. Any one of these tends to create social–emotional pain within us. To avoid the pain of rejection we may stop being receptive to the child's experience of us. Then, like a robot, we try to go through the motions without feeling the pain. Yet, we know that being a robot will never help the child to learn to trust us. What do we do then?

- Do we listen to ourselves and the pain we feel?
- Or do we respond to the child's behavior and the indifference it seems to reflect?

If we are able to hold the nature and source of the child's trauma in our mind, we are more likely to be fully present with them, regardless of the pain we might be feeling when they reject us.

Imagine that we succeed in providing all we believe the child needs to resolve the trauma. And yet the child:

- avoids and fights against sources of safety
- avoids all opportunities to experience comfort
- avoids experiencing joy with us and other good and committed adults
- denies all responsibility for the problems that are occurring

TIME FOR REFLECTION

Our friend and colleague, Jon Baylin, says, "If a child doesn't show it [their trauma and its impact], you got to know it." What does that mean to you?

- Is it sufficient to know the facts of the child's history of trauma?
- If not, what else do you need to know about the trauma?
- If you need to know the child's experience of those facts, how do you go about gathering that?

It may be that we need to truly *not* know what the child's experience of the trauma was in order to begin to learn about their experience. In this way we both come to know it in a new way.

If we are able to engage the child with PACE (described fully in the next chapter), we can discover qualities of the child that provide worth and resilience, not shame and fear. Supported by our attitude of PACE, the child is encouraged to actively engage in experiences consistent with a secure attachment, intersubjectivity, and interpersonal neurobiology. Developmental trauma deprived the child of these experiences. DDP (psychotherapy, parenting, and practice) provides an opportunity to experience them anew.

A SECURE ATTACHMENT

Infants are born with few abilities to keep themselves safe. To survive they need the active support of adults who are available, sensitive, and responsive to their cues. Attachment theory explores the role of adults as attachment figures responding to cues of distress and restoring a sense of safety for the infant.

Attachment principles are universal, while the particular expression of these patterns will vary. For example, variations regarding the respective emphasis on individualization and socialization occur among cultures. Children learn to safely engage adults in every culture, but the emphasis regarding nonverbal and verbal communications, initiatives, and responses may be different between cultures. The DDP practitioner needs to be aware of these cultural variations and to engage members of the family in ways that demonstrate cultural sensitivity and respect.

Some of these cultural differences are less well understood because of a bias in the research. As we consider the relevance of attachment theory, we need to keep in mind that research informing psychological models and theories is largely based on data generated from Western, middle-class participants. Henrich (2021) coined the term WEIRD to describe Western populations (Western, educated, industrialized, rich, and democratic). These populations are psychologically and behaviorally unusual. Cross-cultural research reveals that they differ in terms of spatial reasoning, memory, attention, patience, risk-taking, fairness, induction, executive function, and pattern recognition. The Western participants lie at an extreme end of the distribution on these dimensions. And because those considered "Western" represent less than 12% of the world population, we must be cautious when making assumptions about the non-Western global majority (Arnett, 2008).

Western psychological models and theories are helpful because a universal repertoire of attachment behaviors is likely to exist across cultures. The selection, shaping, and interpretation of these behaviors over time, however, are culturally patterned (Harwood et al., 1995). We need more research exploring how universal aspects are influenced by different cultures.

For example:

- Sensitive caregiving leads to secure attachment. Sensitivity is demonstrated differently among cultures.
- Secure attachment results in social competence. Social competence is viewed differently by different cultures.
- A secure base fosters exploration. A secure base is provided differently in different cultures.

The DDP practitioner therefore needs to know and understand the culture of each client, as well as learning about those cultures from research, to ensure that any interventions are tailored to the unique needs of the family.

With this proviso in mind, research in attachment patterns indicate that securely attached children differ from children who are insecurely attached in many ways, including that securely attached children:

1. are more successful in engaging in reciprocal relationships with both adults and peers;
2. are more able to regulate their affective states;
3. demonstrate higher levels of reflective functioning and mentalization abilities; and
4. are more able and willing to engage in interactive repair.

Traumatized children are unlikely to manifest attachment security and thus are at risk of not developing these important social–emotional skills. It is crucial that the DDP practitioner assist the child in developing these skills within the therapeutic relationship and via the caregiver.

Similarly, attachment in the growing child is likely to be more secure when the parent evaluates only the child's behavior and not their sense of self. When the child does something that their parent disapproves of, they will experience realistic guilt, but not shame. This is because the self of the child is accepted.

In DDP, the practitioner provides interventions that aim to resolve the traumatic experiences of the child while also facilitating their ability to develop healthy relationships.

These interventions include:

1. utilizing and integrating nonverbal and verbal communication
2. follow–lead–follow: Engaging in ways of relating that encourage both taking initiative and responding to the initiatives of others
3. affective–reflective dialogue: Utilizing both affective and reflective modes of experience and communication
4. interactive repair: Attending to and accepting routine breaks in attunement within relationships and engaging in relationship repair to restore attunement, which maintains and strengthens the relationship
5. allowing space for both enjoyable and stressful experiences to be understood and integrated into a coherent narrative
6. focusing on a descriptive rather than evaluative understanding of the traumatized child's experience, which we describe as discovering stories or narratives of experience.

Through all these interventions, the attitude of PACE is held by the practitioner and the parents. This attitude—characterized by playfulness, acceptance, curiosity, and empathy—increases the child's sense of safety and security. Central to PACE is the experience of unconditional acceptance: The child will be cared for *no matter what.*

When encouraging the adoption of PACE as a way of being within DDP interventions, the practitioner also needs to hold in mind cultural variations in the way this attitude will comfortably be expressed. Cultural variations will be in line with the values and beliefs of the community. This includes differences in the way children are encouraged to be dependent or interdependent, leading to differences in the development of characteristics such as emotional expressiveness and mentalization (Keller, 2022). The DDP practitioner understands these differences adapting the way that they demonstrate PACE to be sensitive to the cultural values of the family they are working with.

CULTURAL VARIATIONS IN THE ATTITUDE OF PACE

(Cultural variations informed by Keller, 2022, and Lancy, 2017)

Play is a feature of parent–child relationships with a predisposition to explore being universal. A family's context and culture will determine how this exploration is encouraged and which times it is discouraged. For example, the Aché Indians of Paraguay carry their infants until they are two, not allowing them to touch the ground, because of dangers in the environment. In many Asian and African cultures, children explore through observation rather than touch, with more interest in people than inanimate objects. The focus in individualistic societies is more on play with toys, and the focus in sociocentric societies is more on engaging the child in household chores.

Unconditional acceptance is likely to be important across cultures throughout the world, as children are universally loved and valued. The expressions of love and valuing are, however, open to cultural influence, which is shaped by ecological conditions as well as the social history of the community to which the child belongs. In an Eastern country such as China, for example, love and value are expressed implicitly through the actions of the parents, whereas in a Western country, such as America and England, where Dan and Kim grew up, parents are more likely to explicitly communicate feelings of love and valuing.

The expression of curiosity is also likely to vary more between cultures. For example, cultures differ in the value given to mentalizing the internal states of self and others. Where there is a cultural model that values and encourages psychological autonomy, there are assumptions that individuals own their own mental states. Within these cultures, parents will come more naturally to a state of curiosity about their children's internal worlds. Where individuality is less valued and the self is understood as part of a community, the internal world of the child will be given less attention than the child's connections with others. All facilitation of curiosity within these parents needs to be based in an understanding of this context.

Similarly, encouraging expressions of empathy will require the practitioner to understand context of the culture the family lives within. Empathy can be demonstrated through words and through actions. In cultures where individuality is less valued and self is viewed as part of a community, talking about individual emotions is considered inappropriate. For example, the Indigenous Australians consider the expression of negative affect to be disrespectful to elders and is likely to reduce social harmony. They will share more nonverbal gestures in their communications, and this will impact how empathy is expressed.

With cultural variation in mind, the DDP practitioner attempts to discover the traumatic events of the child's life with special regard to their attachment relationships. The practitioner supports the child to reflect on the times when they experienced various forms of abuse and neglect. From there, the child's experience of these events will be explored.

For example, a child may have concluded that they were not worthy of being loved, that they were a selfish person and did not deserve comfort. This might have led to avoidance of stressful emotional states. They feel vulnerable when these feelings of unworthiness emerge, and thus adopt an extremely self-reliant pattern of behavior. Changing the caregiver does not lead to change in this avoidance because the child is certain that they can't trust *any* adult's commitment to caring for and comforting them and because they believe they are unlovable.

With time, the affective and reflective experience of the child's relationship with the DDP practitioner (and the current caregiver) can help the child to question this original trauma-induced story. Together they can develop a new story that includes the possibility that they do have worth, that particular adults can see this, and thus these adults are worthy of trust.

The practitioners and caregivers also have their own attachment and relationship history that can impact this work with the child.

REFLECTIVE EXERCISE: RESPONDING TO ANSWERS ABOUT ATTACHMENT HISTORY

Children and parents can be reluctant to respond to questions about their attachment history. Worksheet 2.1, at the end of the chapter, provides an opportunity to explore how you might respond to this.

If you were traumatized by your parents as a child, you are at risk of having your experience activated by similar traumas experienced by the child you are working with. At these times, you may not be able to respond in a manner that is best for the child because your own experience intrudes.

This can lead to less helpful interventions, such as:

- suggesting that the child try harder to avoid upsetting their parent
- suggesting that the child spend more time out of the house
- suggesting emotional or cognitive strategies that you used to cope with your experience

Reflecting on your own history, having confidence that you have resolved the impact any traumas have had on your development, and experiencing the value of comfort and joy in your own life may enable you to stay focused on the child's events and experiences, to see the differences between their trauma and yours, and to discover together what is best for them in their situation.

Suppose your history was fairly uneventful and you think your relationships with your parents are satisfactory. Your attachment history might still have an impact. For example, even if you do not feel traumatized by your parents, you might have developed a dismissive or preoccupied attachment pattern. You might subsequently perceive a child with developmental trauma through the same lens that you developed, failing to see important aspects in their attachment history. Reflecting on your own attachment history will help you be fully open and engaged with the child when exploring their attachment history.

TIME FOR REFLECTION

Reflect on aspects of your history and how they may influence your engagement with a traumatized child.

In DDP, the practitioner tries to intervene with follow-lead-follow. Does your history influence your leading?

Consider whether any of the following statements are true of your own development and how they might influence your engagement with a traumatized child:

1. You tended to be quite independent and self-sufficient.
2. You were quite assertive in expressing your mind if you thought someone was taking advantage of you or others.
3. You found it easy to "let it go" and focus on things that you found satisfying.
4. You avoided conflicts and people you had conflicts with.
5. You found failure to be difficult, so you tended to take the easy way in many situations.
6. You seldom cried/you cried a great deal.
7. You were the "good child" in the family.
8. You seldom admitted to making a mistake.
9. If you were raised by two parents, you counted on one parent when upset, never on the other parent.
10. You worked hard to please your parents, and you seldom admitted to being wrong.
11. You would become quite angry and defiant if you thought that your parents were being unfair.
12. You did not share thoughts and feelings that were different from your parents', wanting to avoid their disapproval.

If you sense that you might be leading the child into your solutions, coping strategies, values, and interests, you might reflect on:

- Is the child feeling that their being liked is conditional, not unconditional?
- Is the child focusing on what you want rather than discovering what they want?

- Are there signs that the child is not wondering enough, not reflecting enough?

In these cases, consider if the child is likely to be too focused on your mind and not enough on their own.

INTERSUBJECTIVITY

Just as we do with attachment theory, as we consider bringing intersubjectivity into our DDP interventions, we bear in mind that this theory developed within Western psychology. Though we consider intersubjective connections to be universal, the way they are enacted within different cultures will vary. The DDP practitioner explores and understands these cultural differences so that they can adapt the interventions while continuing to find ways to help the child discover safe connections.

Attachment behavior is not reciprocal. The child turns to the parent for safety. The parent does not reciprocate by turning to the child for safety. In contrast, intersubjective relating is reciprocal. The practitioner (or parent) has an influence on the child, and the child has a reciprocal influence on them.

Infants begin to form a sense of self when experiencing their parents' experience of them.

- Parents are interested in them: They are interesting.
- Parents love them: They are lovable.
- Parents take delight in them: They are delightful.

These experiences are primarily communicated nonverbally—in the parents' facial expressions, voice prosody, gestures, and movements, all synchronized with the child's nonverbal expressions. This is obviously true for the nonverbal infant, but it is also true for the older child and even the adult. Much of the other's experience of us is communicated nonverbally.

If the infant is seldom able to affect the parent, the parent is emotionally neglecting the infant. The infant needs to matter, needs to be special, needs to be enjoyed by the parent; otherwise their psychological development is going to be impaired. When psychological development is impaired, intersubjective experiences are central to facilitating the child's developmental recovery.

For this reason, the DDP practitioner takes a very intersubjective stance in therapy. This contrasts with the more traditional neutral stance, wherein the practitioner's experience of the child tends to remain ambiguous.

The child who has experienced developmental trauma is likely to avoid intersubjective experiences—the anticipated nonverbal communications involved are too negative and rejecting.

- The neglected child has little sense of self (other than being unimportant) because their parent attends little to them.
- The physically abused child has a sense of self as being bad or evil because most communications are of anger and violence.

In these circumstances, the child is likely to begin to avoid looking at the face or attending to the voice of their parent. It is too painful to receive those communications. This avoidance continues when they enter other relationships.

New DDP practitioners might hesitate to express their intersubjective experiences of the child for fear this method of engaging is unprofessional. They may wonder if they are being too casual, too informal. Since therapy is considered to be an important professional activity, they may think that they should relate in a way that reflects the seriousness of the content, and they feel drawn to practice the way they were trained, which is more formal and objective. And when the child, too, seems uncomfortable with this manner of relating, they may conclude that intersubjectivity is not right for this content, setting, or child.

DDP is a model that places importance on helping children to experience safe intersubjectivity so that they can recover from the impact of past unsafe relationships. Gently, slowly, and persistently, the DDP practitioner provides the child with intersubjective experiences of interest, acceptance, and enjoyment, though at times these are hard for the child to receive. The practitioner accepts the child's anxiety during positive intersubjective experiences, while helping them to wonder about their anxiety. Gradually the child learns to trust these experiences, one small step at a time.

Uncertain practitioners may struggle to maintain intersubjective experiences with the traumatized child if they are providing positive nonverbal communications without modifying them when the child expresses discomfort. For example, they show nonverbally that they like engaging with the child and that they enjoy their time with the child; the child communicates back that they are anxious and feel the need to defend themselves from such a close, spontaneous relationship; yet the practitioner continues to express and animate their enjoyment in spite of the child showing that they do not feel comfortable with these expressions.

When the engagement is truly reciprocal, the practitioner shows that they enjoy the child, but when the child shows that they are anxious, by withdrawing from the affective engagement, the practitioner moves to a lighter, more reflective manner of engagement. This shows complete acceptance of the child's wish for less affect in the engagement. The practitioner is following the child's lead, and the child realizes that they are having an impact on the practitioner. By following the child's lead, the practitioner is communicating that what the child wants is important, that they will follow the child's lead and not relate to them in the animated, intense manner that they initially led with. The practitioner might then gently lead the child back into affective engagement, being ready to follow again if the child is still not ready.

Intersubjective experiences have three primary characteristics:

- matching the child's affective state,

- joining the child in joint attention directed toward a particular object or event, and
- maintaining complimentary intentions

All three of these characteristics are important in DDP.

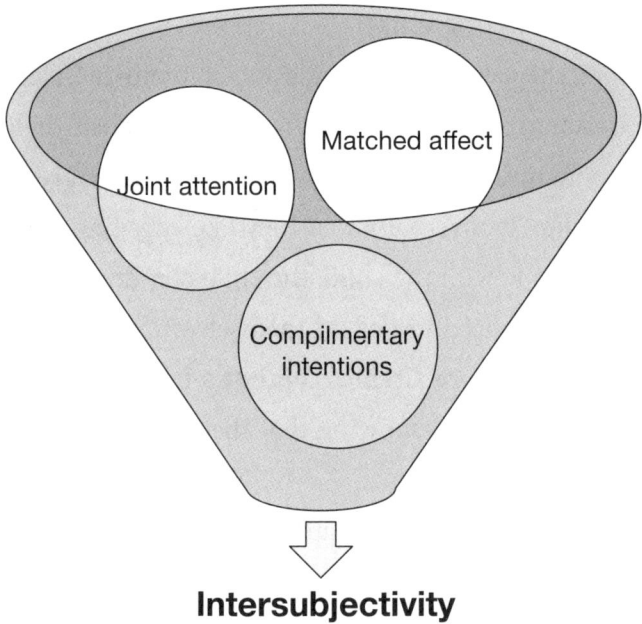

Figure 2.3 Components of Intersubjectivity

1. The therapist's affect matching the child's affective experience and expression is also known as affective attunement. Both therapist and child are having a similar affective experience of an object or event. Affect is considered to be the body's expression of an emotion. If the child is angry, it is shown affectively in their voice, face, gestures. When the therapist matches the affective expression, without having the emotion itself, the child feels that the therapist understands and "gets it." By matching the child's affec-

tive expression of the emotion, the practitioner is coregulating the child's emotion, helping the child to stay regulated. Developmentally, experiencing coregulation precedes the ability to auto-regulate. When the practitioner is attuned to the child's affective experience of the emotion, the child is less likely to avoid the emotional experience out of fear of dysregulation.

2. In DDP, joint attention helps the child reflect on an object or event that was traumatic. The child is not alone in the experience. Together with coregulation of an associated affective state, joint attention often leads the child to explore difficult themes that they usually avoid thinking about. As difficult emotions are regulated, the child can engage in the process of developing a story about the event. The practitioner holds the child's attention to the story through adopting rhythmic, affectively varied voice prosody. This story is likely to have much less of the fear and shame associated with their first story of the trauma. The child develops resilience as the trauma is integrated.

3. Complimentary intentions support the child to explore difficult themes with the practitioner. If the practitioner intends to "fix" the child by modifying their behavior, the child is likely to resist that therapeutic intervention. If the practitioner intends to accept and understand what the child has experienced, to get to know all aspects of the child, the child is much less likely to resist. Traumatized children tend to be very lonely children who often avoid thinking about their life. When practitioners communicate that they want to get to know the child, with no strings attached, many traumatized children find themselves wanting to be known. They actively participate in the process of becoming known; intentions become complimentary.

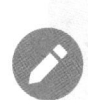

REFLECTIVE EXERCISE: ENGAGING CHILDREN INTERSUBJECTIVELY

Worksheet 2.2, at the end of the chapter, offers an opportunity to explore ways to respond to children. This explores how to maintain intersubjectivity when talking about stressful themes.

INTERPERSONAL NEUROBIOLOGY

Research on neurobiology has increased dramatically over the past few decades, in large part because of advances in technology. There is increasing evidence that the human brain is designed for safe relationships but will adapt when encountering unsafe relationships.

When the infant is experiencing safety, the region deep in the infant's brain known as the amygdala is instantly aware that there is no imminent danger, and the primitive need for self-protection through fight, flight, or freeze is not needed. When sensing safety, the infant's cortex is activated to make sense of the immediate situation, learn from it, and become engaged with it.

Over the first six months of life the infant repeatedly experiences safety through their parents' caregiving behaviors in response to their cues.

The infant also experiences safety within countless nonverbal, synchronized, intersubjective experiences. These provide them with the foundation of social-emotional learning, building on their core regulated biological states and leading to advances in more verbal and cognitive abilities.

One area of such neurobiological studies involves the Polyvagal Theory developed by Stephen Porges (2011). Dr. Porges's findings indicate that:

- When the infant feels safe, the ventral vagal circuit in the autonomic nervous system is activated.
- When the infant experiences threat, the dorsal vagal circuit is activated.

Safety further activates a complex neurological circuitry within the infant that Dr. Porges calls the social engagement system. This enables the infant to develop the social–emotional skills that are crucial if they are to have success as a social mammal. These skills are primarily nonverbal and involve the ability to make sense of voice prosody, eye contact, gestures, and movements and to join the adult in synchronized nonverbal communications.

These communications are present throughout human development and are crucial if the DDP practitioner is to help the traumatized child to trust an adult sufficiently to become engaged in a joint process of shared experience.

Dr. Porges has found that when two people are interacting with each other, they tend to become synchronized either in expressing safety through social engagement or expressing threat through defensiveness. If one person is defensive, the other person is likely to also become defensive to ensure their safety. However, if in response to the first person's defensiveness the second person is able to inhibit their tendency to become defensive and instead remains open and engaged, the first person is likely to gradually join them in this open and engaged state.

The traumatized child will often react defensively to an open and engaged practitioner. The DDP practitioner strives to remain open and engaged despite the child's defensiveness to help the child slowly begin to experience safety and thus become open and engaged also. When this happens, the practitioner then has the opportunity to help the child, who is now allowing themself to begin to trust someone. The therapist can guide the child toward engaging in a developmental relationship.

REFLECTIVE EXERCISE: UNDERSTANDING YOUR NERVOUS SYSTEM

This is a study group exercise to explore your own nervous system when it is exposed to cues of danger and safety. You will reflect on neuroception in action! This can be an emotional exercise so please look after yourself.

If you are alone, you might reflect on a recent experience when you were neurocepting cues of danger and how your nervous system responded.

Keep in mind the image of the autonomic ladder provided by Deb Dana (2018).

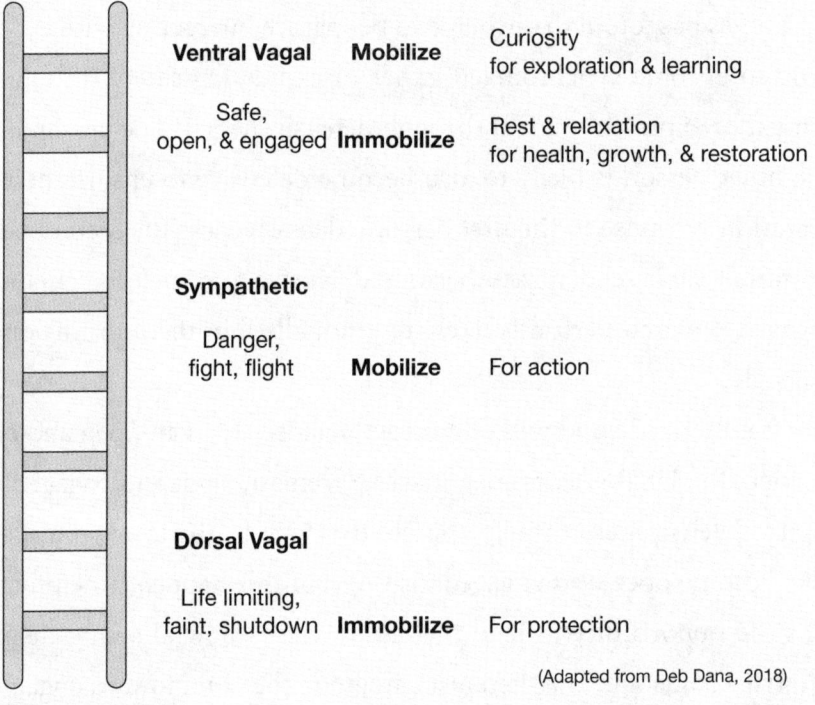

(Adapted from Deb Dana, 2018)

Figure 2.4 The Autonomic Ladder

We are also drawing on Deb Dana's (2018) concept of a ventral vagal anchor—an image, memory, or experience that, when savored, allows you to settle into your ventral vagal state.

1. Focus on a ventral vagal anchor: Bring to mind an image that makes you feel relaxed and balanced, such as from nature, a person, or pet. Savor this experience for twenty seconds as your breathing slows and you relax.

2. Now send nonverbal cues of danger to each other within the study group for one minute. Notice what is happening within your nervous system as you send and receive these signals.

3. Refocus back onto your ventral vagal anchor for another 20 seconds. Notice any changes in your nervous system.

4. Reflect together. Notice the pull on your nervous system. Where did you go on your autonomic ladder? You might notice an urge to move away or react (sympathetic) or an urge to hide or shutdown (dorsal vagal).

5. For the next minute, send cues of safety to each other non-verbally. Again, notice what is happening within your nervous system as you send and receive these signals.

6. Reflect together on this experience. Were there things that made it hard to remain socially engaged? What helped you to remain or to return to being socially engaged?

A related body of research demonstrates how various brain circuits are activated when the amygdala is sending signs of safety. These circuits are central in social-emotional learning, which enable the child to learn to differentiate cues of safety from cues of threat.

This research has been extensively studied by a colleague, Jonathan Baylin, PhD. Here is part of a long conversation that Dan had with Dr. Baylin.

Dan: Jon, tell me about the neurological foundations of blocked trust, which tends to be a response of the child to being abused and neglected by their primary caregiver.

Jon: Children with early histories of developmental trauma are at risk of developing blocked trust, a survival strategy that helps them to suppress their inherent need for relationships, for connections with other people. Helping these children to shift from this nonrelational state of mind toward a relational state of mind is not a simple process. It requires adults—therapists, parents, and teachers—to appreciate how mindless and automatic self-defensiveness is for maltreated kids.

This mindless mistrust is supported by an over-developed brain circuit called the innate alarm system, a system dedicated to processing small bits of information about another person within about a tenth of a second to determine which action to take: unmodulated fight, flight, or freeze and dissociate. As long as they are streaming defensively using this fast and furious brain system, children with blocked trust will not be able to learn from their "relational" experiences. In order to change their minds about the trustworthiness of others or about their own self-worth, they need to have experiences with adults during which they are engaged enough to pay attention to what is actually happening. For this learning and change to occur, we need to help these children shift into relationship, into intersubjective connection with another human.

Dan: Jon, I'm interested to hear how you would describe intersubjectivity from a neuropsychological perspective.

Jon: In relationship, adult brains can get in sync with children's brains, a dyadic process we can now actually see in action in research using a process called hyperscanning. This growing body of research shows, in a lovely way, that when two people are in connection, they are both activating a brain circuit in which a major hub is the TPJ, or temporoparietal junction. In brain terms, it is a goal of DDP to promote this brain-to-brain synchrony. This mutual engagement constitutes the "relational enrichment" that enables and sustains the shift toward a trust-based strategy of living.

Dan: So, what might the DDP therapist be aware of to help abused and neglected children begin to trust?

Jon: In order to have a chance to enable the child to shift from automatic mistrust toward trust, we need to help these children use their brakes, hold their horses, in short, pause and interrupt the automatic stream of defensiveness. Pausing amid an emergent defensive reaction requires the activation of a brain circuit that literally connects the famous amygdala, which is orchestrating those "fast and furious" reactions, to a higher brain circuit that engages a region called the dorsal anterior cingulate cortex, or dACC for short. When the dACC and amygdala are in connection, this circuit supports the process of opening a window of attention while inhibiting a "prepotent" impulse, such as the urge to hit or throw or run. The dACC region can help to increase attention and to suppress defensive behavior through its strong connections with other brain regions.

With the pause circuit on, even for half a second, the child has a chance to look around, to take in more information about the person they are with, to shift, literally, from disengagement toward engagement even as they are continuing to feel the push or pull of that automatic defensive reaction.

Dan: Do you have any thoughts about what the DDP therapist might do to facilitate this process?

Jon: In DDP terms, we need to PACE THE PAUSE. This means helping the child to utilize the pause by coregulating the process of putting on the brakes and then expanding their time in the window of engagement. We, the adults, need to appreciate the value of the pause so that we can respond in a positive way to the child's hovering between still being ready to defend against connection and having a glimmer of possibility to choose to connect.

Dan: Thanks, Jon, for providing us with this excellent summary of this research.

In attachment theory terms, the pause reopens the original state of tension or conflict the child experienced earlier in life, when the beginnings of disorganized attachment were setting in. That's when the child was experiencing the irresolvable conflict between the need for the caregiver's comfort and fear of the caregiver. When we help these children pause in the midst of being mindlessly defensive, we give them a second chance to learn to resolve the original dilemma of disorganized attachment by choosing connection over disconnection.

The practitioner may activate the pause with surprise, through communicating unexpected compassionate responses to the child's defensiveness. In DDP, such responses are most often described as PACE, namely being playful, accepting, curious, and empathic. Blocked trust causes children to automatically predict negative responses, especially when they are in the midst of an emergent defensive reaction. Brain scientists have found that the most powerful learning occurs when our brains encounter something that is unexpected, surprising, demanding of attention, and, possibly, curiosity toward a rising need to understand something that is unusual.

How can we help to activate these "positive error" signals that trigger an automatic pause? By being prepared to respond in a caring, curious, compassionate way to a child's defensive reactions. We're going for the "That's weird," reaction, an attention-grabbing way of relating to the child that can help to open the pause window, making it possible for the child to shift from defensiveness to an emerging intersubjective connection.

Dr. Baylin's description of neurological theory and research shows how the human brain is designed to facilitate development through experiences that are highly congruent with attachment and intersubjectivity theory and research (Baylin & Hughes, 2016). Keeping this in mind helps practitioners who are searching for ways to facilitate trust with a child who does not trust relationships. Without such trust, the child will remain alone in their efforts to resolve past traumas.

In a final note regarding neuropsychology, we want to acknowledge the default mode network (DMN). The DMN refers to how the brain is firing when we are at rest, when our mind is wandering and not focused on any specific task. This pattern of neurological impulses occurs between the anterior and posterior cingulate cortex. These impulses occur in a rhythmic manner; organized, not random. Of interest to us is that neurologists theorize that this neural activity is crucial for the development and integration of our sense of self. It appears to be more integrated and robust when we are experiencing safety and more fragmented when we are under stress and if we have a traumatic history. It is of particular interest to the DDP practitioner that the DMN is more active when we are engaged in storytelling, both the telling of stories and actively listening to stories as they are being told.

The way the DMN functions is consistent with attachment theory and research. The adult who is autonomously attached (the adult equivalent of the securely attached child), manifests a life story—an autobiographical narrative—that is coherent, comprehensive, consistent, and concise. Within attachment theory, an adult who has developed a coherent autobiographical narrative—regardless of the amount of relational trauma that they have experienced in their developmental years—would be considered to have resolved this trauma (Siegel, 2020).

The DDP practitioner needs to understand the nature of the traumatic events the child has experienced. The therapeutic work then needs to involve understanding the nature of the story the child developed to try to make sense of the trauma as it relates to their life. Finally, the practitioner needs to actively cocreate with the child a new story that will help the child resolve and integrate the trauma while developing a coherent narrative.

WHERE SAFETY BEGINS

Safety begins with the DDP practitioner.

Before the session, reflect on your emotional state. Are you feeling safe? If not, leave the office, go for a walk, do what it takes to ensure that you can be open to and engaged with the child when the session begins. Without the practitioner having a sense of safety—present, lost, regained, again and again—the traumatized child will not begin to experience this thing that they have seldom experienced before—their own sense of safety.

You cannot assume that you will be safe when you are in the presence of a traumatized child. You will need to reflect on this and again and again. The traumatized child you invite into your office needs to be sure of you. They need to be sure that you are safe in their presence so that they can discover what safety is like. For this to happen you need to remain safe:

- when the child ignores you
- when the child shows their trauma
- when the child screams at you

You don't need to be perfect! When you become defensive, stop, pause, repair, and create safety again for both of you.

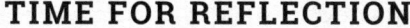

TIME FOR REFLECTION

We invite you to reflect on the following points in your efforts to create, maintain, and regain safety in your engagement with children who have experienced trauma and their families. Do not forget that this is hard! Your brain's default position is to move you toward defensiveness in the presence of a mistrustful child who attacks you or shuns you both physically and psychologically. Be patient with yourself.

1. Your own attachment and trauma history cannot be ignored.
   - Reflect on how you have addressed and resolved or could address and resolve any past relational trauma and/or difficult attachment experiences going back to your childhood.
   - How have friends, colleagues, or therapists helped you to reflect on your history?
   - Notice ways that this has reduced the negative impact of your history on your helping relationship with a traumatized child.
   - If you haven't sought support in this way, reflect on what has stopped you. If you truly value the therapeutic method for others who have been traumatized, you need to value it for yourself.
2. Reflect on your present life.
   - How have you addressed and managed sources of distress in your own life?
   - How has this helped you to remain present with a traumatized child?

- Whatever—apart from your therapy relationship with the child—is causing you some distress needs to be left at the door. If you have trouble leaving it at the door, reflect on what is making this difficult for you. Pause. Take care of yourself. Open the door only when you are ready.

3. You will become defensive within a split second of the traumatized child pushing against your sense of safety and its wobbling.
    - Notice how this shows itself for you. Try to notice your defensiveness within another split second, pause, become open and engaged again, and invite the child again (with PACE) to enter your safe presence.
    - After the session, reflect on this experience. Notice how easy or difficult it has been to pause and what has helped you to become open and engaged again.

4. Providing care for a traumatized child is often difficult. How do you ensure that you are cared for—both in your personal life and in your professional life—so that you are able to continue to provide care for someone who finds it difficult to receive your care?

Making mistakes is hard. We like to get things right, to be successful, to feel a sense of pride about our accomplishments, and to be recognized for our skills.

TIME FOR REFLECTION

Recall some times when you have made a therapeutic mistake.

- What made it difficult to address what you did and fix it?
- What helped you to do this?

Everyone finds making mistakes hard, and therapists are not immune, even though this is our area of expertise.

Mistakes are hard when they trigger a sense of shame. We conclude that it was more than a mistake, that it was a sign of our incompetence. Not that we *got it* wrong, but that we *are* wrong. When we minimize our mistakes, blame our client, make excuses for what happened, and get angry when someone questions us about it, we are experiencing shame. These defensive responses allow us to avoid the experience of looking at ourselves and finding ourselves lacking.

Shame is a pervasive experience among those who have experienced developmental trauma. Maybe it is also an all-too-common experience of those of us who try to assist those who have been traumatized.

If shame is a common part of our life, we can seek to understand what it might represent. For example:

1. Our parents may have related to us from the outside in. Namely, when they attended to us, they mostly focused on evaluating our behaviors and lost sight of our need for the attachment relationship with them to be based on unconditional acceptance of the self. They—and we—then lost sight of the difference between self and behavior. As a result, when we make a mistake, we experience our self as being wrong or lacking.

2. Our parents may have habitually taught us "right" and "wrong" through mixing their efforts at discipline with their relationship with us. Consequences for misbehavior may have consistently involved expressions of anger (even verbal assaults) and/or avoidance (even shunning). This experience may have created a sense that relationships are conditional and routine mistakes are a threat to the relationship.

3. Our immediate family, and possibly our whole community, might have been highly competitive and/or perfectionistic. There was little room or readiness to accept mistakes.

4. We may be marginalized or excluded within our immediate community because of our race, religion, gender, or disability. If, simply by being alive, we are "less than" many others in our community, we are at high risk of experiencing habitual shame.

5. Conflicts, like mistakes, are a natural part of any close relationship. Possibly, in our experience, anything leading to a conflict required someone being right and someone being wrong. This can lead to a tendency to minimize or deny mistakes to avoid the experience that there is something wrong with us.

6. Mistakes require acceptance of the value and need for relationship repair after having made a mistake. If we haven't experienced this, we may have difficulty acknowledging and initiating a need for repair.

CONCLUSION

The foundation of DDP and our understanding of developmental trauma are based on attachment theory, intersubjectivity, and neuroscience, all of which ensure that our therapeutic interventions are not dominated by the cognitive models of the mind which are so characteristic of Western psychology (Kinouani, 2021). As a result, DDP is highly affective and relational, ensuring that the narratives that emerge in the sessions as well as in DDP-influenced home care is both experiential and reflective, blending verbal and nonverbal ways of engagement. Relationships based on these principles provide safety and open and engaged ways of exploration and discovery.

Still, DDP primarily adopts a largely Western worldview. As our knowledge expands through cross-cultural research, our knowledge of attachment, intersubjectivity, and neuroscience is likely to do so as well, further guiding the development of DDP interventions into a wider range of cultural applications.

Worksheet 2.1

 Reflective Exercise: Responding to
Answers About Attachment History

Here are some brief dialogues within which a parent or child has responded to questions about their attachment history. Consider what you might say in response to each.

1. From what you've said, your parents were quite strict with you. It sounds like they were not patient if you did something wrong.

   A. **Teen:** *That's just how it was. I lived with it and didn't think about it, so it doesn't really affect me now.*

   _____

   _____

   _____

   _____

   B. **Parent:** *I know that I get angry too much with my kid! I'm not going to make excuses by blaming it on my parents!*

   _____

   _____

   _____

   _____

C. **Child:** *I used to hate them for it, and maybe I still do at times. But I don't see any value in going back and dwelling on that stuff again! Just tell me what to do now!*

2. When you lived with your parents, and your dad would beat you and your mom would ignore you, how did you make sense of that?
A. **Teen:** *When I thought about it, I figured that I must have deserved it, even if I also thought that I didn't. So, I stopped trying to figure it out.*

B. **Teen:** *I knew that I was just a rotten kid and if I'd stop acting like a jerk, they'd stop treating me that way. I still do sometimes. And I'm afraid if I have kids, they'll turn out just like me.*

C. Child: *How do you think I made sense of it! I hated them, and I still do, and nothing you say will make me forgive and forget that!*

---

3. Your life has been so hard in so many ways! What would you say has been the hardest for you?

A. Child: *I try so hard to make a better future for myself and forget the past! And you just want me to go back there and then I feel that it's hopeless, nothing will ever change!*

B. **Parent or Teen:** *The hardest is when jerks like you keep bringing up my past even though I tell everyone that I don't want to talk about it!*

_____

_____

_____

_____

C. **Parent or Teen:** *The hardest is that nobody really gives a damn. You have to talk like you care, that's your job. But nobody, including you, thinks about me when I'm not around.*

_____

_____

_____

_____

 Reflections on Worksheet 2.1:
Possible Responses

1. From what you've said your parents were quite strict with you. It sounds like they were not patient if you did something wrong.

A. Teen: *That's just how it was. I lived with it and didn't think about it, so it doesn't really affect me now.*

Response: And its hard stuff to think about, so if you believe that it won't help, I can see why you wouldn't want to do it. It might seem different if you told me about it and we understood it together. Maybe seeing it differently now might help you to see yourself and your life in a way that brings some hope for change.

B. Parent: *I know that I get angry too much with my kid! I'm not going to make excuses by blaming it on my parents!*

Response: So, you won't blame your parents and you're left with blaming yourself. Maybe if you could make sense of why they were so hard on you—not blame them, just make sense of it all—it might help you to see your son differently and have a different relationship with him.

C. Child: *I used to hate them for it, and maybe I still do at times. But I don't see any value in going back and dwelling on that stuff again! Just tell me what to do now!*

Response: I'm afraid "that stuff" is informing what you do now, and it sounds like you feel hopeless that this will ever change. Maybe it seems hopeless because you're all alone with it now, just like you were then. Let me be with you in it and maybe we can figure out how to make it change.

2. When you lived with your parents, and your dad would beat you and your mom would ignore you, how did you make sense of that?
    A. Teen: *When I thought about it, I figured that I must have deserved it, even if I also thought that I didn't. So, I stopped trying to figure it out.*

Response: So, you tried . . . and couldn't really make sense of it. And you still can't. Maybe together we can. And I suspect we'll see that it says a lot more about your parents than about who you really are.

> B. **Teen:** *I knew that I was just rotten kid and if I'd stop acting like a jerk, they'd stop treating me that way. I still do sometimes. And I'm afraid if I have kids, they'll turn out just like me.*

Response: It must have been so hard—being hurt like that and also thinking that you were a rotten kid. I wonder if there were other reasons why you did what you did, and you and your parents never figured out what they were. Maybe reasons to do with being all alone, discouraged, and angry that no matter what you did, it seemed that your parents still saw you as being rotten, and you were left believing them.

> C. **Child:** *How do you think I made sense of it! I hated them, and I still do, and nothing you say will make me forgive and forget that!*

Response: I'm so sorry that you think that I want you to "forgive and forget"! I didn't say that very well! I want you to be able to see yourself more like I and your foster carers see you, not how your parents do. If someday you stop hating them, it will be your choice, not mine. Maybe you won't have time for hating them because you're discovering what is good about you.

> 3. Your life has been so hard in so many ways! What would you say has been the hardest for you?
>   A. **Child:** *I try so hard to make a better future for myself and forget the past! And you just want me to go back there and feel that it's hopeless, nothing will ever change!*

Response: The things you're trying to forget are still there, still blaming you! If we can make sense of them together, maybe they'll start to leave you alone. And then you might be able to discover a future that is not held back by your past—a future you can build, not the one your parents wanted to give you.

> B. **Parent or Teen:** *The hardest is when jerks like you keep bringing up my past when I tell everyone that I don't want to talk about it!*

Response: I get why you're angry with me—I have heard you say you don't want to talk about it, and I then ask about it anyway! Why, you think, am I still bringing it up? My reason is to help you make sense of it, so it stops dragging you down! So you can build a life without it contaminating you.

> C. **Parent or Teen:** *The hardest is that nobody really gives a damn. You have to talk like you care, that's your job. But nobody, including you, thinks about me when I'm not around.*

Response: Oh, you're so alone, and you've been so alone all of your life. Why would you think that your foster mother or I will be any different? No wonder it's hard to trust us . . . hard to believe that you are more than a job to us.

Worksheet 2.2

 Reflective Exercise: Engaging Children Intersubjectively

Here are some comments from a child in response to a stressful theme being introduced by the practitioner. Consider some responses that you might use to facilitate the active engagement of the child using matching affect, joint attention, and complimentary intentions.

1. **Practitioner:** Help me understand what was so difficult for you yesterday when you swore at your mother.

   Child: I don't want to talk about it! You don't understand, and you never will!

   _____

   _____

   _____

   _____

2. **Practitioner:** What was it like being all alone and seemingly ignored by the other kids at the game?

   Child: When I got home, I watched an incredible show on TV! I had been waiting a long time to see that.

   Practitioner: But what was the game like for you?

   Child: I've been thinking about asking my dad if he'll take me into the city this weekend. There are some cool shoes on sale that I really want.

_____

_____

_____

_____

3. **Practitioner:** Lately you and your mom seem to be having a hard time getting close. I wonder how you might approach that?

   Child: And I wonder how my mom might approach that. And I also wonder if you'll ask her that too or if it's all on me to make it right.

_____

_____

_____

_____

 ## Reflections on Worksheet 2.1: Possible Responses

1. **Practitioner:** Help me understand what was so difficult for you yesterday when you swore at your mother.

   Child: I don't want to talk about it! You don't understand and you never will!

Response: (Involves matching affect) Of course you wouldn't want to talk about it if I wouldn't understand what you were going through! Of course not! Just one more person who doesn't get it, who thinks you were wrong!

2. **Practitioner:** What was it like being all alone and seemingly ignored by the other kids at the game?
   Child: When I got home, I watched an incredible show on TV! I had been waiting a long time to see that.
   Practitioner: But what was the game like for you?
   Child: I've been thinking about asking my dad if he'll take me into the city this weekend. There are some cool shoes on sale that I really want.

Response: (Involves facilitating joint attention) And that's something that you'd like to do with your dad? Do you think he'd think they're cool too? Are you close to your dad about stuff like that? . . . Thanks for letting me know about your dad. When you're having a hard time with some of the other kids, is he someone that would understand . . . that you might want to talk with about it?

3. **Practitioner:** Lately you and your mom seem to have had a hard time getting close. I wonder how you might approach that?
   Child: And I wonder how my mom might approach that. And I also wonder if you'll ask her that too—or if it's all on me to make it right.

Response: (Involves complimentary intentions) Ah! It seems to you that I want to know what you can do because I think that there's something wrong with you! That I think you messed up and that it's my job to get you to please your mom! Is that what it seems like? If so, I understand why you wouldn't want to talk with me about it. You figure I'm not really listening to you and I'm just trying to fix you because I believe your mom has nothing to do with your not being close.

IN CONVERSATION ONE

Kim met with Elizabeth Studwell, Alexia Jones (a pseudonym), and Lewis Maskell to talk to them about their experiences growing up in care or as an adoptee.

Elizabeth is an international and transracial adoptee with a doctorate in clinical psychology. Elizabeth says: "My primary area of knowledge and focus is working with adoptees and their families. I am very passionate about supporting children who have gone through significant life losses and traumas and helping parents and families who adopt these children to more fully understand their inner lived-experiences and to learn how to best support them toward a healthy developmental path with love and deep connection. May this discussion encourage you to slow down and put yourself into the child's experience, to gain a glimmer into their inner world before you make any decisions about them."

Alexia grew up in foster care. At the time of this conversation she was a trainee psychologist. Kim and Alexia wrote *A Tiny Spark of Hope* together (Golding & Jones, 2021). Alexia says: "I feel incredibly proud to be in the privileged position to represent and amplify the voices of those who have grown up within the care system."

Lewis grew up in foster care. He is a qualified social worker. Lewis says: "It is my pleasure to share my experiences and thoughts regarding DDP and the social care system along with the important role that it had throughout my life and development. I am passionate about ensuring children and young people within the care system have the correct support and understanding of professionals around them so that they can develop and progress the best that they can at their own pace. I hope my and my colleagues insights within the conversation will help you understand how to engage with children and young people who have experienced the care system."

Kim: I'm really interested to hear about your experiences of being brought up in foster care and adoption and what you would want DDP practitioners to know about this experience.

Elizabeth: The thing that really jumps out for me is that practitioners need a deep-rooted sense of the complexity of our identity experience. The complexity of "Who am I and where do I belong?" I think this is particularly true in a transracial experience, when so many pieces of your identity change: your name changes, your language changes, your religion changes, your culture changes, the food you eat changes. So many things are different. Understand what it feels like on the inside when you look different and are identified as different and for children who move from family to family and each of those families have their own identity, maybe even their own racial background. For example, they might spend time in a family that's fully Spanish speaking and then spend time in a family that doesn't speak any Spanish at all. I feel like it's an existential difference from somebody who knows, and doesn't ever have to doubt, that this is my family, this is who I am. I think that's really hard for clinicians who have never experienced it to wrap their head around. It certainly is for adoptive parents too.

Lewis: What really resonates with me is the sense of not belonging, not knowing where you fit in. Comfortable as I was in my foster family, I experienced the pull to go back to my parents, it's quite a powerful thing. Do I belong here? Do I belong there?

Kim: And there can be a big difference in socio–economic status, the class differences, from your birth family to your foster family.

Lewis: Yes, there are differences. My mom's quite confrontational, quite aggressive, which has come from her own experiences. In my foster family things are a lot more conversation based, with encouragement that you can do it.

Alexia: One of my first memories of my foster family was that I was convinced that we were millionaires. Looking back, I think it's quite adorable, but also kind of sad. We lived in a standard Victorian terraced house in the city. Coming from a house with a room with one sofa and nothing else in it and my bedroom pouring water when it rains just due to the nature of the council house[2] that I came from, I was utterly convinced that we were millionaires. It was such a big difference, going to a house that was full of stuff and full of food. It just felt so different to what I was used to. Smells for me are really big. Everything is so different in a foster family. The smell when you walk in, the smell of the cushion or the smell of the bed clothes. It's just fundamentally different right down to that kind of level. I wonder if it would be easy for practitioners, who may or may not have this level of lived-experience, to forget how huge this is. Then there is the fear that you could lose this; it's hard to feel safe. While I might seem to be doing well, feeling safer and becoming more secure, I think there's always one eye that is looking for any hint that something is changing or a sign that I'm going.

Elizabeth: When you're adopted as an infant, that first house shift hap-

---

2   A council house is a house owned by the local government and rented out.

pens when you're teeny tiny. And when you mentioned the senses and that smell, it really struck me for infants too. Each family has their own smell. This might seem a little weird, but I'm the only one I know who smells like me, because I've never met anybody in my immediate biological family. Infant adoptees have to adjust to all new sensory perceptions. They have to adjust to new sounds, new tastes, and new smells. Our brains have to do a lot of adjusting really early without any understanding or awareness of the change. It took me many more years to wonder who I would have been. What I would have been like. Where do I belong? Am I safe? I experienced that too. That fear of closeness because the loss, even if I don't remember it, still feels really palpable.

Lewis: And safety is so important for DDP practitioners to provide. It's building that relationship. You don't start with, "Right now, we're going to look at your past." It's very much, "Let's have this chat." Understand as much as you can about that child before you start trying to unpick what are some really big feelings and experiences that the child has gone through.

Kim: Yes, it's what we say in DDP all the time, you have to slow down. You can't do this too quick.

Alexia: I think it's really important for people not to assume that because you've been in a foster family for 15 years, you feel safe and you trust all the adults. That couldn't be further from my experience. And I think that speaks to thinking about working with a DDP practitioner. I was watchful, waiting on Kim for a long time. It took me many, many years to realize that I could approach her for some support as a young adult. That was the level of mistrust that I had to contend with. It was that idea of "Is she safe enough to approach?" Don't underestimate that; it was huge for me.

Kim: Yes, and this has taught me that we never know what seeds we're planting early on and when they will start to flourish. That experience of us coming in and out of your foster home and supporting your foster carers was all building up to something so many years in the future. I think it's really important to hold onto that. It's not all going to happen now. You know, this is a lifetime journey.

Alexia: And there's something for me about choice. As a child, do you really have a choice of going to your therapist? I was sniffing out people being in charge of me a mile before they were. That's been part of my survival, and that meant that as a child I probably couldn't engage in something that I'd been taken to or was being encouraged to do when it wasn't led by what I wanted.

Elizabeth: Can I ask a question, Alexia? Because that seems so spot on to me and I think DDP clinicians should know this. How would you want a therapist to handle that situation? So, let's say the therapist was able to really deeply know that this child is coming against their will. How can I accept that and still work with that? Maybe it's that we have to slow down and do our best, but I'd be curious to see if you have any thoughts about what would be helpful for a kid going through that.

Alexia: My first thought is, "Whose agenda is this? Who wants the child to be in therapy and why?" I don't think we often trust in our clients to know themselves as well as they do and to be guided by them. I wonder how often we really listen to the children. If they're not engaging, they're not engaging for a reason. We need to listen to that. And then we need to think about how else we can intervene, because direct intervention isn't the only intervention. Can I offer this in other ways? What is the pressure on me, as the practitioner, to offer this to this child? Is it in the child's best interest, or is it another many leveled system problem that is being put on the child? And bringing it back to your question, I would say, meet me where I'm at. If you get into a battle trying to make someone do something that they don't agree with, you're not going to get anywhere anyway.

Lewis: It's about going at the child's pace. They might not want to engage straight away, but that comes down to the skill of the practitioner at building the relationship. I do think there should be more [of an] element of choice, but if the child has been brought to you,, you have to do what you can and sow those seeds [to be] ready for the future.

Elizabeth: I know DDP says it everywhere, but the relationship does actually have to come first. It's OK if we're not talking about a full level of trust. Maybe that shouldn't even be expected. Meeting kids where they're at by going at the child's pace. Allowing kids to be the ones that are setting the agenda and guiding. This is family focused. We want to first support parents to be able to slow down enough to hear what their child is saying. It's OK to be who you are. That's what helps settle the nervous system as much as possible.

Alexia: Time also needs to be put into exploring the foster carers'
barriers, blocks, experiences, patterns, and responses. When
you think it's enough with a parent, there's probably always
some more that can be done. It's so easy to put stuff on the
kid. I think there was a lot that I felt shame for and that
could have been worked out with my foster carers.

Elizabeth: I couldn't agree more that there's so much work that can and
needs to be done with parents. It's so important because the
children need to be seen as children. Finding where we can
slow down to help the insight come just feels so important.

Kim: Those parents often come to us thinking that we're going to
fix their child. How do we get to a mindset where they see
support for them as their right? It's not about fixing them.
It's not about fixing the child, but it is about exploration so
we can do better for each other.

Elizabeth: Parents can be woefully unprepared, especially if they have
never been a parent before, and then they're adopting a child
who has a challenging attachment-based history. I would
want more practitioners to be aware of just how the multiple
changes, the early attachment difficulties, and the loss make
it really hard to connect. Adopters need to be prepared not
to expect attachment quickly. It takes years, actually.

Alexia: This feels like a bit of a paradoxical thing, but I want to think
about the idea of "good enough." What is good enough, and
what is more than good enough? Good enough to somebody
like me, who hasn't had anywhere near enough, feels almost
intolerable. So, imagine what perfect would feel like. That's

just run-for-the-hills time! Imagine it as a number of bricks. If you've come from having a couple of bricks, and all of a sudden you are expected to be open to 20 bricks, that's overwhelming for their physical nervous system. It doesn't have to be shiny and perfect, good enough is OK. The most important thing is repair. I can't over exaggerate how important that is. And not once: repeated micro experiences of things being tricky and then things being OK, things being tricky and things being OK.

Lewis: I'd like to echo what you're saying about repair. Even when you have had repair, you still don't get it, that you are valued and will be taken care of. I remember I was having trouble recently, and I just went straight to thinking about how I was letting my foster carer down, worrying that she's going to hate me. I know it's not true, but still, even as an adult, it's there. I see therapy like a spiral. You're going to have that one point in the spiral that you're always going to revisit.

Elizabeth: That's something I've thought a lot about and noticed more and more as I've gotten into my adulthood, as I've done my own work. How much support is it possible to take in at any given time? Different kids need different amounts, their nervous systems are able to take in very different amounts. For some kids, hardly any at all is tolerable. At different times you can only tolerate so much. What's right for this kid is going to be really modulated based on what this child needs now. Oftentimes a sense of pain and discomfort comes along with the comfort. I physically experience pain and even become tearful when I'm receiving extra comfort and support. That's so complex because you both yearn for it and then it can be physically uncomfortable.

Lewis: I think it's the same regarding praise. I hate when people say, "You've done really well there." It's really hard to accept that actually I did a good job.

Alexia: I was going to say something about praise too, Lewis. As you were talking about it, I could feel that "ick" in my body; I could physically feel it. It's really uncomfortable. And yet attempts by the carer to connect and provide, they don't go amiss either. I might not respond. In fact, the more important it feels, the more I might not respond, but it wouldn't go amiss. I would notice and probably be grateful for that. And if you are really grumpy, name it. If there's something going on, name it, because I will know a million seconds before you, and if you hide it, I will still know. I have had to survive by knowing what adults feel and what is going on for them. Just be as authentic as possible.

Kim: That feels like a really important piece of advice to end on. Thank you so much everyone.

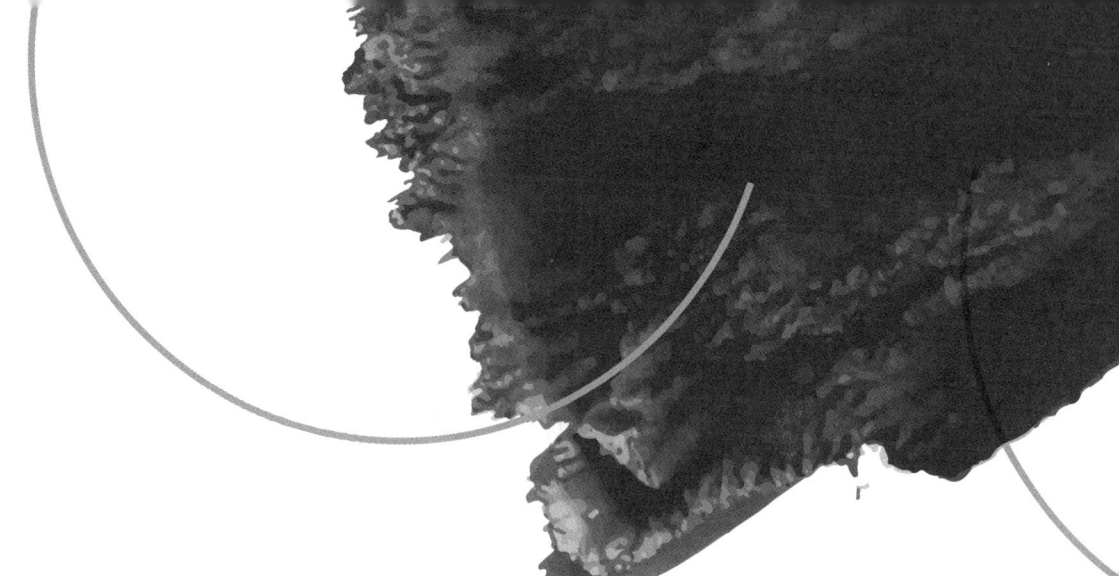

Chapter 3:
PACE: The Foundation of Safe and Healthy Relationships

PACE is where trust begins, allowing mistrust to exit. Mistrust is a tricky character, however. It continues to reappear. Only when PACE accepts mistrust too will it hand over the stage to trust. PACE is therefore a way of being toward the child in all her parts. As the child experiences being deeply accepted by the adults, she can come to accept herself. This is the beginning of learning that she is a good person and that parents can be trusted after all. (Hughes et al., 2019, p. 29)

REFRESHER

PACE is an acronym described by Dan based on observations of adults and infants interacting. This denotes qualities of playful connecting, acceptance of the child's inner world, curiosity about the meaning underneath behavior, and empathy for the child's emotional state. PACE is at the heart of emotional connection with infants and is central to the development of attachment and intersubjective relationships. Experiencing PACE leads to a sense of being unconditionally loved, the building block for security.

TABLE 3.1 PACE

P = Playful	This is the experience of joy in relationships. We don't need to try to be playful. Instead discover a liking for and enjoyment in the other. Playfulness will follow. Playfulness also expresses a lightness that conveys a sense of confidence in the child, the relationship, and the future, regardless of the immediate problem.
A = Acceptance	This represents a deep acceptance of the inner world of the other. Feelings, thoughts, beliefs, and wishes are not evaluated but are accepted as neither right nor wrong; they just are. We may not want a child to feel the way they do. What they need from us is to be with them in this uncomfortable experience.
C = Curiosity	To truly connect with another we need, through curiosity, to understand their experience. Curiosity seeks these stories that will deepen our understanding. This curiosity comes from a place of not knowing and is nonjudgmental. We wish to understand, not evaluate. We are asking, "Who are you?" and "Will you let me get to know you?"
E = Empathy	We communicate our understanding of, acceptance for, and enjoyment in our relationship with the other through our empathy. This involves us experiencing the other and their experience so that they truly feel felt by us. With empathy, we resonate with their experience as if it were our own, though it is not.

Children and adolescents who have experienced relational trauma have missed out on opportunities to experience secure attachment and the reciprocal connections described as intersubjectivity. PACE is therefore an important way of being to help these young people experience and benefit from healthy relationships and thus to start the healing process.

PACE is the central therapeutic stance and relational attitude within DDP. All adults—therapists, practitioners, parents, and educators—are encouraged to communicate their deep interest in and understanding of the child or adolescent through this way of being. Furthermore, adults are encouraged to relate to themselves and each other in this same way.

Although written as an acronym, PACE is not a linear process, it is a whole way of being (Figure 3.1). Within PACE, acceptance and empathy are ever pres-

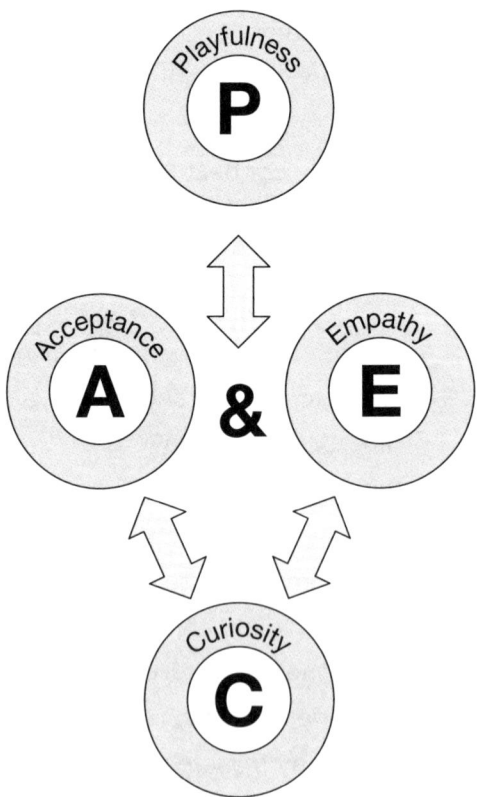

Figure 3.1 PACE

ent. Acceptance, curiosity, and empathy interweave to carry the momentum of the story we are discovering forward. Playfulness comes in and out as appropriate, displaying our enjoyment in our relationship with the other.

PACE represents a deep acceptance of the other alongside our curiosity about who the other truly is. The experience of being understood and accepted begins the process for an individual of developing self-acceptance and learning to trust both self and others.

Notice that PACE is a way of being, not a technique. We are not seeking to change the other, we are simply actively getting to know them and being with them. As we get to know them, we share their experience and, in turn, they deepen and organize their own understanding of their experience. We cannot change the other, but we can change the way we respond. Through this process, change might emerge for them, but this is based on the healthy experience of a relationship and a joint discovery of who they are rather than by an act of will on our part.

When we bring our attitude of PACE to therapy, we provide a relationship based on understanding the other's experience. We cocreate their story together. Alongside this, our presence provides coregulation so that the emotional experience of understanding this story does not overwhelm. PACE also helps us to slow down when we are exploring a behavioral problem with a child. It reminds us that we need to understand and accept what the behavior means before we explore what, if any, intervention we might consider to address the behavior.

When we bring our attitude of PACE to parenting or to other arenas, such as when educating the child, we develop a relationship upon which other things can be built. Kim calls this "PACE-plus." The security that PACE offers can help us when we need to figure out a way forward (problem-solving); to let the child know we experience them differently (affirmation); to increase the child's understanding (teach); and to provide the child with support to behave differently (discipline). The "pluses" will be more successful if built on a foundation of PACE. This will be considered further in Chapter 7, which explores parenting of children.

EXPERIENCING PACE

For the rest of this chapter, we are going to explore PACE together. Let's dive deep into this way of being, developing our understanding and appreciation for this attitude that will be so central to all our DDP interventions.

THE PLACE OF LOVE IN PACE

When we are training, we are often asked what has happened to love. Is there a PLACE for love?

Love is, of course, central to the relationship between a child and parent. All children need to feel unconditionally loved by at least one person in their life. This is the basis for their own sense of lovability. Love however is a state rather than an attitude.

Love is also expressed differently in different families. For example, Chinese colleagues have told us that Chinese parents are less likely to express love verbally, but to demonstrate it through caring acts. Between and within cultures families will express love in different ways. The DDP practitioner needs to understand these differences so that they can adjust their interventions for the unique family they are working with.

Dan and I choose to see love as surrounding PACE rather than sitting within it. If the attitude of PACE is surrounded by love, however this is expressed, the child will have what they need for security and trust.

Incidentally, we also prefer not to include "S," for security, as part of PACE. That would be SPACE—a neat acronym; but security is the outcome, it is not part of the attitude. Here we stick with PACE, as Dan originally conceived it.

Let's start exploring PACE by thinking about the experience of receiving PACE. What is it like when someone has or doesn't have PACE for you?

TIME FOR REFLECTION

We invite you to imagine that you are struggling with a difficult moment in your life. Perhaps, an issue at work with a boss. You feel unappreciated and undervalued. You confide in someone about how difficult this has been.

Reflect on the scenarios below. How would each leave you thinking and feeling?

Notice the difference between support that is not PACEful and support that is. How do these differences show up in your body? How relaxed or tense do you feel, how are you breathing, what is happening in your heart and in your stomach?

If you are reflecting on this with others, you might role play these two scenarios.

Scenario One: Your confidante listens to you as you relate what has happened. They seem sympathetic and then tell you about a similar situation that they experienced. They make a joke about bosses and tell you that you will be fine. You are a good worker and maybe if your boss doesn't realize that, it is time to find another job. They urge you to go back into work after the weekend with head held high, as you have done nothing wrong.

Scenario Two: Your confidante listens to you as you relate what has happened. They seem sympathetic and ask you some questions to find out more about what happened. They agree with you that this sounds very tricky and wonder how it has left you feeling. As you respond, they are accepting of your feelings and empathic to how you feel. They don't offer any solutions but acknowledge that it is going to feel hard going back into work after the weekend.

We wonder if, like us, you experienced these imagined scenarios very differently. In both, the confidante is trying to be supportive. In the first, they try to make you feel better, possibly to relieve their own sense of discomfort, by offering reassurance and solutions. This can leave you feeling tense and not fully understood. You want your confidante to really get you, to know that this has rocked your sense of who you are. Without this, it can feel like you are being dismissed and your issue minimized. In the second scenario, the confidante sits with you with an attitude of PACE. Your feelings are accepted; you experience their empathy and interest in you and in how this issue has affected you. They understand you and what you experienced. This feels emotionally safer and can help you to find more clarity about your experience. They have not offered a fix, but you may still be left seeing the way forward more clearly. The support you have experienced can leave you motivated to carry on and face whatever is ahead with more confidence.

TIME FOR REFLECTION: A DAY IN THE LIFE

It is helpful to imagine being a child or adolescent who is being related to with and without PACE. Within DDP trainings, we do an exercise called "A day in the life." Kim includes some examples in the *Foundations for Attachment Training Resource* referenced in the list of resources.

We include a new example at the end of this chapter in Worksheet 3.1 for you to reflect on.

STRENGTHENING THE ATTITUDE OF PACE

We all respond differently when being introduced to PACE. Most DDP trainees agree that it is not as easy as it looks! Some people find it comes more naturally to them; it fits with their natural style of communicating. Others need to work at it; it is a very different way of relating, and they find themselves quickly falling back on more habitual ways of communication.

REFLECTIONS FROM KIM

Kim grew up in a Western culture. Victorian England attitudes still resonated with a leaning toward authoritarian parenting, a "do as I say" mentality. Within her family, there was little curiosity about the emotional world of family members and instead a focus on achievement and acquiring wealth, the latter a hangover from her father's Jewish heritage; his ancestors came to England as refugees. Money meant some security against the expectation that they would have to move again. Her mother, a Yorkshire woman who grew up in an emotionally cold home, suffered from lifelong depression, which was little talked about or made sense of. Unconscious racism existed in both sides of the family; the Yorkshire person's distrust of the outsider and the Jewish person's need to be accepted as part of the "in crowd" led to discouragement of positively noticing or embracing difference in others. This upbringing did not foster curiosity about others or their experiences.

PACE was not a central attitude in Kim's family. This cultural mix led to some elements of conditionality within her upbringing. While she always felt loved, she also knew that approval would come from achievement. Training as a clinical psychologist facilitated this approval, but this cultural upbringing impacted the type of psychologist that Kim became. For Kim, successful interventions meant moving away from emotional struggles. Parenting support appealed to her because it is more about doing than being. Kim had developed the central features of any good therapist—developing a therapeutic alliance with empathy and positive regard (Norcross & Wampold, 2011)—but her family and community culture had not prepared her to deepen these. She still lived under the instruction to "do as I say," and she carried unconscious biases, which meant that she did not notice or seek to understand differences in her clients, whether via class, race, sexuality, or disability. She cared about them and wanted to support them, but she stopped short of stepping into their shoes.

When Kim was introduced to PACE by Dan, it is fair to say that it felt like a foreign language. It was to transform the type of psychologist Kim endeavored to be. While Kim was empathic, her empathy was not deepened by a bedrock of truly understanding the inner world of the other. Kim needed to awaken her curiosity. She could be playful but lacked the spontaneity that comes from truly enjoying the other.

One day, Kim was listening to the radio. A man was talking about his love of trees, especially the shape revealed in the winter when the trees are bare. Kim never looked at winter trees the same again. The loss of leaves was no longer only a harbinger of the cold, wet weather to come, foretelling muddy walks with her dogs! Suddenly Kim saw the beauty that was revealed. Something clicked, and Kim understood the power of curiosity. If it is powerful with trees, how much more so with people! Curiosity reveals stories, and these pave the way to deeper understanding, to increased enjoyment and truly accepting and empathizing with others. It is different for everyone, but for Kim, unlocking curiosity was a key to developing a PACE way of being.

REFLECTIONS FROM DAN

Dan grew up in a city in the northeastern region of the U.S.—Pittsburgh—within an Irish-Catholic family and community. His family consisted of his parents, maternal grandmother, and seven children. His community and the parish priests had a major influence on how people thought, felt, and behaved. Dan experienced being accepted by his mother and grandmother, which greatly tempered the impact of their disapproval for his sometimes-challenging behaviors. Achievement was not important, as few in the community went to university, but proper behavior was expected at his Catholic school. Dan was certain that no matter what he did wrong, his mother and grandmother would still accept him and that after a short scolding, they would be as engaging and available as ever. Dan's father worked long hours and was a more quiet and distant man. At times Dan wondered what his father thought about him; he was very supportive the few times that Dan caused some more significant behavioral problems at school.

When Dan entered a seminary to become a priest, he hoped to be a missionary in Africa. However, during his three years in the seminary, he became increasingly aware that for him the rules of the Catholic Church were much less important than the attitude of unconditional acceptance and love that is central to the Christian way of life. Bringing such a way of living and relating became his goal. Ensuring that what he did was within the Catholic faith seemed much less important. Dan decided to leave the seminary and study to be a clinical psychologist. At this time, he realized that during his childhood and teen years, conflicts and disagreements were not addressed very well; much was not talked about. His mother's attitude of acceptance made it easier for him to live with the stress of conflicts and the loneliness that came from not having much opportunity to share his thoughts and feelings when they differed from Catholic teachings. He knew less well how to address and resolve conflicts or share with others his unique thoughts and emotions.

For Dan, PACE emerged as a therapeutic way of engaging that began with acceptance. Acceptance came easily for him, and it tended to grow from how his parents managed his behavior with problem-solving, suggestions, and consequences. He soon realized that his parents' responses were not enough. Gradually, being faced with the problems of the children or adults he was meeting with in therapy, he wondered about the meaning of their challenges— opening the door to curiosity. This was still not enough—one day in therapy a 10-year-old boy said, "I feel sad when you talk like that." He was referring to Dan's tone of voice, which conveyed, "I get what you are going through." This was followed by the realization that, for this boy, empathy was the core therapeutic experience that led to new ways of him being with others.

Along the way, Dan realized that for acceptance, curiosity, and empathy to have an impact on his clients, they had best be integrated into a conversation, not presented in a formal or detached manner. There had to be a natural flow in the conversation, a flow that might best be described as relaxed and connected. Dan found that the momentum of conversation was ensured when there was a lightness and storytelling tone to it. He came to experience this tone as involving playfulness. Playfulness gave expression to a sense of optimism and confidence that, through having a conversation together, Dan and the client would be able to make sense of whatever challenge was being explored and discover new ways of understanding and engaging successfully with most situations. When Dan began to describe his therapeutic attitude as PACE, he became more able to maintain that attitude and with increased confidence that the elements of PACE were very helpful in regulating whatever distress was being experienced and in discovering more healing and transforming ways of experiencing the troubling events.

Developing PACE as a way of being is a journey that all DDP practitioners go on. This is often influenced by our own upbringing, our culture and heritage and the various relationships we have encountered throughout our life. These impact the person we become and how we develop as a practitioner (Figure 3.2). We need to be compassionate with ourselves as we work on developing our PACE attitude.

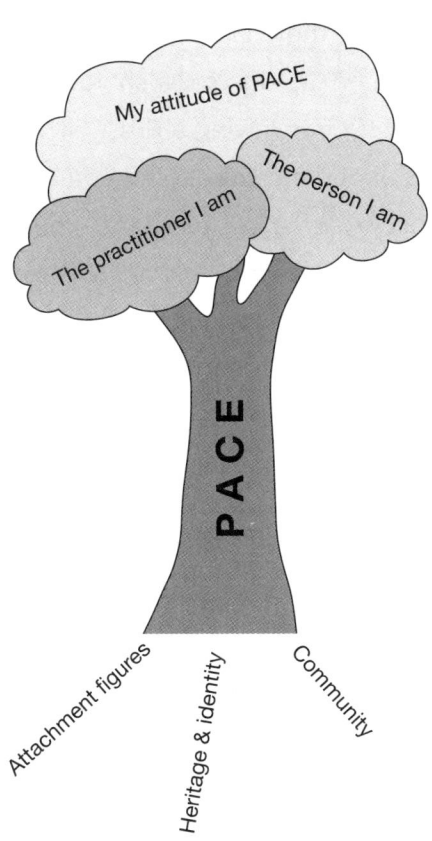

Figure 3.2 Developing The PACE Attitude

TIME FOR REFLECTION

We invite you to reflect on the cultural and family influences that you have experienced.

1. What was your experience of PACE while you were growing up? Can you think of examples of interactions or events when you were supported without PACE? Do you have memories of being supported with PACE?

2. Reflect on the attachment figures you had while growing up. Think about their heritage and identity and how it intersected with your heritage and identity, including race, sexuality, gender, disability, class, and religion. How do you think this impacted the way they related to you?

3. As you explore PACE, do you wish you had more experience of attachment figures having a PACE attitude with you?

4. How has this experience impacted you as a person?

5. How has this experience impacted you as a practitioner? What has it been like embracing PACE as an attitude? What has been difficult? What changes have you seen in yourself as a consequence?

Kim and Dan both recognize ways that their culture and upbringing have influenced their adoption of PACE as a therapeutic attitude. As we explored in Chapter 2, we also need to think about how we introduce and encourage PACE when working with parents from cultures different from our own. For example, Hwang proposes a psychotherapy adaptation and modification framework specifically for Asian American immigrants. They describe a case example where they adapted therapy for a Chinese-American child with the awareness that many Chinese clients can be uncomfortable talking about feelings, such as anxiety, and are more at ease exploring physical symptoms (Hwang et al., 2006, as cited in Bernal et al., 2009). Understanding such differences will influence how a DDP practitioner works with a family. Practitioners and parents can come to a shared understanding of how the child displays emotional distress and think together about how to support this distress, while ensuring that this is adapted to a cultural practice of PACE that feels comfortable for the parent.

Within DDP, we think that there is a good fit with the Australian Aboriginal practice which takes a "both ways" approach (Ryan, 2011). This approach lends itself to remaining curious about the identity, experience, and culture of the parents we are supporting. *Kulini*, which in the Pitjantatjara language means to listen, also encompasses the importance of understanding. If you don't listen *and* understand, it is described as *pina pata* (literally "closed ears"). By working together with parents both ways, we will listen deeply and respectfully to each other.

For example, when working with same sex parents, the both ways approach reminds us to slow down and make sure we understand the lived experience of the parents. What are the daily challenges that these parents face? For example, what attitudes do they encounter when they take their child to school? How are they supporting the child when peers ask questions about their parents?

TIME FOR REFLECTION

We invite you to reflect on the cultural and identity influences that you have experienced within the families you have worked with.

1. How do you ensure that you have collaborative goals for what you want to achieve together?
2. How do you reach a shared understanding of PACE and its potential when parenting a child with developmental trauma?

3. How might you introduce and adapt PACE so that it feels comfortable for the parents you are supporting?

EXPLORING PACE THROUGH THE LENS OF A THERAPY SESSION

In this section, we are going to explore the four elements of PACE within conversations, illustrated here through a therapy session.

TIME FOR REFLECTION

As you read through the example that follows, reflect on the therapist's attitude of PACE with both Crystal and the foster mother, Katherine.

Katherine and ten-year-old Crystal have arrived for a therapy session with some unfinished business from home still bubbling up.

Crystal is in a long-term placement with Katherine, whom she calls *mom*. Bonny, the therapist, has prepared Katherine well to support DDP therapy with Crystal. Katherine is generally reflective with a robust attitude of PACE. They have agreed that Katherine will share any difficulties that occur between sessions so that Bonny is aware of issues that could arise. Unfortunately, a situation arose the morning of the session, and Katherine did not alert Bonny to it before the session with Crystal started. Thus, Bonny begins the session unaware of what has happened, though she does notice nonverbal signs of the tension between them.

TIME FOR REFLECTION

Consider the options that might run through your mind as you meet with this child and her foster mother. You have a decision to make.

You could leave Crystal in the care of a colleague while you have a chat with Katherine. This would help you to find out what has happened, give Katherine the support she needs and ensure she is regulated enough to support Crystal in therapy today.

Alternatively, you could continue with the session, allowing issues to arise as you chat with them and trusting in Katherine's resilience and her response to your PACE attitude.

What decision do you make in that moment as you greet them?

We are going to imagine that Bonny chose the second option and is continuing the session with Crystal.

"P" IS FOR PLAYFUL (WHILE ALSO HOLDING "ACE" IN MIND)

Bonny decides to engage in some light connect-and-chat. She hopes that this will settle them all and bring Katherine and Crystal into a better connection. Here is the start of the session:

Bonny: Another new hairstyle, Crystal. I wonder how long it took to get those plaits in place like that.

(*Crystal sits looking grumpy, with head down.*)

Katherine: (*speaking gently*) Come on Crystal, we're here now. Let's put it aside for later.

Crystal: It's not fair. You've been totally mean to me, and now you just want me to forget about it. I don't want to do therapy today. Can't we just go home?

Bonny notices Katherine's attempts to support Crystal to engage in the session. She therefore decides to engage in some playfulness to shift the mood and hopefully engage Crystal, feeling confident that Katherine will support this. Crystal usually responds to playful initiatives. Perhaps some reciprocal enjoyment can help repair the parent–child relationship that seems to be needed right now. In this way, Bonny hopes to create some optimism that the family can get through tough times, building on the strengths of this parent and this child.

TIME FOR REFLECTION

How might Bonny engage in playfulness at this moment, without undermining the sense of injustice that Crystal is clearly feeling? You do not want to minimize Crystal's experience. However, you also want to avoid getting pulled into the conflict.

Bonny: Crystal, I can see you don't want therapy today (*with a smile*)—well that's not what I was expecting when I was looking forward to seeing you. And I had a brilliant guess about how many rabbits you would have sneaked in today (*referring to a game they commonly play where Bonny guesses how many pictures of rabbits Crystal has on her clothing*).

(*Crystal starts to smile and looks down at the rabbit socks she is wearing.*)

Katherine: Yes, there is nothing more important than counting rabbits in therapy. (*Mom tries to take the sting out of this with a smile, but Crystal's glare says the comment has found its mark.*)

Crystal: Now you're making fun of me. (*Looks at therapist.*) See how mean she is?

TIME FOR REFLECTION

The therapist's attempt to introduce a light, playful start to the session has fallen short. There is an obstacle to playfulness that has shown up in this short dialogue. Perhaps the mother intended to join in the playfulness, but the sarcasm in her comment reveals the difficulty she is having right now. What is signaled to Bonny at this point? What PACE might Katherine need, and how could this be provided? How might Bonny recover and move forward?

We are wondering if Bonny, in using humor, was avoiding the distress that is so clearly present. The elephant in the room has not been named! Perhaps she hopes that if she focuses Crystal on their usual game, the conflict can be left behind. This could be experienced as minimization by this dyad. Katherine is perhaps feeling angry with Bonny. She was hoping for a bit of support with what has been a difficult morning. She tries to join in the playfulness, but with a touch of sarcasm that was actually directed at the therapist. But Crystal experiences this as being made fun of—further evidence of her foster mother's meanness toward her.

Bonny notices the response to her playfulness, and her mistake in not acknowledging what is going on between them. She is also aware that she is feeling frustrated with Katherine, who is not putting Crystal's needs first. All this is leading Bonnie to feel defensive, something that could further derail the session.

TIME FOR REFLECTION

If you were the therapist, how would you take care of yourself so that you could stay open to and engaged with this dyad who clearly need that right now? How could you provide some PACE for yourself to stay PACEful in the session?

Bonny checks her breathing and allows herself a moment of self-compassion, accepting and having empathy for the feelings arising in her. She makes a mental note to be curious about this in her next supervision session. She hopes that PACE and relationship repair with both of them will help them to regulate and engage with her. She judges that she feels regulated enough to use some self-reflection to help this repair.

Bonny: I see you both have strong feelings today. I am sorry that I didn't acknowledge these. I thought being playful might help us all to feel a bit more connected. You're both letting me know that we shouldn't avoid these strong feelings. Boy, did I let an elephant come into the room.

(They have shared this metaphor before when something isn't being talked about. Bonny still thinks some playfulness might help, but not in a way that avoids the issues. Bonny brings out an elephant puppet.)

Bonny: Hey, Crystal, what do you think the elephant is going to tell us today?

Crystal: *(taking the puppet)* The elephant says, "Make Crystal and

Mom a hot chocolate." We need to talk about our feelings and hot chocolate always helps!

Katherine: (*with a genuine smile this time*) What a great idea. Hot chocolate, and then down to business!

Bonny: Well, look at you two. I knew you would both get me back on track. The elephant is quite right. Let's make the drinks, and then you can tell me what has been so hard today.

"A" IS FOR ACCEPTANCE (COMMUNICATED WITH EMPATHY):

With cups of hot chocolate in hand, Bonny wonders what has happened to lead to such big feelings. She learns that Crystal had been found trying to connect with her half-brother, Jake, through Facebook. Katherine is not sure who Crystal has messaged, as Jake is too young to be using Facebook himself. Feeling alarmed, she removed the computer until she could talk to Crystal's social worker.

Bonny: Crystal, wow, you've found your brother Jake. I remember that you've never met him. He was born after you came into care, wasn't he? (*Crystal nods.*) I'm guessing you might have lots of confusing feelings about this. And then your mom discovered you'd been on Facebook and removed your computer. You were so angry. I get that. You'd just found Jake and now you had lost your computer. I can see that it would feel unfair that your mom took your computer away.

Katherine: Yes, but Crystal isn't allowed on Facebook. She knows that. She can't just contact family members. There are all sorts of risks in doing this. I thought she was old enough to know this.

TIME FOR REFLECTION

Both Katherine and Crystal are experiencing intense emotions. How might you start to communicate your acceptance of these before curiously exploring Crystal's experience further? How will Crystal experience your acceptance of her anger toward her mom and, perhaps, her shame in being caught using the computer in a way that was not allowed? How will you let Katherine know that her hurt makes sense to you without it feeling like you are siding with her against Crystal?

Bonny: Mom, I'm hearing you. I'm also noticing Crystal right now, and I think she knows she's messed up. It's so hard to know there are siblings out there that you don't know. It's tough living in foster care.

Katherine: Yes, of course. I know this time is for Crystal and I think I need some help in knowing how to support her with this too.

Bonny: Crystal, I need to take care of both of you today. Do you remember Jesse? (*Crystal nods.*) Well, I'm going to ask him to come in and do some drawing with you while I have a chat with Mom. I remember you did some great drawing together last month. Is that OK? (*Crystal smiles and says "yes."*)

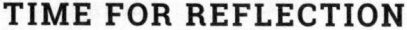

TIME FOR REFLECTION

Here is part of the conversation between Bonny and Katherine. If you are working through this as part of a study group, you might explore this through role play. Alternatively, you could explore the session following this one, which will be with Katherine alone.

Bonny and Katherine chat together for around 20 minutes. Bonny listens as Katherine tells her how angry Crystal became when she removed the computer. She was furious that she couldn't check to see if she had a reply to her message. She accused Katherine of racism and trying to keep her from her brother, whose father is Black African. Katherine felt very stung by this and retaliated by telling Crystal that her computer is now removed for a month! A rash decision that she is regretting.

Bonny: Oh, Katherine, how difficult for you. I can understand that you're feeling angry with Crystal; hurt too I'd guess.

Katherine: Yes, I am. I'm also worried. What will the social worker say? Crystal shouldn't have been on Facebook. I think she'll be cross that I let this happen. I don't blame her; I'm cross with myself.

Bonny: That sounds like a huge worry. I can see how much you feel you've let Crystal down. What is your biggest worry right now?

Katherine: Well, mainly how hurt Crystal could be if contact with her brother is not planned and supported. She's too young to manage this on her own. That's why I was so cross with her.

Bonny: Yes, that makes sense. You want to protect her, and she's making this so difficult to do. Your motives are spot on. I think this is making it hard for you to focus on Crystal's feelings about her brother and her shame for having disappointed you.

Katherine: Yes, I really lost sight of Crystal didn't I. I was so worried about what she'd done. And then when she called me racist. What does that say about me as a foster carer? I feel I've let us both down. Removing the computer wasn't helpful. I think I knew I hadn't handled this well. Maybe that's why I didn't let you know what had happened. I thought I'd be OK, but clearly I wasn't. I've let you down and ruined Crystal's session too!

Bonny: Wow, Katherine. So many worries. I'm sad to see you being so hard on yourself. Crystal is such a closed book and so self-reliant. She makes it hard for you to support her. I can understand how worried you are for Crystal, and yes, it's hard to think that others will be judging you. You've had a big emotional response to this. This has really triggered doubt and self-blame. Maybe we can think more about this when we next meet.

Katherine: Yes, that would be good. Now we need to focus on Crystal. I knew Jake was dual heritage but hadn't thought to talk with Crystal about him. She deserves to know about her brother.

Bonny: That sounds like a good place to start.

As Bonny listens with acceptance and empathy, Katherine feels supported. Katherine is now able to focus on Crystal and how difficult this has been for her. She is keen for the session with Crystal to continue and assures Bonny she will be able to support her.

"C" IS FOR CURIOSITY
(HELD WITH ACCEPTANCE AND EMPATHY):

Now that Katherine is ready to accept and have empathy for Crystal's experience, it is time to wind up the curiosity. They all settle back into the session, with Crystal sharing the drawing she has been doing. They all enjoy looking at the drawing, and then Bonny leads Crystal back to the difficulties.

Bonny:	I'm glad you enjoyed drawing with Jesse. Are you ready to think with me about what happened this morning?
Crystal:	It's not fair. She's taken my computer from me. Now Jake will think I'm not interested in talking with him. She's ruined it all.
Bonny:	Wow, Crystal, what big feelings you have. You're feeling really cross. Any ideas about why Mom has taken the computer away?
Crystal:	See, I knew it. You always take her side. I guess you'll say I shouldn't have the computer back for a year! All adults are so mean.

TIME FOR REFLECTION

This does not exemplify a good start at bringing curiosity in. There are certainly some obstacles to helping Crystal stay curious. What do you notice? What would you suggest to Bonny here?

Bonny has chosen to focus on Crystal's behavior and her experience of the consequence. Not only that, the focus is on Katherine: "Why do you think she did that?" rather than staying with Crystal's experience: "What was that like for you?" The result, more shame.

Notice also that Crystal has offered a theme within this dialogue that Bonny has not picked up: that Jake might interpret her silence negatively. Let's explore what would happen if that theme was followed and the focus was moved away from Crystal's behavior.

Bonny: Oh Crystal, I get it now. Losing that computer is really, really hard. I'm sorry, I missed what you told me. You're worried that Jake might respond to you, and you won't be able to answer him. What is he going to think if you don't get back to him?

Crystal: Yes, he's going to think I don't care. He might give up and decide I'm not worth bothering about. He might think I'm racist and that's why I'm not answering him. She's ruined it all!

Bonny: Those are some major worries. You really want to connect with Jake. I guess you were already wondering if he would respond to you, and now you might not even know. Your anger toward Mom is really making sense to me right now. (*to Katherine*) Your daughter is being so brave, letting us know what her fears are. I'm understanding more now why she got so angry.

Katherine: Yes, I hadn't thought about whether Jake would respond or not. I can see that Crystal needs to know that. It's a big step, trying to find her brother, and Crystal did this all by herself. (*turning to Crystal*) I'm sorry I got angry. I just want you to know that I can help you with this. Jake is your brother and of course you want to find out about him.

Bonny: (*to Crystal*) This is hard, Crystal, I am glad you've got a mom who can help you. Can you tell me a bit more about Jake?

Crystal: I didn't mean it when I said Mom was racist. I was just feeling so cross. I wanted to talk with Jake, and she was stopping me.

Bonny: Thank you Crystal. I think mom is happy to hear that. The racist thing has come up a couple of times. I am wondering about that. Jake is dual heritage, I think.

Crystal: I saw his photo on Facebook. He looks Black, but my birth mom and me are white. I don't understand.

Bonny: You didn't know that Jake's father was born in Africa and is different from your dad? Many children have parents who come from different heritages. Your mother's heritage is white English, and Jake's father's is Black African, so Jake has both white English and Black African heritage.

Crystal: No, I didn't know that. I thought it couldn't be my brother when I saw the photo, but his name is right. I was shocked, and then I worried that meant I was being racist. We learned about that at school. My dad was racist—he was always calling Black people names. I'm worried that maybe I'm like him.

Bonny: It sounds kind of confusing and worrying. Lots of worries about your dad too. We can chat about this some more, but is it alright if we focus on your brother just now? (*Crystal nods.*) You knew you had a brother, right?

Crystal: Yes, and that he went to live with his grandparents. He's a few years younger than me. I wanted to see what he was like. That's why I looked him up.

"E" IS FOR EMPATHY (DEEPENED THROUGH OUR CURIOSITY AND CONVEYING OUR ACCEPTANCE):

As a session progresses, it is not uncommon to move from reflective with light empathy to a deeper affective–reflective dialogue. The role of empathy becomes even more important as the affective experience of exploring the story is shared.

TIME FOR REFLECTION

Empathy and acceptance have been present throughout this curious exploration. It is now appropriate to deepen this empathy, allowing Crystal to experience her story affectively and reflectively.

Reflect on the experience of the therapist. How might curiosity lead Bonny to deeper acceptance and empathy for Crystal? Think also about how Bonny might communicate this to Crystal.

Crystal needs to experience Katherine's acceptance of her story. She began to feel this acceptance when Katherine sought to repair the rupture in their relationship, apologizing for being angry and signaling that she would help Crystal connect with her brother. How might you continue to bring Mom in, allowing Crystal to communicate directly with her and supporting Katherine to respond to what she has heard?

Bonny: Yes, I see. You knew you had a brother. I think your social worker told you that when he was born. He went straight to live with his grandparents, didn't he? I guess you've been wondering about him for a long time. Then you wondered if you could find him on Facebook. You did a search and there he was. I am wondering what that was like. Kind of exciting maybe, and perhaps a bit confusing. He didn't look like you were expecting. I guess you knew that Jake had a different dad, but not much about him.

Crystal: I didn't know anything about him.

Bonny: Oh Crystal, how sad. You've been told so little about Jake. What a shock then. Jake wasn't what you expected. I am wondering what that was like. I would have felt so confused if that had happened to me and so sad that I'd not known him for all these years.

Crystal: (*crying quietly*) I wanted a baby brother, but I wasn't even allowed to see him. The social worker told us when he was born. That was all. He went to live with his grandparents a long way away. I overheard my social worker talking to mom. They mentioned his grandparents' surname, and I remembered it because it was such a strange name. I wasn't even sure if he would be on Facebook. I know he is still little. I found him through his older cousin's page. His cousin may not even pass my message on. I just want to talk to him. He's my brother.

Bonny: Crystal, I'm so sorry that you were told so little about him and no one helped you to be in contact with him. You're such a resourceful girl, finding him all by yourself. You learned to be strong when you were little. I guess you learned to do things by yourself, and it's hard to trust that adults will help you. I get that. You found him, and then what a surprise. He wasn't what you expected.

Crystal: I was surprised. I want him to like me. I don't know if he will though. He might not reply. Maybe he'll even be cross with me for messaging his cousin.

Bonny: Such a lot of worries, Crystal. Finding your brother is a big deal, and of course you want him to like you. We need to help you now. We need to find out much more about your brother, where he is living and who he is living with. I bet you have lots of questions, let's see if we can find some answers. First, I want to check in with mom. Shall we tell her what we've been talking about?

Crystal: You tell her.

Bonny: (*to Katherine*) Mom, Crystal has been so brave talking with us today. I think Crystal has waited a long time to find out about her brother. Crystal has lots of feelings right now. So sad she has a brother she never got to meet. So confusing to find him in another country. His life must seem very different. And lots of worry about Jake being Black and she white. Will he like her? Will he want to talk to her? Big worries. And she has been learning about racism at school. Maybe this got her remembering her birth dad being racist. I guess that is a worry and confusion too. She worries that seeing Jake and being shocked that he is Black means she is like her father. What big fears.

Katherine: Yes, I understand now why Crystal accused me of being racist. I think she was telling me her own fears. I'm sorry I didn't listen very well. Crystal is such a kind girl. She is friends to everyone. I think she would make a great big sister for Jake.

(*Bonny notices Crystal moving close to Katherine. She is looking tearful, and Katherine looks ready to comfort her.*)

Bonny: (*to Crystal*) I'm going to talk for you. Let me know if I get it wrong. OK? (*Crystal nods.*) Mom, Crystal has given me permission to talk for her. She has a lot of feelings right now, and it's hard for her to talk.

Katherine: OK.

Bonny: (*as Crystal*) Mom, I'm feeling sad right now. I wanted to find my little brother. I want to know him. It's not fair that I never got to meet him. So, I looked for him. I thought if

I could send him a message maybe he would talk to me. I didn't know he was living in another country. I didn't know he was Black. I thought he would look like me. I was shocked when I saw his photograph on his cousin's Facebook page. I sent a message, and then I got really scared. What if his cousin was cross with me and didn't pass my message on? What if Jake doesn't want to talk to me? What if he thought I was racist for being shocked? What if he was disappointed that he had a white sister? It's so confusing, Mom.

Katherine: Oh, Crystal. How hard this has been for you. I hadn't realized how much you missed your little brother. (*Crystal cuddles into her foster mom.*) It must have been so confusing for you, finding him like that. I am sorry we didn't tell you more about him or make sure we had some photographs of him for you. I realize now how important this is for you. I'll find a way of helping you connect with him. I don't know if Jake will want to know you, but we will find out together. First thing, we need to see if your message has had a response (*Crystal gives Katherine a big smile*).

TIME FOR REFLECTION

Do you think this is a good point to start to end the session? Maybe some lighter chat and some playfulness before winding up? What would that look like?

You will be meeting with Katherine next week. What are the themes you will want to pick up with her?

And what else might you wish to explore with the network?

Bonny will want to explore the way Katherine was triggered and the self-blame that arose, her feelings of failing and of letting Crystal down. Bonny also has lots of questions about why Crystal was not told more about her brother and why some contact had not been maintained by the social workers. She wonders whether Jake's heritage has contributed to this. She also wants to know more about the lessons at school. There is a lot of confusion for Crystal, and they will need to work with the school and the social care team to help her.

TIME FOR REFLECTION

Additional reflections:

1. Think about how the attitude of PACE was conveyed.
   - How did PACE support Crystal? Reflect on the four elements of PACE and how they were interwoven through the session.
   - Katherine was not feeling safe with Bonny. She feared Bonny's judgement. This impacted Crystal's safety. Notice how Bonny held PACE for Katherine as well as for Crystal.
   - Bonny needed to take care of herself during this session so that she could stay open and engaged with both Crystal and Katherine. Reflect on the themes of this session that might have led Bonny to feel more defensive. How could she provide a PACEful attitude to herself within the session and afterwards?
2. We chose a scenario which included a white child discovering that her half-brother has dual heritage. Reflect on how the themes of race and racism emerged.
   - How might this impact the way that Crystal is supported?
   - How might the situation have been different if the characters had different racial identities?

- Imagine this scenario with you as therapist, and reflect on how your identity might impact the way you provided this session.
- Consider the possibility of institutional racism as a reason why Crystal was not helped to know about her brother and to have some contact with him. Might this have been different if Jake had been a white child? How might you take this forward, while holding PACE for the network?

PACE RESPONSES TO CHALLENGES

As the example illustrates, it is hardest to respond with PACE when the child or parent is challenging, defensive, and/or dysregulated.

REFLECTIVE EXERCISE: RESPONDING DEFENSIVELY AND PACEFULLY

There is an opportunity to explore the differences between responding defensively and with PACE in Worksheet 3.2 at the end of this chapter.

CONCLUSION

Developing PACE as a way of being can be challenging for all of us. It is an attitude that comes so easily when talking to an infant but seems to slip from our grasp when talking to older children, adolescents, and with each other.

PACE can so easily get lost when we provide reassurance to move away from the emotional experience of the child. The same is true if we move too quickly into problem-solving or provide discipline without the curiosity that leads to a deeper understanding of the child. Reassurance, problem-solving and discipline all have their place in parenting. However, applying them alongside the emotional connection of PACE generally leads to much more effective communication and action.

"Slow down to get there quicker" has been adopted by the DDP community to emphasize the importance of taking the time to look after ourselves, to coregulate with others, and to seek understanding of their emotional worlds. This allows us to remain open and engaged, able to offer an emotional connection facilitated by the attitude of PACE, which can stay strong through whatever ensuing struggles may come.

Worksheet 3.1

 Time for Reflection:
A Day in the Life

Imagine being a child or adolescent who is being related to with and without PACE.

On your own: Try reading the script through with just the ordinary responses. Reflect on how the child is left feeling. Next read it through with the PACE responses and notice any difference that this makes.

In a study group: Assign roles to each of you from the list of characters. Any extra people will be observers. The "child" sits in the middle, and the script is read through, ordinary responses first. The child then reflects on how that felt. Repeat this process with the PACE responses.

We have chosen an example of a family parenting a child with a physical disability. If this example doesn't address the issues or challenges you want to reflect on, consider writing your own "A day in the life" script. You can choose the age, identity, experience, and family type of the child and each character to fit with scenarios that you are interested in exploring.

Manda is 14 years old and lives with her **Mother, Father,** and older brother **Derek**. Manda is affected by cerebral palsy and has a left-sided hemiplegia. She attends the local high school, where she is placed in regular classes (middle sets), probably an underestimate of her abilities which would place her in AP classes (top sets). She enjoys swimming and music.

Other characters are **narrator, design & technology (DT) teacher, games teacher,** and **swimming coach**.

NARRATOR

It's a school day, and everyone is running late. Derek has been sent to tell Manda to get up. Manda has had a restless night and does not want to go to school. She enjoys seeing her friends, but school is stressful. She is already worrying about the taxi ride. The taxi driver always talks slowly to her with a jolly voice, like she is a little kid. Just yesterday he was really patronizing, telling her to smile and that she didn't look so bad. He even told her that it could be worse, as she could be in a wheelchair!

DEREK

ORDINARY RESPONSE

Manda, you're going to make us all late. You know how long it takes you to get dressed. Mom says if you don't get up now, there will be no time for breakfast. She has asked me to see you into your taxi, but I can't miss my bus and be late for college. So get up now.

PACE RESPONSE

Come on sleepy head, time to get up. (sits on the edge of Manda's bed) What's up? Don't you fancy school today? Oh, are you still not sleeping well? It sounds like you have a lot on your mind. That taxi driver sucks. I need to see you into the taxi before my bus goes so that I'm not late for college, but I tell you what, I'll blow a raspberry at him as he drives away, that should give you a giggle!

NARRATOR

Reluctantly Manda gets up and into the clothes her mother has left out for her. She walks to the kitchen but refuses breakfast. She sees her specially adapted boots by the door and scowls. She hates the way they look, so different from her friends', never mind the blisters they are giving her.

MOTHER

ORDINARY RESPONSE

Don't be silly, of course you're going to have some breakfast. You can't go to school without eating something. Now come on, I still have to help you into your boots. You know how long it takes, and I should be on my way to work by now. There's no need to look at me like that, you know those boots are for your own good.

PACE RESPONSE

Oh, Manda, I know those boots don't look nice. Seeing the other girls with their smart shoes is really hard for you. I guess you wonder if the gain from wearing them is really worth it. We can sort out the blisters though. I'll talk to the pharmacy and see what else we can try, and maybe the boots can be adjusted. I want you to wear them to school, but you're going to the cinema this weekend. You can wear your shoes then. Now what are you going to have for breakfast?

NARRATOR

Manda has arrived at school, where her friend Mia is waiting for her. The morning starts well with an English class. Manda enjoys literature. The teacher can see her potential and is encouraging her. Manda and Mia then have a DT lesson where they are learning soldering. Manda struggles to manage the soldering iron because of her movement difficulties, so Mia comes over to help her. They are giggling together when the teacher comes over.

DT TEACHER

ORDINARY RESPONSE

Mia, will you please return to your own bench. I didn't tell anyone to pair up for this lesson. I want you to do this by yourself. Now, I don't want to hear another sound from either of you.

PACE RESPONSE

Now girls, what is all this giggling about? OK, that solder does look a little strange. I'm sorry, Manda, I should have thought that you might need to pair up for this one. Thanks, Mia, for helping. Next lesson I'll put you all in pairs and you can have another go. Keep the noise down now, the other girls will think you are having far too much fun!

NARRATOR

The day gets worse. During lunchtime Manda has to manage the spitefulness of a particular group of girls who seem to delight in mocking her. Thankfully she and Mia find a quiet place to sit. Then they have to go to different classes. Manda has a games class. She has to join her peer group to plan for the upcoming sports day. As they walk across to the games hall, the other girls are walking quickly and Manda struggles to keep up. When she finally reaches them, she discovers they have put her name down for the 1,500-meter race. She tries to point out the unfairness of this, but none of the other girls want to do it. They are arguing about this when the games teacher comes over. Manda tries to tell him that she can't run 1,500 meters.

GAMES TEACHER

ORDINARY RESPONSE

Well it looks like you have drawn the short straw, Manda. You'll just have to manage. Come on, I need the list, and I do want you to spend time actually doing some activity today. Manda, you can go out on the track and get some practice. Which of you are going to join her?

PACE RESPONSE

OK, let's have a look at your list. I can see the problem. You're right, Manda; the 1,500-meter race doesn't suit you. I am wondering why you girls decided to allocate the events out this way. Ah, I see. I take it that no one wants to run 1,500 meters, but I think you're going to have to think this through again aren't you? I want you to do something active now, so you will have to finish this at break. Manda can have first choice, and the rest of you will fit around her. Does that sound fair?

NARRATOR

The school day finally comes to an end and Manda is pleased to see her father, who will take her to swimming club. They are having a friendly competition with another group, and Manda is looking forward to racing the able-bodied girls. She enjoys the freedom of swimming, where she is at less of a disadvantage. As they drive to the club, Manda tells her father about the girls putting her down to run the 1,500-meter race.

FATHER

ORDINARY RESPONSE

Well for goodness sake, what was the games teacher thinking, letting them choose? Of course you can't do the 1,500. I will email the school and tell them to get their act together and figure out something you can actually do. Don't look at me like that. I know you don't like me talking with school, but they do need reminding that you are disabled. It makes me so mad that they don't take your difficulties into account. It's like they have no brains.

PACE RESPONSE

Those girls can be really mean, can't they? Do you want me to email the school about this? No, I won't get angry. Maybe we need another meeting to look at the support you're getting at school. You have so much ability, they need to figure out how to help you use it. It sounds like school has been really tricky today. Let's get you to swimming, and you can relax in the pool.

NARRATOR

The swimming competition goes well, and Manda is pleased when she comes in third in the freestyle. While she is getting changed, the mother of another swimmer comes up and congratulates her. She tells Manda how inspiring she is. Manda grimaces and turns away. Later she complains to the coach. It's not fair: at school she is expected to do the impossible, and here she is treated as if there is something wrong with her. Why can't she just be treated like a normal person just living her life?

SWIMMING COACH

ORDINARY RESPONSE

The mother was just being kind. You did well today, you deserve to have this noticed. If you want to go on to some of the competitions you'll have to get used to the attention. It's not likely that there will be other children with cerebral palsy competing, after all.

PACE RESPONSE

Is that difficult for you, being told you are inspiring? I suspect she meant it as a compliment. Help me to understand. Ah, OK, I hadn't thought about it feeling patronizing, and then I go and expect you to respond positively to her comment. It must be hard when you are treated differently. I can understand how painful it is when people mock you, like that time a couple of weeks ago. Now I see that this is equally hard. It must really build up when you are experiencing things like this every day. Thanks for helping me to understand.

NARRATOR

Back home, after dinner is over, Mom sits down to talk with Manda. She has had a letter from the physiotherapist suggesting some new exercises. The physiotherapist is asking them to immobilize her right side so that they can work on the weaker side. Manda protests that this is barbaric. She remembers them doing something similar when she was in her first school, and she hated it.

MOM

ORDINARY RESPONSE

I think we should give it a try. If it makes it better in the long run, it will be worth it. The physiotherapist knows what she's doing. I know it will be a bit uncomfortable, but imagine how well you will do when that left side gets stronger. You might even win some swimming competitions then.

PACE RESPONSE

Well I guess the physiotherapist thinks it will be better for you in the long run, but I can see it must feel barbaric. It doesn't seem fair when the treatment is worse than what you are experiencing now. Strengthening your left side does seem important to me. Any ideas how you might do this? Piano lessons, OK that sounds like a good idea. You'll need to use both hands together to play the piano. Let me talk to the physiotherapist and see what she thinks.

NARRATOR

Manda relaxes for the rest of the evening, unwinding from the day. She and Derek even agree on what TV program to watch! It's time for bed, and Manda thinks she will have another restless night worrying about what might go wrong tomorrow. Mom brings in a new milk drink to try. It has valerian and honey in it to help her sleep. Dad lets her know that he has talked to the special needs teacher and that he didn't get angry. The teacher is going to arrange a meeting so that they can think together about how to better support Manda in school.

Worksheet 3.2

 Reflective Exercise:
Responding Defensively and PACEfully

Here are some scenarios of responding to children and parents. Explore how the DDP practitioner might respond defensively or with PACE. Notice the differences and how the PACE elements in the second response are missing from the defensive response.

Scenario One: A child feels anxious as the therapist seeks to understand their experience.

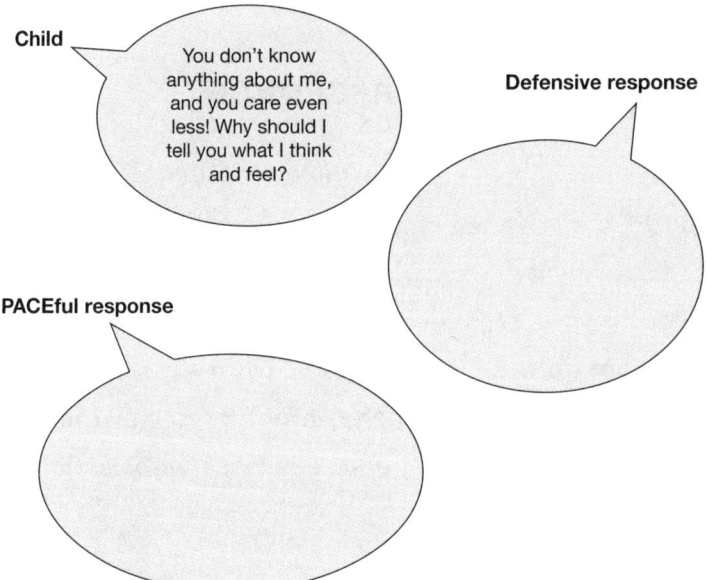

Scenario Two: A parent meets with a therapist following a session with their child. The parent is feeling undermined by the therapist.

Scenario Three: A child distrusts the therapist's acceptance of them.

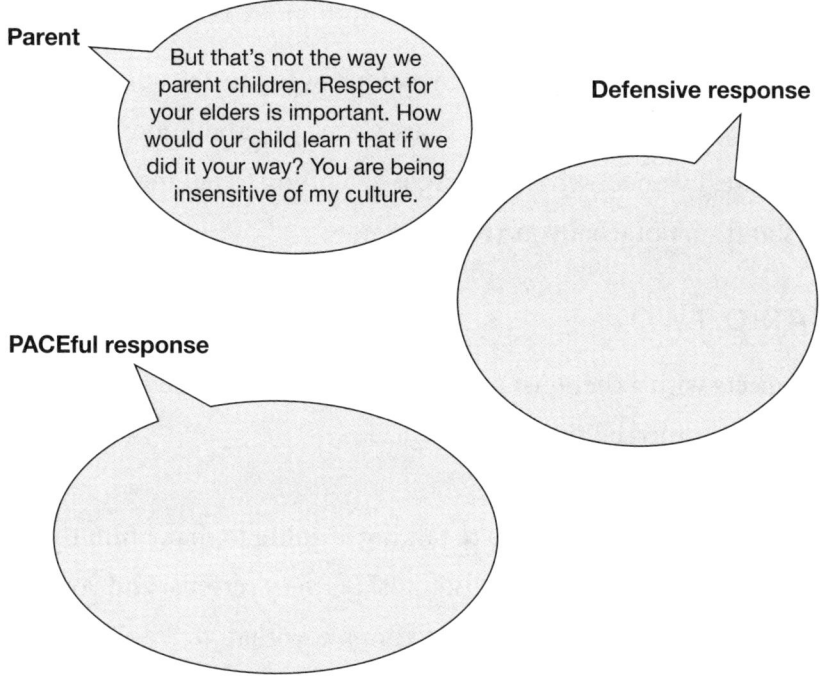

Parent

But that's not the way we parent children. Respect for your elders is important. How would our child learn that if we did it your way? You are being insensitive of my culture.

Defensive response

PACEful response

Scenario Four: A parent and therapist are meeting for a parent support session. The parent feels uncomfortable with the parenting ideas being offered, which are very different from the way they were brought up.

Reflections on Worksheet 3.2: Possible Responses

SCENARIO ONE

A child feels anxious as the therapist seeks to understand their experience.

Child: You don't know anything about me, and you care even less! Why should I tell you what I think and feel?

Defensive Response: I am asking you so I will know more about you. I think if you tell me it will help you to handle your challenges better!

PACEful Response: Of course you wouldn't want to tell me things that are important to you if you think I don't care about you and know little or nothing about your life. I wonder what you might be willing to tell me that will help me to understand a bit of what you are facing now.

SCENARIO TWO

A parent meets with a therapist following a session with their child. The parent is feeling undermined by the therapist.

> **Parent:** The way that you're talking is going to make him think this is not important! But it is! It's very serious, and you need to support me in making him know that!

Defensive Response: If I do what you want me to do, Judith, he'll never talk to me at all. Please let me say it my way, as it is likely to be more effective!

PACEful Response: Oh, Judith, if I have communicated to him that this is not important, I am very sorry! Of course it is! Thanks for letting me know your concern. If I see him thinking it is not important I will find a way to show him that I think it is, even if he disagrees with you and me about it!

SCENARIO THREE

A child distrusts the therapist's acceptance of them.

> **Child:** You think there's something wrong with me just like everyone else does! You're just paid to pretend you don't feel that way!

Defensive Response: I don't think there is anything wrong with you! You just made some poor choices, but you can learn how to make the right ones.

PACEful Response: You think that I'm pretending! Oh, Tom, that would make it hard to trust me . . . to believe anything that I say! If I were not pretending, not thinking there is something wrong with you . . . how would you know?

SCENARIO FOUR

A parent and therapist are meeting for a parent support session. The parent feels uncomfortable with the parenting ideas being offered, which are very different from the way they were brought up.

Parent: But that's not the way we parent children. Respect of your elders is important. How would our child learn that if we did it your way? You are being insensitive to my culture.

Defensive Response: I am sensitive to your culture. Your child will learn to respect you, but we need to help him to feel more secure too. Try it. I think you will be surprised how your child responds.

PACEful Response: I really apologize. I did not intend to be insensitive, and I'm sorry that's how you felt. Please tell me more about your culture and how you help children to learn respect. Perhaps if I understand better, we can think together about how your parenting can both help your child to feel more secure and to learn respect.

IN CONVERSATION TWO

Kim met with a group of DDP practitioners, Benjamin, Julie, Gill, and Georgia, who identify as LGBTQIA+.

She witnessed their conversation and experienced the ambivalence associated with wanting to be heard while also fearing the risks of being seen. After careful thought, they agreed that Kim could share some of this conversation and they helpfully drew out the themes that arose during their conversation, identifying how these might help DDP practitioners.

1. Individuals versus community

LGBTQIA+ covers a range of individuals and communities. People grouped together under this acronym can be very different from each other. What brings this vast incredible mix of people together is what they share in navigating life outside what most perceive as conventional, acceptable, and, often, legal.

> **Kim:** Thank you so much for inviting me into your space. I am interested in hearing about your experience as a group of people from within the LGBTQIA+ community who are involved in the DDP world.

> **Benjamin:** There's a lot of discussion around gender, generally, at the moment, the history of gender, what gender is, how gender is perceived, which is really changing a lot of people's ideas about their own gender, particularly within the queer community.
>
> One of the things that is important to me is how the elements within the wider LGBTQIA+ community are all quite different. They inhabit different spaces and places. The conceptual and ideological backgrounds can vary in terms of how they exist, where they go, what they fight for, and

what they think about. LGBTQIA+ cultures cover a really wide range.

Kim: Thank you. That is important to remember. LGBTQIA+ is not a homogenous group, and there are differences between sections of it. We need to bear in mind that this group can't speak for the whole continuum.

HOW CAN THIS HELP DDP PRACTITIONERS?

A place to start is acknowledging each individual's experience and how different parts of these communities are. One person can't speak for others. Much of the published work and mainstream media coverage is from a white perspective, one that has largely ignored the impact of intersectionality, including how gender and sexuality, race, ethnicity, culture, disability, and neurodiversity interact.

2. Safety

Many individuals who identify as LGBTQIA+ share the common experience of not feeling safe in many environments, including with family. Feeling unsafe can become such a common experience that differentiating between when one is safe and when one isn't becomes difficult. Constantly code-switching[3] (scanning all aspects of each situation to check for risks) to get by in a world where you are not noticed, not recognized, or you are stigmatized—feeling and being under threat of intimidation or violence—means living in survival mode. This dynamic becomes so habitual that one ceases to be aware that they are living like this every day.

Georgia: DDP is about connection and intersubjective experience, and the ability to have these absolutely depends on your

---

3 Code-switching, in this context, describes the ways in which a member of a marginalized group adjusts their voice, language, mannerisms, behavior, and appearance to fit into the dominant culture.

life experience. When you live in the world as a minority, of any sort, you will experience times when you haven't felt safe. DDP is about safety, so this might be a common thread within all elements of the LGBTQIA+ community. How do we, as DDP practitioners, stay open to that? How do we enable people to bring their full selves, and how do we connect with them?

Kim: There's something in what you're saying about making sure that we don't assume someone feels safe, or maybe that we should assume they don't feel safe. I anticipate that you will not feel safe in this space between us, whether this is a training space, a therapy space, or a parent's support space. How do we come into these spaces and create that sense of safety while accounting for people's different experiences in the world?

Benjamin: This really rings true. A lot of the time, I might not realize that I don't feel safe because it's such a common feeling. The identification of feeling safe or not safe isn't straightforward. How often am I feeling unsafe without really spotting it? And if you don't know, then you have to feel a bit unsafe in order to protect yourself. I think this happens a lot in the queer community.

Kim: Yes, creating safety is a complex process that needs a lot of time and attention. It goes back to understanding the experience of the other, sitting alongside them and building safety at a pace that they can manage, being careful about making assumptions, and truly getting to know the person or people you are working with.

Julie: We live in a world where anyone can say what they want about us. We are trying to survive in a world where who you are is not noticed or recognized. If you accept this and you accept nonsafety, then the issue is how do we create safety. Organizations need to proactively create the conditions that support a shift from survival to some sense of belonging. Trainers and consultants need to attend to creating safety so that practitioners experience how to do this within their own DDP interventions, starting at Level One training. DDP, for me, is a model where all the components are there to enable this to happen, to help people go beyond survival into something else. This can be emotionally overwhelming for people who are accustomed to and familiar with living in their survival zone. If not prepared, experiencing someone recognizing them when they are not expecting it can be like, "Hang on, I'm used to being in a space where nothing like this is talked about. If you shift that, I have to think because I then have to decide how I respond or join in."

HOW CAN THIS HELP DDP PRACTITIONERS?

Recognize the impact of feeling unsafe all the time. Anticipate that someone might not feel safe in the space they are sharing with you, whether a training space, a therapy space, or a parent support space. Be curious with individuals about ways they have found to protect themselves and their families. Find ways to manage your own worries about how to come into these spaces so that you can create a sense of safety while accounting for other people's different experiences.

Talk with others and share ideas and experiences about how to connect with people who are within the LGBTQIA+ community. Find ways to become knowledgeable, ask organizations for training, help, and support about what might be relevant for the adults and young people you are working with.

Work on providing conditions that allow individuals to shift from survival mode to feeling a sense of belonging. The DDP model includes core components that enable this to start to happen. Recognize that PACE, as a way of being, is just the beginning. PACE on its own is not enough to build the level of trust needed to begin to offer safety for all marginalized people.

Recognize that feeling safe can be a long, slow process, despite your best efforts. Anticipate that clients of all ages, supervisees, and training attendees, need to observe you and assess how you will be with them before possibly experiencing the safety you are offering. While this is likely to be true for anyone coming into a DDP intervention, this process is more complex and needs more time for those who have grown up in minority groups, who have encountered oppression and discrimination.

3. The melting pot of shame and pride

The word *pride* has been associated with LGBTQIA+ over the past 50 years. Pride and shame involve a complex, powerful, and scary mix of emotions.

Benjamin:	My thinking has been influenced by reading *The Velvet Rage*, written by therapist Alan Downs (2012). It's a book about the experience of cis gay men and includes a discussion on the experience of shame that growing up different from peers can bring. He suggests that gay men go through three states, moving back and forth between them. The states he names are denial, then an overcompensation for the shame experienced in this first state, and then acceptance and a sense of peace with one's identity. I have found this helpful to hold in mind to understand the different ways people manage and express feelings of not being safe. We can see this in the behaviors of the young people we work with. There is often some kind of defense against the shame of denial. And then you hope that they are going to get to a point where they feel

comfortable enough with themselves to live authentically, whatever that means to them.

HOW CAN THIS HELP DDP PRACTITIONERS?

The DDP practitioner needs to understand the different ways people manage and defend against feelings of shame and lack of safety, which can be combined with feelings of pride at how they negotiate an uncertain and, at times, frightening world.

While a stage model can help us understand the person in front of us, it is also important to remember that each person is unique. Not everyone feels shame around their gender or sexuality, and each will create safety in their own way.

4.   Family and day to day life

Parents take the lead in helping their children negotiate the world. Children must engage with schools, and this has an added layer of difficulty when the child is in the minority in terms of sexuality and/or gender and/or is living with parents who are in this minority. These children have to learn a language, a way of being, a back story not just about being fostered, adopted, having a birth parent hospitalized etc. but also about the gender and sexuality of themselves and/or their parents.

Julie:	Cisgender, heterosexual practitioners can fail to understand key experiences of their clients because of their fear of getting it wrong, of seeming insensitive, or because they make incorrect assumptions, which gets in the way of curiosity. This is not the world and family life these practitioners have experienced, and they often voice how challenging it is for them to talk about the experiences that their clients—adults and children—are encountering every day. It is important to stay curious. One small example: Think about an adolescent, living with a same sex couple, who doesn't invite friends

around. Perhaps this is because they don't know what to say about having lesbian or gay parents.

Kim: I can see how important it is to check our assumptions, to get to know the person in front of us and their unique experience. This is so central to DDP. It is very disturbing to notice that we can make assumptions and curiosity can fail when working with different marginalized groups. We have to be more curious than we are at the moment about the person in front of us.

Gill: To some extent, we can choose our own community and stay safe in it. We choose where we live, where we interact, and where we go. Whereas when you have a child, they have to go into the "normal" world because we don't have lesbian or gay schools. You can choose to have a community around you that accepts you and your child, but they also have to venture into areas where it isn't their community, where it isn't safe. They have to learn a language, a way of being, a back story. They have to learn stuff to survive.

Georgia: Family life is a small world at first, but then when the child goes to school, it's much wider. They might be the only child in that class with two moms, and they might be the only child in that class who's adopted, and they might be the only child in that class with dyslexia. There can be many layers through which they are navigating.

Kim: This is so important for DDP practitioners to understand.

Gill: Think about parents' evening. Who goes? We had a friend whose child said, "I only want one of you to come to parents' evening because I don't want you both to come in." So, she hid one of her parents. She said, "I can't manage the repercussions of you both turning up and being who you are."

Kim: I am hearing the importance of finding community and a feeling of belonging and how these can be threatened. Heterosexual children who live with gay parents and children who are discovering their LGBTQIA+ identity and live with heterosexual parents can all struggle to feel safe.

Julie: Even going to the school gate every single day. Think about that daily interruption to being safe. Imagine what that's like for the child. This is one tiny example of a day-to-day routine in which safety is regularly compromised.

HOW CAN THIS HELP DDP PRACTITIONERS?

Children may have many layers through which they are navigating. Within DDP interventions, we need to be able to articulate, and we need to help the parents and children to articulate, what it feels like in the worlds they inhabit.

Find ways to wonder what it's like to live where, for many moments of many days, you're thinking to yourself, "Am I going to tell this person? If so, what shall I say? Will they talk to me again or see me in the same way once I've told them? How will I act this time so that it looks like this does not affect me? Or shall I make a point, and is it worth it?"

Find the words, practice, or role play with others so that you can ask directly, matter-of-factly, and without judgement about the experiences the LGBTQIA+ individual has had.

There are so many things to be curious about with children and adolescents.

- Ask about the language used to refer to and describe family and caring relationships both inside and outside the home.
- Ask how they define or see themselves.
- Ask how they tell their story to friends, partners, teachers.
- Be curious about whether their parents and carers know this about them. Do they ask them about this? Do they help them to figure this out?

For parents and carers, consider the added complexity of feeling that you can't let your community down. For example, if a parent is experiencing extreme difficulties raising their fostered or adopted child and the child has to leave their family, they will experience this additional shame on top of the feeling that they have failed as a parent to this child.

5.   Gender, sex, nonbinary, history, and politics

People within the LGBTQIA+ communities are usually not born into their community. They must actively seek this community as they grow up. In addition, these are communities that have been impacted by trauma, such as the Aids crisis, over generations. These two phenomena are connected. If you are not born into your community, then the history might be lost. Children may not be growing up with the stories that profoundly affected previous generations.

| Julie: | The forgotten history can lead people to think that the community is a whole lot safer now for the children that they're adopting, fostering, and giving birth to. Just because people now know not to say things about beliefs they still hold doesn't mean that the world has changed. We might feel comforted when we act as if things have significantly changed in our country, but we still need to help children navigate a world that will discriminate against them because they don't fit. |

HOW CAN THIS HELP DDP PRACTITIONERS?

Most DDP practitioners live in a binary world where heteronormativity and binary concepts of gender and sex are assumed. Curiosity can fade when working with LGBTQIA+ communities. Practitioners need to find ways to stay curious about the person in front of them and how their experience interacts and intersects with the norms of the heritage, culture, and religion of their childhood and the environment they live in now.

Be interested in the history and the current legislation where you live and work. For example, being homosexual (usually linked to men) is illegal in 77 countries, in some, it is punishable by death. U.K. Conservative government laws associated with not promoting lesbian and gay family life (Clause 28 in the 1990s) are considered recent history, but similar policies have even more recently been enacted in some U.S. states.

It's not about being all knowing, it's about developing an interest in history, politics, culture, and religion. Coming out as lesbian, gay, trans, or nonbinary will always be significant. Foster a stance of curiosity to make sense of the impact this has on the context the person has lived in.

In countries where legislation is more accepting, keep in mind that safety still depends on making choices, such as code-switching and how to respond to microaggressions, every day.

Kim: I'm hearing about the importance of finding community and a feeling of belonging and how these can be threatened. Heterosexual children living with gay parents or children discovering their LGBTQIA+ identity while living with heterosexual parents can all struggle to feel safe.

Julie: Yes, that's the world that these children navigate from almost the day they're born. Certainly from the time they go to play school or meet people in the street. It doesn't start when they go to secondary school or make a legal commitment, such as a civil partnership or marriage. When the outside world puts a whole way of being onto you, it's a life you constantly navigate. People often don't know what they don't know. Many DDP practitioners are open about feeling that they don't know what to be curious about or what words to use, and they would like help to deepen their understanding. Without this, we live in a world that continues to be separate.

6.   The importance of compassion

Alok Vaid-Menon talks eloquently about our urgent need for compassion. As a gender non-confirming person, Alok emphasizes how we do not need to understand someone to have compassion for them. (For example, see *ALOK: The Urgent Need for Compassion: The Man Enough Podcast*, https://www.youtube.com/watch?v=Tq3C9R8HNUQ.) Compassion is more important than ideology, because we need to value what is and not what should be. When we try to understand in order to find compassion, we are doing it backwards. We need to start with compassion.

Benjamin:	The concept of compassion rather than understanding as a starting point is so important for DDP practitioners. I think it is the same as acceptance and empathy in many ways. This can free people from being worried that they can't work with someone because they don't know about the entirety of queer history or all about the specific issues queer people face. I know my own therapist was very clear with me about being unsure she could work with me for that reason, but she has turned out to be great.
Kim:	Well, thank you so much for inviting me into your world today. I will continue to stay curious and keep listening, and I hope others reading this will do the same.

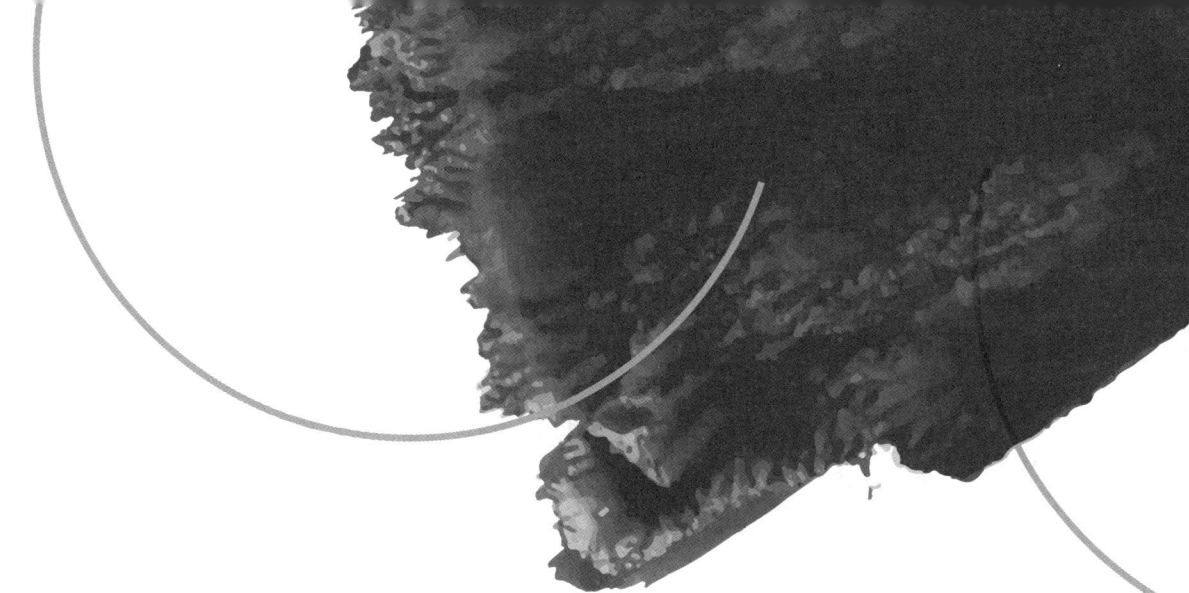

Chapter 4:
The Experience of Dyadic Developmental Psychotherapy

Through synchronized conversations, there is an increased ability and opportunity for the child to develop stories about the current events in his life. As he is more comfortable with this new storytelling skill, he is able to wonder about deeper meanings and begin to be curious about the possibilities presented to him now. He is also likely to be more able to contrast the stories that are being cocreated in the present with the therapist and adoptive parents and the past stories that had largely been created for him by those who had traumatized him. (Hughes et al., 2019, pp. 68–69)

REFRESHER

The experience of being human develops within the self–other dyad in which the experience of self (A) is embedded in the experience of other (B) including the other's experience of self (A; Figure 4.1).

This is quite evident in the infant's experience of self, which is barely present. The infant does experience the parent experiencing their world, especially the parent's experience of them. This self–other dyadic experience is present

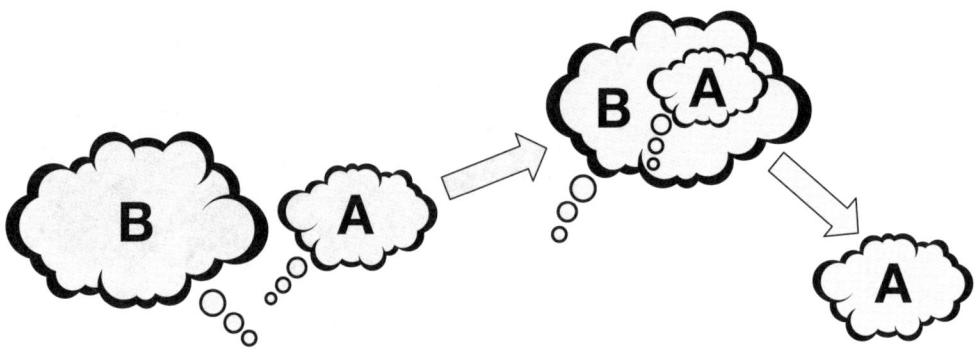

Figure 4.1 Self–Other Dyad

over the entire developmental trajectory; though, as the child matures, especially in some cultures, the "self" component of this dyad is emphasized while the "other" component moves into the background.

Humans are even able to create an illusion that the self is entirely independent of the other. This is the case in individualistic societies where individual identity is valued at the expense of identification with the group and its unique rituals and meanings. This contrasts with sociocentric cultures where the understanding of self is embedded within the social group (Keller, 2022).

Dyadic developmental psychotherapy (DDP) is modeled on the relational activities of the infant and parent that are central to the infant's integrated emotional, social, and cognitive development and that lead to their emerging autobiographical narrative. To get things started, the infant—and parent—need to experience a sense of safety. Without safety, there is little energy to discover each other within the relationship because the child's energy is instead devoted to creating self-protective defenses, such as dissociation and pervasive control.

With safety, initial patterns of synchronized nonverbal interactions begin to emerge between parent and infant, which are the foundation of all subsequent interactions. These conversations gradually include words, enabling them to expand from the here-and-now into the past and future.

These conversations provide the structure and experience that allows the child to begin to develop stories that hold the meanings of the experiences that they are having together. Through shared interests and joint activities, the stories form the child's emerging sense of self, reflecting the organization of the physical, emotional, social, and cognitive skills that they are developing. Patterns of experiences develop, and these become the child's evolving autobiographical narrative.

These abilities and activities are characteristic of relationships at all ages and are crucial for an individual's continuing psychological development.

Relationship is fundamental to the development of a person. The practice of DDP involves developing and then using the relationship that we observe in the securely attached infant and their parent.

DDP is characterized by safety and reciprocity. The two selves are engaged in a relationship that involves matched affective states, joint interests, and highly cooperative intentions. Distant goals of therapeutic change will still be present but not central in the relationship. These goals are within reach because these living conversations develop stories. These stories begin with the stories of trauma, which were shaped by pain, fear, and shame. They are then joined by stories influenced by the relationship, including the practitioner's experiences of the child's trauma as well as the child's challenges and strengths that emerged from the trauma.

These conversations—the core of the DDP sessions—provide the words and meanings that create jointly developed stories of the child's resilience, strengths, and capacities for discovery and joy, eventually providing the child with a coherent narrative.

DDP was developed for the treatment of children and youth who had experienced developmental trauma. Frequently, children who have been abused and neglected are unable to resolve the traumatic relational events that they have experienced or to develop secure attachment relationships with new caregivers. They are isolated, with limited ability to enter into the healing and restorative conversations necessary to develop new relational stories that can enrich and support them. They are locked in their fragmented sense of self and others, which is permeated with fear and shame. The developmental abilities that they need for an integrated sense of self and a coherent narrative are not in place. The intent of DDP is to facilitate the development of these core skills.

Children who have experienced developmental trauma have great difficulty engaging in relational activities. Focusing on either defensive self-protection or attacking the other, they avoid synchronized nonverbal and verbal conversations, regardless of the topic.

- Without such reciprocity, their social and emotional world is limited, and they have little sense of being able to affect the world in a way that is good for both self and other.
- Without these successful conversations, they are unlikely to develop joint stories about self and other and are likely to have little sense of the mind and heart of their parent.
- Without these intersubjective stories, their ability to develop an integrated sense of self is impaired.
- Without the predictability of an integrated sense of self, their ability to form a coherent autobiographical narrative and to relate with others in a cooperative, reciprocal manner is restricted. This lack of coherence is the core feature of disorganized attachment patterns.

COMPONENTS OF DDP

The components of DDP are essentially the qualities of these therapeutic conversations.

PACE—described in detail in Chapter 3—is likely to be present throughout most of the treatment sessions. These four ways of engaging are especially helpful in creating intersubjective experiences central to therapeutic change.

When the DDP practitioner is relating with playfulness (when appropriate), acceptance, curiosity, and empathy, the mind of the child becomes engaged and the conversation will be a dialogue, not a monologue.

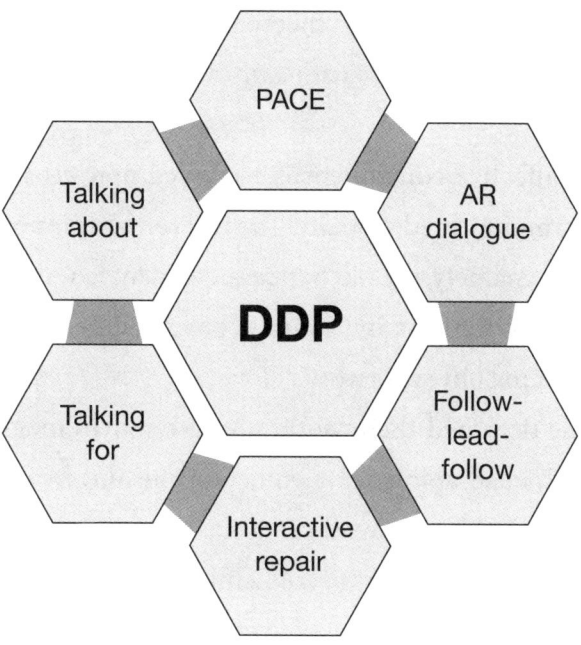

Figure 4.2 Components of DDP

Within PACE, the practitioner's mind is holding the child's mind along with their own. The experiences of both minds must have a place in the conversation if it is to lead to therapeutic change. As the practitioner is aware of—and expressing—the content of their own mind, they are also aware of—and receptive to—the content of the child's mind. It is not a question of either/or; neither is it about right/wrong. The two minds are present as both/and. How the two become interwoven and related represents the intersubjective realities that open the minds of each to new perspectives and possibilities.

Affective–Reflective dialogue (AR dialogue) refers to the need for the conversation to contain both affective and reflective components.

- When we have only affect, this is catharsis.
- When we have only a cognitive component, this is intellectualization.

Neither of these alone is likely to be therapeutic. Like good conversations with friends over lunch, conversations with our clients contain both affective and reflective features.

Much of the affective component is conveyed nonverbally, while most of the reflective is communicated verbally. The nonverbal component includes the prosody of the voice; namely, the pitch, stress, segment length, tone, and intonation. These patterns of rhythms and sounds convey subtleties of personal meaning that are difficult to convey by words alone.

Too often, the detached therapeutic stance removes much of the prosody from the voice and, in so doing, leaves much of the affective meanings ambiguous. While this might be ideal with certain clients and therapeutic models, it is not desirable in DDP with traumatized children. Here, clarity of meaning is seen as important to creating both a sense of safety for the child and a rich form of intersubjective learning.

REFLECTIVE EXERCISE: EXPLORING AR DIALOGUE

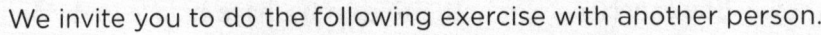

We invite you to do the following exercise with another person.

Think of a descriptive paragraph about a stressful event in a person's life. Hold it clearly in your mind so that you are able to say it out loud and not have to read it from a script.

Now describe the event to a colleague or friend in two ways:

1. As much as possible, remove the prosody from your voice. Try to speak with little rhythm, inflection, or variation of pitch.

2. Speak in as natural a way as possible, including the prosody that is evoked by the meaning of the story that you are telling. Ensure that your intention is to fully convey the affective meaning of the event.

Now discuss with your friend/colleague their experience of listening to the story under each condition. Reflect on your own experience of telling the story in these different ways.

Did the story have a greater impact on you both under the second condition?

We expect that you and your friend were aware of being touched by the story more under the second condition. Bringing "A" together with "R" is a more impactful experience.

Follow-Lead-Follow. In keeping with the goal of making the dialogue into a conversation, DDP is neither a directive nor a nondirective intervention, which allows a story to be created and told about the life of the child or parent.

The practitioner is an active participant in the story's development in various ways:

- The practitioner might introduce or follow a particular theme, connect it to a related theme, and engage in the process of exploring its implications for other areas of the client's life.
- The practitioner's active curiosity demonstrates a fascination with the events of the person's life and the meanings that might be present. As the practitioner wonders about aspects of the client's life, the client often experiences them more deeply than if they had reflected alone.
- When the practitioner actively expresses empathy for the stressful events in the story, the client feels those events more fully and with a greater sense of safety and a stronger felt-sense that what happened is able to be understood and accepted.

As the client experiences the practitioner's genuine interest in and active exploration of the emerging story, the therapeutic conversation that emerges is truly dyadic.

When only one person is telling the story and the other is passively listening, the story itself tends to be compromised. The following may then occur in the mind of the child or parent and/or in the mind of the practitioner:

1. The listener is likely to lose the plot of the story. What is its meaning? Why is it being told?
2. The speaker is likely to go off on a tangent. The story is less able to hold the mind of the listener, the speaker, or both and their minds are likely to wander.
3. They are likely to become disengaged from the meaning of the story.
4. The listener is less likely to buy in to the purpose of the story.
5. The story is less likely to be integrated into the lived-experience of both the speaker and the listener.

REFLECTIVE EXERCISE: EXPLORING STORY CREATION

Three people are needed for the following exercise. The parts they will play are indicated by X, Y, and Z.

1. X tells an interesting story of a recent event. Y and Z listen to the story. Y then recounts to the other two the story that they heard from X.
2. X tells the story, and this time Z tells the other two the story that they heard from X.
3. X tells the story, and this time Y and Z jointly tell the story that they heard from X.

After the exercise, reflect on the differences between Experiences 1, 2, and 3.

- What differences in telling the story were evident when Y and Z jointly told the story?
- Did the joint telling evoke greater interest and engagement for both?
- Did more questions about possible meanings and implications emerge?

Interactive repair refers to any action that the parent (or practitioner) takes to attend to and repair a breach in the relationship. When a parent initiates such a repair, it doesn't necessarily mean that the parent made a mistake in how they related to their child. Rather it simply means there is a breach and the parent is committed to repairing the breach. The child may have asked to do something and the parent denied the child's request. The child becomes angry, leaves the room, and is distant from their parent to show their displeasure. If their parent then approaches them in an open and engaged manner and shows in their attitude that they are inviting the child back into a closer relationship, the parent is engaged in interactive repair. This would not include "I'm sorry" if the parent did not do anything that they thought was a mistake. It would simply acknowledge the breach and indicate that they are not annoyed with the child and are open to supporting them with any upset they are still feeling.

The repair might sound something like this:

"How are you feeling? You were upset with me for not letting you visit your friend. I could see you really wanted to see her! Anything I can do to help? Let me know if there is. I'm planning on baking later if you want to join me."

TIME FOR REFLECTION: EXPLORING INTERACTIVE REPAIR

Do you think there are reasons to engage in interactive repair in these situations?

1. You communicate an evaluation, rather than acceptance (e.g., "*Why* did you *do* that?").
2. You are told, "You should have listened better!"
3. You were distracted and misheard what the child said.
4. The child said they just wanted you to listen and understand, but you gave advice.
5. You forgot something important that the child told you in the previous session.
6. The child questioned what you said, and you became defensive.

The important thing to remember is that needs for repair are not limited to times you believe that you made a mistake. It is important that you simply take the initiative, showing that the relationship is important to you and that you will attend to it whenever there is a conflict, regardless of who, if anyone, is right or wrong. Considering this, you can see that a repair would be appropriate in all the above examples.

Suppose you suggest that the parent's preoccupied behavior may have been a factor in their child's angry outburst, and the parent then exclaims:

"Are you blaming me? Are you saying it's my fault that they can't control their anger? So, I have to be the perfect parent all the time?"

You may conclude that the parent was projecting onto you their own feelings of shame or their past experiences of being blamed by their parents who they felt were never satisfied with them. Yet, there is still a breach in the relationship. The DDP practitioner addresses and repairs the breach by saying, without becoming defensive, something like:

"I'm sorry if you experienced me as blaming you and thinking that you should be perfect! No wonder you seem annoyed with me. That was not my intention, and I truly don't think you should be aware of what's on your child's mind all the time."

Or, if the practitioner does not want to suggest they made a mistake by saying they are sorry when they believe they didn't, they could say:

"I regret that I said it that way, if you feel that I'm blaming you. That was not my intention, nor do I believe you were in the wrong."

Would there be value in addressing the parent's apparent projection or triggering of past experiences? Certainly, there would be if there was a pattern in their responses to the therapist's comments. The practitioner might say:

"I have noticed that a number of times you have experienced me as blaming you when I'm pointing out something that is occurring. At these times, I was not aware of myself blaming you. Could we explore this and see if we might both understand it better?"

In DDP, the practitioner is responsible for initiating repair just as the parent is in the family. By initiating repair, the practitioner is not denying that a conflict or problem may be present in the relationship. Rather, through interactive repair, the practitioner is communicating that the relationship is more important than the specific problem or conflict.

Speaking For and Speaking About. Since having good conversations is a central goal of DDP, it is important to learn ways to facilitate them.

The practitioner may assist the child in finding words for their experiences by speaking for them based on what the child has communicated verbally or nonverbally.

The DDP practitioner may choose to *speak for* the child when the child is reluctant or unable to verbally speak for themselves. This may provide the child with a bit of momentum to find the words for themselves.

Sometimes the practitioner speaks for the child with great affect through voice prosody. This helps the child who is guarded about expressing the affective meaning of what they are saying.

Whenever the practitioner speaks for the child, they will be tentative, making it clear that they are trying to approximate or guess as to what the child is experiencing. The child alone decides if the practitioner's words are accurate or not.

Alternatively, the practitioner might *speak about* the child. They do this in a way that lets the child know that they are welcome to join the conversation but are also free not to. The child may choose to listen and not add to the conversation when this feels like a safer option.

Here are six reasons why speaking for and speaking about are used in facilitating therapeutic conversations in DDP:

1. Traumatized children often lack the ability to give words to their inner lives of thoughts, emotions, wishes, and intentions. When the DDP practitioner is able to put these aspects of their inner lives into words, the child is often likely to think, and even say, as one 10-year-old girl did, "I don't know how you knew what I was thinking. When you said that, I knew that I really had been [thinking that]. And now I know that I've been thinking that for a long time. I just didn't know it!"

2. Often the goal of DDP is to assist children (and their parents) to go more deeply into the affective states that underly their behaviors. These are often states of vulnerability that the child has consistently avoided exploring. Speaking for a child often safely opens them to these vulnerable experiences.

3. When the DDP practitioner speaks for and about them, the child often begins to sense the practitioners interest in them and that they are noticing them without judgment. The child begins to know that they are safely in the mind of their practitioner, something that they may have seldom felt in their other relationships.

4. Speaking for and speaking about often make the conversation itself more engaging. The practitioner can hold the interest of the child longer when they periodically guess what the child might be thinking or feeling or when they speak about the child as if the child were not there.

5. When the child hears the practitioner speaking about them, they are likely to be listening more openly than if they felt pressure to respond. The child knows that there is no expectation that they will respond or even listen; it is their choice.

6. When the practitioner is speaking for or about the child, they have the opportunity, through their voice prosody, to convey their non-judgmental curiosity, acceptance, and empathy for the child and their inner life.

TIME FOR REFLECTION: SPEAKING FOR A CHILD

When you speak for a child, keep in mind that your voice prosody will be critical in helping the child to experience what you say as representing their inner life.

Say the following as if you are speaking for a child. Say it twice, the first time using a matter-of-fact tone and the second time conveying what you believe the child's affective experience might be using your voice prosody. (Anger is conveyed in the first sentence; distress and confusion in the second sentence; and sadness in the third.)

"Yes, I was angry with you because you said 'no' to me. It seems to me you often say 'no,' and I think it's because you don't care what I'm thinking. Sometimes I think that you don't care about me and even that you wish I weren't your child."

Did you have a different experience when you heard what the child was saying based on whether voice prosody was present?

TIME FOR REFLECTION: COMPARING SPEAKING TO AND FOR THE CHILD

Speak aloud the following sentences. The first speaks to the child. The second speaks for the child.

1. *"I wonder if you're thinking that your dad doesn't care about what you want when he says 'no' to you. That what you want is not important to him."*
2. *"I wonder if you're thinking, 'When you say "no" to me, I just don't think that you care about what I want. Sometimes I think that what I want isn't important to you!'"*

Reflect on how the child might experience your words differently based on whether you were speaking to or for them.

Speaking for the child often evokes a more complex experience, making it more intersubjective for the child. Your experience of them becomes more vitally a part of their experience of themselves.

TIME FOR REFLECTION: COMPARING TALKING TO AND ABOUT THE CHILD

Speak the following sentences. The first speaks to the child. The second speaks about the child, using her name, Joan.

1. *"You might have been really confused, since she said that she would not tell anyone and then you heard her tell her sister. Maybe you wondered if you could trust her with things that are important to you."*

2. *"I imagine Joan was really confused when she heard her friend tell her sister what Joan had told her. Joan might have wondered if she could trust her with things that are important to her."*

Reflect on how the child might have experienced your words differently based on whether you were speaking to her or about her.

When speaking about, the child might listen more openly, not having to prepare an answer. They might also have more confidence that you were seriously thinking about their situation with acceptance, that what you were saying was more than just words to you.

The practitioner thinking out loud may be a variation of speaking for or speaking about the child. This helps the child to be safely and quietly receptive to what the practitioner is saying. Here, the theme is broader than speaking about the child, though it might be similar.

For example, the practitioner is speaking about the child when they say:

"I wonder if Avery begins to worry about whether he is that special to his mom when he asks her to go out to eat with him and she says 'no.'"

The practitioner is thinking out loud when they say:

"I've noticed over the years how hard routine disappointments are for the adopted child who has experienced a major rejection before being placed for adoption. When the adoptive dad says he is too busy to do something with him, the child often begins to doubt how much the adoptive dad cares about him."

In the first example the child might feel a need to deny the practitioner's guess. However, he might be more able to entertain the possibility for some adopted children, without having to acknowledge whether he feels the same way.

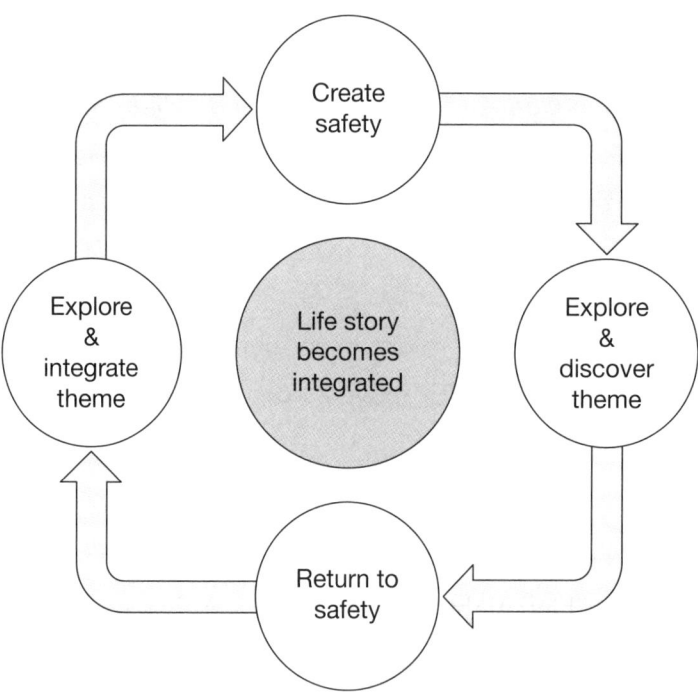

Figure 4.3 Cyclical Process of DDP

THE CYCLICAL PROCESS OF DDP

The process of DDP over the course of therapy is a cyclical one. This process involves:

- creating safety
- moving through exploration and discovery of an important theme
- experiencing a threat to safety
- reestablishing safety
- further exploring stressful themes so that they become integrated and no longer are a threat to safety
- discovering and addressing another theme

It might seem that the same themes are explored again and again, but with each completion of this cycle, the life story becomes more integrated and comprehensive, with fewer fragmented bits of fear and shame. This cyclical process is a deepening one, leading again and again to greater safety and awareness of self and other.

SAFETY

In Chapter 2, we discussed how central safety is to DDP, and we explored its roots in attachment, intersubjectivity, and interpersonal neurobiology. We will now focus on its development and importance for the child and parent within DDP.

The safety of the DDP practitioner needs to be established and maintained first if the practitioner is to ensure safety for the child and parent.

There are many challenges to establishing and maintaining safety for the child and parent, requiring that the practitioner maintain sensitivity to a variety of issues.

These are:

1. When the child experienced developmental trauma, their core sense of safety in relationships was violated. The child will find it difficult to establish safety in subsequent relationships. When it is established, it is likely to be easily lost. This is because the child remains vigilant and overly sensitive to potential signals of danger within the relationship; they perceive signs of disappoint-

ment, rejection, and abandonment even when these phenomena are not present.

2. Traumatic themes need to be explored in DDP if the child is to be able to resolve and integrate the trauma and ensure that it no longer impedes their healthy development.

3. The experience of exploring past traumas will cause the child to be vulnerable. Most likely, the child has learned to defend strongly against vulnerability in order to maintain some semblance of safety in the face of repetitive traumatic experiences and memories. If the child has a central defense of avoiding thinking about traumatic events, the therapeutic exploration of these events is likely to be stressful.

4. The child's developmental skills of regulation, reflection, trusting relationships, and relationship repair are likely to be insufficiently developed, making it harder to safely address the trauma.

5. The child is not likely to experience trusting relationships with others, outside of therapy, that would be helpful in providing support in dealing with the challenges of therapy.

6. In early therapy sessions, the presence of the child's caregiver is likely to be experienced as a threat to safety, since the child anticipates rejection from them as their family struggles are being explored.

7. The child who experienced developmental trauma is likely to experience pervasive shame. This shame is likely to undermine the child's sense that they are safe to explore and express their inner life.

The DDP practitioner needs to be aware of these threats to the child's sense of safety and to ensure that safety is established and reestablished again and again and that the challenges to safety are being explored.

Safety can be enhanced in many ways:

1. The open and engaged state that is central to Stephen Porges's (2011) Polyvagal Theory is also central to creating and maintaining safety within the session. For the polyvagal state to be experienced by the child, the practitioner needs to convey acceptance, not evaluation. The practitioner's voice needs to be spoken with rhythmic prosody, not as monotone.

2. The practitioner needs to keep in mind that with each bit of progress, there are likely to be new threats to the child's sense of safety. For example, as the child begins to trust their caregivers more and explore their challenges and trauma more fully, the child is likely to experience new reasons for why they might be rejected. As they express more experiences embedded in shame, their beliefs that they may be unlovable and bad are likely to increase initially.

3. The DDP practitioner, sensing that the child has many self-doubts and insecurities, may be tempted to frequently praise the child, hoping that such recognition will help the child feel more confident. However, such praise will often create more uncertainty. The child may experience it as conveying pressure to always be good or right. Praise is an evaluation and is likely to lead the child to feel that they are always being evaluated. If that is the case, they may feel certain that they will eventually fail. The anxious child needs to feel accepted and to gradually develop confidence that the practitioner's positive attitude toward them is unconditional rather than to receive copious positive evaluations.

4. The DDP practitioner communicates that the child will never be trapped into exploring trauma regardless of how they feel about it. Safety will come from knowing that the practitioner will defer to their judgment if they believe that they need a break from exploring any theme.

5. The DDP practitioner needs to be alert to the child's nonverbal signs that they are not feeling safe. This may be evident in their

facial expressions, gestures, or an increasing intensity in their voice prosody. At the first sign that the child may be about to dysregulate, the practitioner must assist the child in remaining regulated by changing the topic, reducing the intensity of their own vocal expressions, reflecting on the conversation, or talking about the child/talking to themselves, all of which tend to reduce the affective component of the conversation.

6. The practitioner may notice that the child's caregiver is adopting a judgmental attitude in response to the child's expressions. The practitioner may address that through conveying acceptance of the child to the caregiver, talking with the caregiver about the need to understand the child's perspective, talking about the child in a nonjudgmental manner, or changing the focus of the conversation. If this becomes a pattern, the practitioner will meet with the caregiver alone and stress the need for PACE so the child can feel safe enough to be actively engaged in therapy. If it is still difficult for the caregiver to be nonjudgmental, the practitioner needs to explore aspects of the caregiver's own attachment history that might be making it difficult.

REFLECTIVE EXERCISE: MAINTAINING SAFETY FOR THE CHILD

There is an opportunity to explore responding to statements that parents can make to their children during sessions in Worksheet 4.1. These need to be made in a way that supports the parents while holding safety for the child.

SYNCHRONIZED NONVERBAL–VERBAL CONVERSATIONS

The findings of infant intersubjectivity, described in Chapter 2, are our guide for developing interactions that enable the traumatized child to engage in synchronized nonverbal–verbal conversations with us.

Conversations are inherently nonverbal and verbal, with the emotional meaning of what is said being carried by the nonverbal expressions that we make as we speak. These expressions involve characteristics of our voice prosody (rhythm, tone, pitch, accent, intonation), facial expressions, gestures, and posture. When someone is "just talking," most likely they are using words with little nonverbal context. Their voice is monotone. One might quite accurately say that psychotherapy is not a "talking cure" but rather a "conversation cure."

Much of what is contained in the therapeutic value of the characteristics of PACE involves their nonverbal components.

- Playfulness is conveyed with a light, rhythmic tone that is both inviting and animated.
- Acceptance is conveyed with an open and engaged attitude. There is no hint of evaluation in the tone; rather, what is being conveyed is being unconditionally received.
- Curiosity has a similarly nonjudgmental tone while also conveying interest, even fascination, with aspects of the other's life.
- Empathy is conveyed with nonverbal expressions of warmth and understanding. "I am with you" is expressed with the eyes, voice, gestures, and possibly touch.

The therapeutic value of PACE is much lower if the therapist expresses themselves with just words, presented in a detached, nonengaged manner.

When the flow of the conversation has been established, the practitioner and child or parent become synchronized. The flow of words alternates from one to the other, often without a pause. There is a similar joining of facial expressions, gestures, and even movements, such as scratching your arm or hair. This synchronized state seems to heighten the sense of cooperation between the practitioner and client, with each holding a complimentary intention. This cooperative state makes it easier for both to focus their attention on the same theme and to enter a matched affective state. In this intersubjective state, time often seems to pass quickly, and those engaged with each other tend to be unaware of surrounding, incidental events.

When the traumatized child does not trust the practitioner and is reluctant to become engaged with them, this synchronized nonverbal state is less likely to occur. The nonverbal rhythms of the practitioner may evoke a responsive, cooperative state that is then strongly resisted by the child's mistrusting attitude. This defensive stance of the child may evoke a similar stance in the practitioner, causing them to abandon their open and engaged stance.

Thus, if the practitioner is not aware of what is happening, the lack of prosody in the child's voice is likely to reduce the prosody of the practitioner's voice. If the practitioner is able to inhibit this tendency toward reduced prosody and to maintain the same degree of prosody as they initially expressed, the child is more likely to increase the prosody of their voice and become more synchronized in the conversation.

However, if the practitioner notices a lack of synchronization between them and the child, they might deliberately reduce their own nonverbal expressiveness to some extent in order to be closer to the child's nonexpressive state. If there is too great a difference between the practitioner's degree of prosody and the child's, the child may be less likely to synchronize with the practitioner. If the practitioner reduces the difference between them, the child may accept the practitioner's invitation to join them.

When the practitioner is engaged in a synchronized conversation with the child, they are establishing a momentum that carries the discussion from theme to theme. This momentum increases the likelihood that the child will continue to engage in the conversation when the practitioner moves from a light and casual theme to a theme that is more difficult, such as one conveying fear and shame. It is the voice prosody of the practitioner that carries the momentum and increases the likelihood that the child will remain engaged. If the practitioner stops the more rhythmic conversational tone and switches to a more sober, serious, monotone when focusing on a "problem," the child is much more likely to disengage from the conversation. If the voice prosody is continuous, the child often remains in the conversation even when the theme becomes more difficult.

When this synchronized state is present, the conversation is felt more strongly and the sense of "we" becomes more real. The relationship itself is often more fully experienced as a fundamental reality, more so than the reality of two separate individuals. The resulting sense of cooperation is not in conscious awareness but rather experienced as the core presence of the dyad.

CREATING STORIES

Within the rhythmic conversations flowing between practitioner and child, stories begin to form that integrate the experiences of both child and practitioner. Early in the conversation, the child is supported by the practitioner to safely explore and express prior stories held by the child, even when these are held outside of awareness.

The practitioner's attitude of PACE creates safety for the child, reduces any sense of defensiveness, and enables them to be open to the practitioner's words. The child gradually develops an awareness of the meanings of their behaviors. Once the shame-based story unfolds, the child gradually becomes engaged with the practitioner in holding other possible stories in response to the particular events being discussed. As they develop a synchronized conversation about that particular theme, the original story is affected by the practitioner's experience and becomes more coherent.

Often in DDP, the practitioner invites the child's current primary caregiver into the conversation so their experience can contribute to the story being developed. The caregiver's empathy is crucial in enabling the child to safely explore their shame-based story, in creating doubts about its validity, and opening the child's mind to the new story.

The facts and events in the child's history are gradually seen as reflecting many possible meanings. The original meaning, often given to the child by the perpetrator, is now seen as more reflective of the perpetrator's raging and shaming behaviors rather than qualities in the child.

TIME FOR REFLECTION

DDP involves moment-to-moment conversations that gather deepening meaning as they go along.

We invite you to reflect on the following conversation between a foster child and his foster parents and to notice how a therapeutic story gradually develops. Pause as you read the conversation to see if the meanings of their experiences of the events are changing.

12-year-old David is foster son of Sara and Ed and has lived with them for the past two years. This is his third foster home since he entered care when he was seven years old. He was physically abused for most of his early years by his father, while his mother failed to protect him. He has much difficulty accepting the rules in his foster home, leading to conflicts that tend to be slow to resolve.

This is David's sixth therapy session with Victor. Both of his foster parents are present. We join it 10 minutes into the session, following a light discussion about an enjoyable family event. David has just hinted at problems between him and Ed.

Victor: I heard that you and Ed had a big conflict a few days ago. What was going on?

David: Nothing different. We fight a lot because he's always on my back about something.

Victor: That would be hard for you both if you have that many conflicts. How do you make sense of that, David, if Ed is always
on your back?

David: Easy, I'm not good enough for him. He's never satisfied with
me. He'd be a lot happier if I was another kid.

Victor: Happier if you were another kid! If that's how it seems to
you, it must be hard to live there.

David: Not hard. As I said, I'm used to it. That's the way it was in the
other homes too.

Victor: Because?

David: Don't you listen! I said, I'm not good enough for him. He
wants someone else, and someday he'll make me leave just
like the other two did. I could tell he didn't want me as soon
as I walked in the door. Everything [at the house] cost so
much and was so neat and clean. If he knew where I grew
up and saw that we had nothing, he'd have gotten rid of me
sooner. I just don't fit in with him and his family. If he wasn't
stuck with me, he'd never make time to get to know me.

Victor: I know that you were really poor, David, but I also know
that your dad used to beat you and swear at you. I wonder if
that's really why you don't feel that you're not good enough
for this family.

David: Duh! What do you want me to say? He thought I was a great kid? OK, he thought that I was just a bad, worthless kid! You happy now?

This excerpt follows a variety of conversations that Victor has had with David and his foster parents covering many episodes in his life. The central story that emerges tells David's way of making sense of all the conflicts that he has with his foster parents, a story that is congruent with his original traumas, involving physical abuse by his father. This story includes his sense that his caregivers are often angry with him because he is a disappointment to them. This led to David forming the belief that he will be rejected by his foster father, just as he had been twice before. His original explanation for the abuse—that he was bad—is only confirmed by the conflicts and anger that he experiences with his foster parents.

David would not have felt safe enough to acknowledge this story with Victor if, in previous sessions, they had not engaged in a number of synchronized, reciprocal conversations about many aspects of his life. As David's current story becomes clear, it is now Victor's task to develop a new story to help him to make sense of these events in his life and give them new meanings.

However, David has added another element to his experience. He believes that he will experience rejection from Ed and Sarah because of his poor background at least as much as because he was abused. Victor is integrating this into the story as well.

Victor: *(with empathy)* Oh, David, again and again it seems that the main people in your life who are supposed to take care of you . . . to care for you . . . are disappointed in you! Your dad abused you, and then your foster parents sent you away! It seems to you that your father's abuse means there is something wrong with you. And your poor background makes you worry that your foster parents will think there is something wrong with you too. It seems to you that everyone finds something wrong with you. How hard that must be, to live with that belief day after day, year after year.

David: How else can I make sense of it?

Victor: I can understand why it seems that way to you! I'd like to see how it seems to your foster dad. Is it OK if I tell him what you just told me and see what he says?

David: I guess.

Victor: Ed, David gave me permission to speak for him and tell you what he just told me. (*Using a childlike and intensely angry voice*) Ed, you always seem to be angry with me, you never seem happy with what I do! And I don't dress like you or eat like you. Sometimes I don't have a clue why something is important to you guys. I do think you're disappointed in me. (*Voice softening*) I sometimes think you feel you made a mistake in taking me and that you're going to want to get rid of me . . . . You won't want me, and no one ever will. I guess I am worthless.

Ed: Oh, David, that would be so hard if you think that I'm disappointed in you . . . that I don't want you . . . and that you think you're worthless and that maybe I do too. So hard.

Victor: (*still talking for David*) You get mad at me all the time!

Ed: I know we get angry with each other a lot, David. And I wish we didn't. I know it's hard for you to follow the rules that I have, and I wish I had understood how hard it was and didn't get so angry. I know you try. And I know that you've been poor most of your life and don't feel you fit in here. I'm sorry if you think that I think less of you because of that. And I know that sometimes you really think that I don't like you and just want you to be unhappy! When you think that, of course you'd be angry about it! Your foster parent wants you to be unhappy! I have to work harder to find a way to show you I get this! That I don't want to make you unhappy . . . and that I don't think you're a bad kid. You've been hurt a lot, and you're angry a lot—which makes sense since you've been hurt a lot—and I have to give you reasons that make it easier for you to trust me. I do care about you and want this to work between us.

Victor: David, I think that Ed was really listening to you and seems to really mean what he just said about you. He seems to want to figure this out so you two can work it out. Maybe so you both can trust each other more. Do you think?

David: I don't know.

Victor: Good for you for being honest. I don't imagine you'll be able to believe him that easily. I think, though, that you both want to try to work this out, to not give up on your relationship. That maybe you're both worth it!

David: I guess.

Such conversations need to be repeated about other stressful events that occur in the foster home. The conversations would need to work toward greater understanding about why David mistrusts Ed, why he had been abused by his father, why he has trouble regulating his emotions and making sense of problems without withdrawing into a sense of shame.

Ed also needs to be more sensitive to how David's poor background is affecting him in Ed's middle-class home. He often feels awkward and ignorant when he does not know something or is not able to do something that Ed and Sara just take for granted.

David will gradually begin to trust the intersubjective experiences that he is having with Victor, and, increasingly, those with Ed and Sara too. These contradict the experiences with his abusive father. David will gradually be able to notice that his poor background does not bother his foster parents the way he fears it does.

David's new story has much less fear and shame, with space to discover a sense of worth, reciprocal interests, and joy.

AN INTEGRATIVE SENSE OF SELF

As stories develop within the therapeutic relationship with safety and openness, not shame or fear, they become integrated with the other stories that are also being formed. Together, they become organized into a coherent and comprehensive sense of self. The self of the child is now developing in a continuous manner that can engage flexibly with the various events that are encountered.

This continuity of self contrasts with the fragmented self that forms when one experiences developmental trauma. As each traumatic event becomes integrated into this holistic sense of self, it becomes understood and resolved. A stressful memory within one's narrative, yes, but not a disorganizing, dysregulating one.

The emerging sense of self is one that can retain its sense of integrity while at the same time be openly, intimately, engaged with the other. Each self affects the other without controlling or competing with them. The child does not have to choose between self and other, but rather knows now that the sense of self is enhanced by such close relationships and that such relationships are also enhanced when each member of the dyad brings to it their own unique qualities.

Attachment theory and research suggest that an organized sense of self is correlated with a secure attachment. This is a protective factor against the development of both externalized and internalized symptoms of mental illness. A disorganized attachment—and fragmented sense of self—is considered a risk factor for the development of mental illness.

When DDP facilitates the development of an integrated sense of self, the impact of developmental trauma is reduced and the resilience needed to limit the impact of any future trauma develops.

TIME FOR REFLECTION

Much has been written about the negative developmental impact of adverse childhood experiences. We know that the more adversity there is, the greater the negative impact. Though this relationship seems logical, there might be value in wondering why.

It may be that an integrated sense of self enables the person to buffer the impact of a traumatic event. This enables the event to become integrated into the self, making sense of it and reducing its overwhelming impact. If there is too much adversity, the self is not able to buffer the impact of the trauma; rather the trauma, along with subsequent ones, impairs the integrated development of the self. The resultant disorganized self not only loses its ability to buffer the impact of trauma but is also poorly prepared to form a more comprehensive, resilient, and resourceful narrative that could provide greater satisfaction and success in one's life.

TIME FOR REFLECTION

Imagine two children experienced the same traumatic event—physical abuse by a caregiver. The first child had, previously, failed to establish an organized sense of self and instead had a self that was fragile and fragmented. The second child previously had established an organized sense of self within a secure attachment with another caregiver.

Consider the possible consequences for each child and how these might differ.

The following are some possible consequences for each child.

1. The child with a fragmented sense of self
    A. mistrusts others to provide safety and care
    B. becomes excessively self-reliant with rigid defenses, along with symptomatic reactions to stress
    C. experiences self with a pervasive sense of shame
    D. shows impairment in achieving developmental milestones
    E. becomes anxious in the presence of opportunities for close relationships, success, and joy
2. The child with an organized sense of self
    A. turns to trusted others for comfort and healing
    B. develops resilience, blending reliance on the self and others
    C. can protect the sense of self from shame, having confidence that the self did not deserve the abuse
    D. can continue to attain developmental milestones
    E. seeks and takes advantage of positive opportunities for growth

The ongoing impact of developmental trauma is greatly influenced by the sense of self of the person who experienced the trauma. It is reasonable to assume that if the impact of a trauma severely and pervasively extends into the future, the traumatized child may well have experienced one or more traumatic events in the past as well. At the time of the most recent trauma, the self may already have been fragmented.

A COHERENT AUTOBIOGRAPHICAL NARRATIVE

Over time, the developing conversations, stories, and an integrated sense of self enable the child to create a coherent autobiographical narrative. No longer are they ashamed or afraid of remembering events from their past. No longer are there gaps in their memory associated with the relational traumas that they experienced. Their memory of those events may well evoke anger, sadness, or fear, but not rage, despair, or terror. They do not lead to emotional dysregulation nor to a complex web of defenses and symptoms that were once needed to maintain some sense of precarious safety and a patchwork sense of self.

When the developing narrative is coherent, it is likely to be strong enough to be maintained in the face of a traumatic event, integrated enough to be able to make sense of apparently contradictory meanings and demonstrate a degree of autonomous attachment needed to withstand relationships that violate the sense of self.

The DDP practitioner's immediate intention is to create and maintain an intersubjective connection with a traumatized child. Their more distant intention is to maintain this connection with the child until they feel safe enough to become aware and elucidate new meanings from the relational trauma. Their ultimate goal is for this connection to lead to the experience of safety within conversations and stories.

CONCLUSION

The experience of DDP is both the same and different for each child, family, and practitioner who engage in it. Universal in DDP are the experience of safety, conversations, stories; an emerging, integrated sense of self; and a coherent narrative. Every time DDP assists a child, who has experienced relational trauma, to develop a coherent narrative within a safe and thriving home, this universal reality is expressed in a manner unique to this individual family.

Worksheet 4.1

 ## Reflective Exercise: Maintaining Safety for the Child

Here are some statements that parents may say to their children during sessions. With the child's safety in mind, suggest a response to them.

1. **Parent:** Don't take that attitude with your therapist! You need to cooperate if you're going to get something out of this!

_____

_____

_____

_____

2. **Parent:** You know that I care about you! My job as your parent is to teach you that you can't have everything you want!

_____

_____

_____

_____

3. **Parent:** You're not a bad kid! I told you that. You just made a mistake!

_____

_____

_____

_____

4. **Parent:** Don't say you don't know! You must know why you did that!

_____

_____

_____

_____

5. **Parent:** You can't keep using the abuse that happened four years ago as an excuse for your angry outbursts now! You're the only one who is responsible for your actions!

_____

_____

_____

_____

Reflections on Worksheet 4.1:
Possible Responses

1. **Parent:** Don't take that attitude with your therapist! You need to cooperate if you're going to get something out of this!

   Practitioner: Dad, would you let me and John work this out together? This is hard stuff that I'm asking him! And I can see it is hard for you too, Dad. You so want us to be able to help him with the challenges he is facing.

2. **Parent:** You know that I care about you! My job as your parent is to teach you that you can't have everything you want!

   Practitioner: Mom, it is important that we understand Robert's experience now. Would you hold off on giving your experience and be with me in just understanding what Robert is saying? I know that it must be painful for you to think that your son sometimes does not feel that you care for him.

3. **Parent:** You're not a bad kid, you're a good kid! I told you that. You just made a mistake!

   Practitioner: Mom, I know that's what you want Sue to feel about herself, but she is saying that she doesn't! We have to understand her experience now, because if she sees herself as a bad kid, that would be very hard for her. Let's just understand her as she is now!

4. **Parent:** Don't say you don't know! You must know why you did that!

   Practitioner: Dad, I think Tom is speaking honestly about how confused he is about why he did that! Not knowing why we do what we do is common.

5. **Parent:** You can't keep using the abuse that happened four years ago as an excuse for your angry outbursts now! You're the only one who is responsible for your actions!

   Practitioner: Oh, Dad, I can hear in your voice how hard it is for you to think that the abuse might still be affecting your son. You want to believe that it could not hurt him that much! But I think it does, Dad, and we have to find ways to help him so that it has less impact on him.

IN CONVERSATION THREE

Kim met with seven Chinese clinicians, trained and supported by Sun Han (DDP trainer), also known as Hannah Sun-Reid, to provide DDP interventions within China. All these clinicians are about to start the DDP therapist practicum. Hannah translated for us.

Following the conversation with the clinicians, Dan and Kim met with Hannah separately.

CONVERSATION WITH CLINICIANS:

Kim: Hello, thank you so much for giving up time to meet with me. Maybe we can start with you telling me about your experience of DDP?

Ye: I think that DDP is quite useful with the birth parents that I work with. I work with primary age children, between 6 and 11 [years old]. I mix DDP with play therapy. The parents want the therapy to be very efficient. They want us to talk, not just play, so that they can understand the children and how they can help them at home. They welcome this style of DDP. The challenge is how to mix together the play and the talk.

Guanning: I find that the parents come because of the children's behavior problems. A challenge is that when they see behaviors improving, they want to stop, although more work is required from our initial assessment.

Hannah: One of the challenges is funding for the therapy. Most schools will provide service, at no extra charge, with the school's in-house counselors, but often the parents must pay for this [service] out of their own pocket.

Guanning: It is helpful knowing how intersubjectivity works. I provide PACE and match affect, and I am more attuned. Very quickly I notice that the parents and children feel safe. They are more connected as their affect becomes regulated. I notice this at work and in my personal life. One example, I work with a family whose child was refusing to go to school. This really bugs Chinese parents, and mom was really frustrated. This mom, because of her own attachment history, did not experience a lot of connection. I helped her to play, interact, and connect with her child. The connection is so much better.

Jing: When I work with adolescents, I focus on the way they express their difficulties and their capacity to express emotions. I prefer a present- and future-oriented focus. In my work, I have experienced some parenting styles that are hard to work with. Some parents believe in a controlling parenting style because of their own educational background or professional experiences. They expect their child to listen, be obedient; they often use teaching, lecturing, or punishment as parenting strategies. It is hard to convince them to accept other communication methods with their kids. I would like to learn more about working with these different parenting styles.

Hanwei: I find the DDP approach is very close to our human nature and human connection. In China, I find DDP and the attachment modality more effective and really useful. It is cross-cultural, how we live, grow, and interact. Even when there are cultural differences, the attachments are cross-cultural. We work with these attachments with families who don't know how to express emotions. I work with younger and older children.

Kim: Is your experience of DDP different when working with younger children compared to with older children?

Hanwei: There are differences. With younger children I use the DDP approach to help the parents understand their child and to learn how to coregulate. With older children, above nine, I help the parents to understand their child and the child to understand their parents. Adolescents start to have their own ideas, and when they have difficulties, they can't communicate with their parents. DDP can help parents to really understand their child and can help the children to understand their parents' intentions. I would like more teaching about how to help the adolescents who, when younger, didn't learn how to make their emotions explicit. Either they become flooded with feelings they can't express and their parents don't know how to connect with them or they are super avoidant and say they don't feel anything. This is the challenge for us.

Peng: I work with highly educated parents. I run a parent group using the DDP approach. In China things are changing very fast. The parents try to parent in the way they were parented and find its not working well. Most of the parents often neglect their own feelings, their own happiness. I try to encourage the parents to say how they feel. This is hard for them and therefore more challenging for their child. I would like more ideas, more resources about how to help parents to tune inward and to be more self-aware. This will improve the parent–child relationship.

Fang: The parents have had little emotional connection when they were young. They are open to new experience but have very little emotional base. When they were little, they were sent to study here and there. They never had the experience of being coregulated by their own parents. Staying with the PACE approach is working well. Gradually the mothers get the experience of what emotion is about and then they are able to be PACEful with their child.

Kim: I am interested in hearing about your experiences developing the use of DDP within China.

Dongmei: There are big differences between moms and dads. The Chinese dad will say that he is the dad in the family and needs to have authority. He wants to tell the child what to do and for the child to listen. When I ask him to accept his child, he worries that he is accepting their behavior and that this is not good for the child. The dads struggle to be accepting and empathic. Chinese moms are the opposite, sacrificing everything for the child. They often neglect their own feelings. They don't express their needs. They cover up how they feel because everything is about the child. I work in the southern part of China, where there are strong beliefs that girls are not as worthy as boys. If these mothers grew up in these families, they were never encouraged to express their own feelings. They just do what they are supposed to do as the dad asserts authority. These moms then don't know how to attune to their child's emotions. They don't know how to coregulate; on the contrary, they expect the child to self-regulate. Hence, children who grew up in this environment tend to be on their own to deal with emotional challenges. It is hard to help the mother to be an emotional caregiver for their child.

Peng: Lots of parents, especially the mothers, are raised to self-sacrifice. So, lots of them have their own problems, their own trauma experiences. When I invite them to be PACEful for their child, they find it really difficult. I want to learn more about how to help the parents to recover and to be able to attune to the parent–child relationship.

Kim: I am hearing of the differences between mothers and fathers and wondering, what is it like for the fathers when the mothers start to parent in ways that are DDP informed?

Peng: It is very typical in Chinese society that the expectation for academic learning is really high. This means parents focus on knowledge and learning more than emotional needs. And there can be an absence of the dads, as they are busy being the breadwinner. They work really hard and expect the mother or grandmother to look after the child. It is hard for them to participate in clinical work.

Dongmei: Once I help the mother to express how she feels, most times the dad is happy to hear his wife's emotional needs. The marital relationship is better. From this point, the dad is more attuned to their child's emotional needs.

Fang: Both parents are devoted, will do anything for their child. However, dads can be very emotionally avoidant. In one family I have worked with, the dad is OK with the mother doing therapy with the child, but as soon as I call on him to do emotional work, he says his son has no problems. That is the challenge to getting very avoidant dads to join.

Kim: I am also thinking about the challenges that you might encounter as female clinicians, again thinking about the differences between men and women in Chinese culture. Are most clinicians female?

Hannah: Yes, most clinicians are female. There are some male clinicians, but not as many.

Fang: Being a female clinician, I work well with mothers, but when the dads come in, I can sense the difficulties there. Dads keep themselves separate and have a hard time connecting. The dads experience a female clinician asking him to work on emotional connection as way too difficult. We need some direction and teaching about how to connect with ultra-avoidant dads. How do we help the dads to know that we are on the same team?

Hanwei: As a female clinician I can work with mothers, female-to-female. I can connect with them easily. The challenge is how to connect with dads and how to get a balance between working with the mother–child relationship and bringing the dads in.

Kim: I am thinking of the importance of getting alongside the dads, to understand where they are coming from, their values, what feels important to them. Explore why it is difficult for them to feel emotion and what they think that means about them. Help them to feel understood, and they are more likely to be open to thinking with you.

Hannah: We are talking about the slowing down?

Kim: Yes, that's right, slow down and trust the process. I think it would be good for the dads to have male clinicians to support them as well.

Jing: In rural areas, there are lots of so-called "left-behind children" whose parents must find jobs and work in distant cities for years. Meanwhile, in the cities, there are some children whose parents are entrepreneurs who are too busy to engage in their children's lives. These children are most likely raised by nannies or by grandparents from infancy. When these children grow older or reach puberty, they present severe behavioral and mental health issues. These children can specify what they don't want their parents to do, but they find it hard to say what their parents can do to help them. This is a challenge for both parents and children.

Kim: So, grandmothers can do a lot of the caring for their grandchildren. I am thinking about the trauma that the grandparents might have experienced, growing up during challenging times in China. I wonder how much their traumatic experience impacts the family.

Peng: Absolutely, their own trauma history impacts how they raise their grandchildren. There is also a confusion of roles. Who is grandparent and who is parent? The whole family dynamic is affected.

All clinicians: We have talked about some unique characteristics of Chinese families we observed in our clinical practice. We want you to know that we love our country and our people. We really want to help children and families to become healthier. The most recent government policy advised schools to give less homework to students and to reduce extra academic programs; instead, schools and parents are encouraged to increase extracurricular activities related to arts and sports and social–emotional activities for the purpose of more balanced development.

Kim: Absolutely, I am hearing this. You have told me what you would like to learn from our book. I am looking forward to you teaching me as well. What you learn about supporting Chinese families will help DDP to grow and develop.

CONVERSATION WITH HANNAH:

Dan: Thanks for talking with us, Hannah. We are interested in hearing about your experience supporting therapists in China and Singapore.

Hannah: Your work has had a huge impact on the therapists. Watching the recordings, seeing how you coregulate the parents and children, how you move them along, and understanding why you're doing that.

Dan: And do they see that they can learn how to do this, that this is possible for them?

Hannah: Yes, I think they do. Right now, a few of them are ready for the practicum. There will be hurdles though. While I'm able to understand Chinese, a second consultant will need subtitles. Another hurdle is cultural. The consultant needs to know a bit about the culture, so that they're not just viewing the recording solely through our more traditional DDP lens.

Kim: Do you have examples, Hannah?

Hannah: Yes, I remember a tape review in which it appears that the therapist is not doing enough to interrupt or redirect the parent from being critical to the child, and that may be seen as the therapist not keeping the child safe. However, knowing the Chinese culture in this case, that therapist needs to be very cautious in how she challenges the parent's authority in front of the child, otherwise they run the risk of the family withdrawing from therapy immediately, even though they had made much progress in therapy. You have to gently coax the parents while being respectful. Another thing is that parents can be very quiet in their emotional reactions. They may have a lot inside, but they're not very expressive in their feelings, especially in explicit verbal expressions of love.

Dan: So, the first consultant needs to be very knowledgeable about a particular culture and to ensure that the second consultant is also sensitive to that culture. Certain themes that are important in DDP have to be addressed in all cultures, but the particular way that this is done needs to be safe for both parent and child in the given culture.

Kim: That leads to questions about how much we, as non-Chinese, are wanting these parents to parent from our cultural viewpoint.

Hannah: Yeah. I agree, Kim, and this is similar to situations in Singapore. They speak English, but there are still clear cultural differences. I don't think I can make them any more affectively expressive, because that's the culture.

Dan: If I was a supervisor, I would really want somebody like you to guide me. I don't want to lead the therapist in the wrong direction, making it less successful with the parents and the child. I have to be very mindful of the differences in how to generate safety when I'm not from that country, that culture.

Hannah: I would really agree. Some of the therapists notice, Dan, that you're very expressive. They say we cannot do that.

Dan: And I think I need to take this more seriously. I tell therapists to do it their own way rather than joining them and exploring how this is a challenge. We need to figure out how it is understood within the culture to really invite greater sensitivity to cultural differences. In the Chinese therapists that you're supervising, are there any consistent concerns they have about DDP, times when they say, "No, not in the Chinese culture, it is not appropriate to use some of the DDP principles or interventions here"?

Hannah: In DDP, and in developing PACE, I really stress how harmful shame is and how PACE is so crucial to reduce shame. I think all Asian cultures tend to shame children into doing something well. Shame is related to the family ties. For example, Chinese parents will say that when you're not doing well, it's not just a representation of you, it also makes us look bad. It makes the whole family look bad.

Dan: Right, they see value in social shame. I'm bringing shame to my whole family. They might see value in raising children with that sense of family shame. Whereas for me shame is individual. I don't see how I bring shame to my parents for something I do. At least I don't experience this in any depth. So, what would you recommend to the therapist who's talking to a parent with these beliefs?

Hannah: We would explore with PACE to accept the parents' pain rather than giving them any suggestions. We have to empathize with their pain from experiencing their child's problem. I think it's coregulating them first and then really making it explicit how they feel shame and how they feel shunned by society. They have to deal with this as well. We empathize with how hard it is to have a child with these difficulties.

Dan: In supporting the parents with PACE, then it'll be easier for them to support the child with PACE. This will help the child's shame. You're helping the parents' shame at the same time as you're helping the child's shame. You're recognizing the parents feel the shame too, much more so than parents do here.

Hannah: Yes. Another thing I find is that we really help the parents to go into curiosity, which Chinese parents seldom do. Often, they have good intentions, but they're not interested in how the child thinks or feels about it. They just say, "We think this is what you need to do." We really want to help parents to be more curious about the child's experience, planting the curiosity seed from the very beginning.

Kim: And how are they at being curious about their own internal experience, or is mentalization not a strong part of the culture?

Hannah: Good question. I would say mentalization about their own and their child's experience is quite weak. They focus more on the need for the child to work hard and succeed.

Kim: So how do they emotionally connect with their children?

Hannah: Parents connect by really caring for their children, making sacrifices for them. They really care about the best nutrition, the best opportunity. They'll sign their child up for extensive, private tutoring. They move their home to where the best school is. They'll go with a child wherever their child needs to go. They say, "Day and night, I'll drive, I'll walk, I'll study with you." Asian culture is more about doing than saying.

Kim: So DDP is asking for cultural change?

Hannah: I would say in a good way. We really work on helping parents to be curious about their affective experience. We work with the parents' affect: "So, what's it like for you when you hear your child saying that? I could see the sadness in your eyes." We are really curious about their affective experience and then curious about the child's affective experience. It's not totally absent, but it's much more implicit. If the parents can have some space for an affective reflection on their experience, then they can connect with the child a little more emotionally. Everyone agrees on this, as a whole society I think we are more aware of this being needed.

Kim: I am also wondering what we can learn from the Eastern cultures we have been discussing.

Dan: I wonder about the emphasis on success. In DDP, at least in America, I think that's sort of set aside. We focus on getting to know the child with acceptance, curiosity, and empathy. The success sort of takes care of itself. I wonder if there's value, in America, to emphasize more the success for our kids. Perhaps we so emphasize the inner life of the child, that we are not doing enough to integrate the behavior with that? We're asking them to integrate the inner life with their behavior. Should we be integrating more of the behavior with the inner life?

Kim: And how can we develop DDP globally without imposing a Western idea of what family, relationship, and connection should look like? How do we adapt and learn?

Dan: I think that if we're really attuned to our Chinese and Singapore parents, we won't push them down paths that are foreign to their culture. We will be aware of how they express things that help their child to feel safe, feel worthy, and be motivated to have a better life within their culture. As long as I have a not-knowing stance, then together we'll find ways to help their child to feel safe and connected. It's going to look different than it will in my culture.

Kim: So, if you were wanting to give one piece of advice to a practitioner, maybe in the U.K. or in the U.S., who is working with a Chinese or Singaporean family, what advice would you give them?

Hannah: I would say, don't rush into what we think is right or wrong, just stay curious and make this expressive. Be curious about, for instance, how come you do this and explore it a bit more. What is your motive? What are you trying to get and why? It's the same principle as in DDP, not jumping into our own judgment.

Kim: That seems like a good point to end on. Thank you so much, Hannah, for spending this time with us.

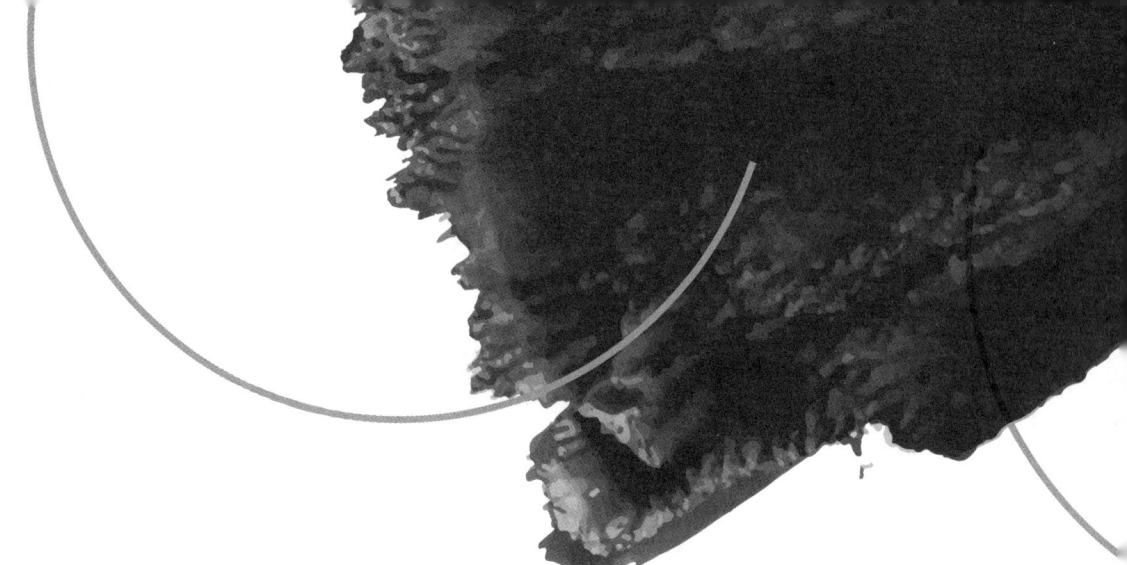

Chapter 5:
The Nuts and Bolts of Dyadic Developmental Psychotherapy

> *Good beginnings, where the more cognitive information-sharing processes take place effectively, create a later context and atmosphere of shared awareness and complementary goals. This enables parent work and therapy sessions to focus on emotional connections and on setting necessary limits to behavior when required. Therapy involves weaving narrative threads together to make one story. (Hughes et al., 2019, p. 120)*

REFRESHER

DDP, especially when it involves working with a child with developmental trauma and their family, is a complex therapeutic journey. The journey for the child is even more complicated. The child's traumatic experience may have occurred years ago, and the impact on their development may have become embedded into their psychological functioning and patterns of relating to family in ways that are difficult to unravel. The child's history may include having lived in more than one family. The source of the child's challenges may have developed long before they entered their current family, creating challenges that these caregivers never anticipated and that may not have been present with other children they have parented.

This complexity means that interventions need to be similarly complex (Figure 5.1).

The expectations of the referring individuals and the child's caregivers may differ from the therapeutic vision of the DDP therapist. These differences need to be addressed clearly before any therapeutic contract or interventions begin. For that reason, the caregivers, and possibly the referring professional, may need to be seen first to ensure that they know what to anticipate and that they are able and willing to engage in DDP as described by the therapist.

The therapist may also meet with the caregivers and child together during this initial assessment phase. Observing the child with the caregivers can

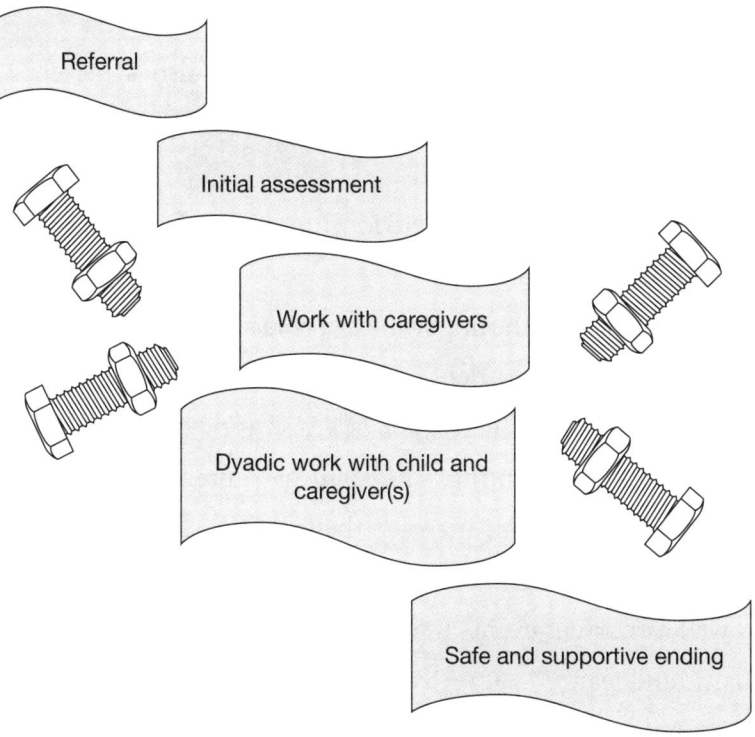

Figure 5.1 Nuts and Bolts of DDP

help inform the discussions when the practitioner begins to meet with the caregivers alone.

There are two phases of DDP treatment; the first involves meetings with the caregivers, without the child. This contact involves establishing an alliance between the therapist and caregiver while getting to know the nature of the family (explored more fully in Chapter 6). This includes the challenges faced by them and the child but extends beyond this into getting to know the strengths of the child and family along with other challenges the family is currently facing. These initial understandings and early interventions regarding the functioning of the family and its members will extend back into the attachment history of the caregivers themselves, since this history will be impacting their current relationship with their child. If there are unresolved issues in the caregivers' attachment histories, these need to be explored before beginning joint sessions, so that these issues will not compromise the child's sense of safety.

When the caregivers are seen alone, they will also experience the DDP approach that will be used with their child.

- They will learn that their relationship with their child is central to their child's progress.
- They will be taught the importance of considering the meaning of their child's behavior before determining how to address the behavior.
- They will be shown the attitude of PACE and how PACE can become a part of their parenting. They will gain preliminary understanding of how PACE can increase their child's sense of safety during therapy while the therapist explores both past traumatic experiences as well as current events that may involve the child's experiences of shame and fear.
- They will learn about their role in providing acceptance and support to their child while the child's challenges are being explored.

They will see how any problem-solving or evaluation of their child's behavior needs to follow the creation and maintenance of the child's safety throughout the session and in the home. This enables the child to explore their challenges without defensiveness and with an openness to new learning.

During the initial period of the DDP therapist seeing the parents alone, they may decide that joint sessions that include the child are not needed. The interventions with the caregivers alone may create the circumstances of effective therapeutic change.

If joint sessions are indicated, the therapist will determine when the caregivers are able to provide the safety necessary for these to begin. After joint sessions have begun, the therapist and caregiver will still have regular, ongoing contact without the child to reflect on the work and so the therapist can continue to support the caregivers.

DDP interventions may take longer than interventions within other, less relational approaches. The therapist will still be working toward an ending. They will:

- notice when there are changes within the family that indicate a reduced need for support from the practitioner
- monitor the development of the coherent narrative child is developing about their life
- notice if the family relationships are developing in a manner that provides consistent support and repair

Endings will then be planned with careful preparation. The child needs to experience an attachment relationship with the practitioner that will continue beyond the therapeutic work. In a good ending, the child knows that they remain in the mind of the practitioner even when they are no longer meeting.

SESSIONS INVOLVING THE DDP THERAPIST AND CAREGIVERS

At the core of DDP are three dyadic relationships: between the therapist and caregiver, between the therapist and child, and between the caregiver and child (Figure 5.2). A strong relationship between the therapist and caregiver needs to be established and then repaired and maintained throughout the course of therapy if the other two dyadic relationships are to develop and promote therapeutic change. We will briefly explore all three dyadic relationships within this section. Building a therapeutic alliance with caregivers is explored in more detail in Chapter 6.

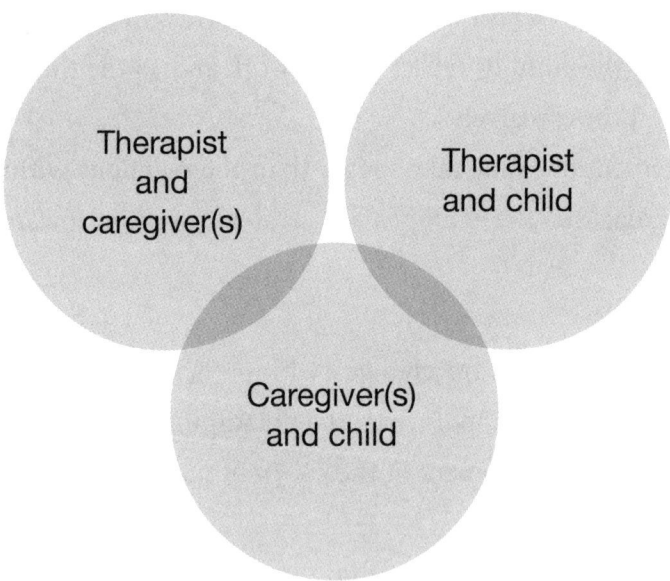

Figure 5.2 Three Dyadic Relationships

The qualities of DDP, which are so central in the therapist's relationship with the child, will be central in the therapist's relationship with the caregiver. These qualities include:

- providing intersubjective experiences that are embedded in PACE
- committing to understanding the relational stories that are reflected in the child's behavioral problems
- attending to the new relational stories needed to create therapeutic change

When the caregivers experience the therapist relating with them in this manner, they will be able to understand the value of the therapist relating to their child in a similar manner.

When training DDP therapists, we emphasize the importance of expressing their intersubjective experiences of the child in the session. These include experiencing the child as being interesting, enjoyable, clever, brave, loveable, and delightful. This same emphasis needs to be given to the therapist's relationship with the caregiver.

We can find that this relational work feels more comfortable with a child than a caregiver, perhaps because we are less used to conveying our intersubjective experiences of our clients within parenting work. Our level of comfort or discomfort can be influenced by the expectations of caregivers, power imbalances between therapist and caregiver, our previous life experiences, and expectations we have from our own training.

It can be helpful to consult with a colleague or trusted supervisor about how our intersubjective experiences can be expressed and to consider differences between us and the caregivers. For example, understanding differences in values can help us to appreciate the parent more.

It might also be helpful to explore aspects of our attachment history, which might make us hesitate to express our experiences of the caregiver.

TIME FOR REFLECTION

We invite you to reflect on what qualities in the caregiver you are open to experiencing and whether you are ready to communicate those experiences to the caregiver.

- Do you find it is easier to convey your intersubjective experiences to a child or to a caregiver? Consider why this might be so.
- Do you feel less safe speaking openly to the caregiver about your experience of them?
- Does your own attachment history impact your experiences of the caregiver and your sense of safety in telling them of your experience?
- Does age, gender, or difference in sexuality, race, religion, class, neurodiversity, or disability cause you to inhibit your expression of your intersubjective experience? If so, how might you address this?
- Would it help to reflect on how the caregiver is likely to experience your expression? Do you have worries that it might hurt your developing relationship with them?
- What additional support might you need for these reflections?

Establishing, repairing, and maintaining a safe relationship with the caregiver is not easy. You are talking about their child, their relationship with their child, and their responses to their child's challenging behaviors, which you are evaluating! You have to work hard to help them stay open to you, to avoid a descent into defensiveness.

PACE is central in DDP, and acceptance is the foundation on which the other aspects of PACE rest. You need to convey acceptance of the caregiver and their journey in caring for their traumatized child. You convey acceptance when you experience them—intersubjectively—as being good people who care deeply about their child and who are doing the best they can to relate to their child; having the child's best interests in mind. Once, that experience is established and communicated in the way you relate to them, they are likely to be less defensive when you evaluate their behaviors toward their children. They are likely to remain open and engaged when you say:

"Your good intentions for your child are obvious to me, though I fear that the way you address their behavior may cause them to get defensive and push back against your wishes. You might try . . ."

If the caregivers are defensive, they are likely to blame the child for any conflict that is occurring. If they are open and engaged with you, they are more likely to explore what they might do to improve their relationship with their child.

At times the caregiver may relate with you in an intense, agitated manner, defending their position and conveying little empathy for their child. Often this is because they do not feel confident that you understand them and will help them in a meaningful, nonjudgmental way. You might try to experience their intensity as reflecting a sense of urgency to be understood and helped with their child. When such a sense of urgency is present, consider responding by matching their affect and intention, conveying your own sense of urgency to understand and help them. This is likely to help them to experience that you are with them and walking alongside them. This can reduce their fear that you are going to place the cause of their child's difficulties on them, diminishing their sense of worth.

REFLECTIVE EXERCISE: RESPONDING TO DEFENSIVE CAREGIVERS

During early meetings, caregivers may react defensively. This may represent a lack of trust in their relationship with you and/or the presence of shame associated with their child's behaviors and their inability to help their child to resolve them. If you respond defensively, there is likely to be a break in the relationship that might be difficult to repair.

Worksheet 5.1, at the end of this chapter, provides an opportunity to explore how to respond, without defensiveness, to the comments that a caregiver might make.

MAKING DECISIONS ABOUT THE RIGHT TIME TO INVOLVE THE CHILD IN SESSIONS

It can be difficult to decide when the time is right to begin joint sessions with the child.

If these joint sessions begin too soon, the child's psychological safety may be put at risk because their caregivers are not able to respond to them with PACE. In DDP, the therapist is saying to the child:

"You are safe here to give full expression to your inner life. You will not be judged or criticized when you tell me and your caregivers what you think, feel, or want."

When the caregiver does not convey PACE for their child's inner life, then the child will feel deceived, and safety is lost, in this session and possibly subsequent sessions as well.

On the other hand, if these joint sessions begin too late, precious time might be lost in providing both child and caregiver the support that they need to be able to strengthen their relationship and to help the child resolve past trauma.

TIME FOR REFLECTION

We invite you to reflect on times you have planned to begin joint sessions by bringing the child in.

Think about the factors that helped you to make the decision during your work with the caregivers.

Finding the right time is a valuable skill for the DDP therapist to have. Indicating factors that will help with this decision are:

1. During sessions, the caregivers are open and engaged in the conversation, rather than defensive, most of the time. When they do become defensive, they consistently engage in relationship repair in a timely manner.

2. The caregivers have been able to remain engaged and regulated when themes and interactions that the therapist anticipates will be challenging in the joint sessions have occurred in the sessions with just the therapist.

3. The caregivers have given the therapist permission to interrupt them during the joint session in front of the child, such as if the therapist thinks that the caregiver is saying or doing something that will hurt their relationship with their child. The therapist feels confident that the caregiver will be able to consistently allow this. The caregivers do not have to be perfect, they will feel defensive at times, but they are willing and able to rely on the therapist's lead for direction when the joint sessions become stressful.

4. The caregiver can relate to their child successfully with PACE. They can stay open to their child's distress and criticisms, and the therapist has confidence that they will do this in the joint sessions. The actual presence and words of their frightened or angry child might cause dysregulation and defensiveness. If this seems likely, the therapist might role play with the caregiver an imagined conversation with the child, or at least have them consider examples of what their child might say and do. If these experiences are hard for the caregiver, then further sessions alone are likely to be indicated.

TIME FOR REFLECTION

Consider reviewing your DDP cases with regard to how many sessions you met with the caregivers alone before beginning the joint sessions.

Do you feel that you generally spend a long or short time on these joint sessions, before bringing in the child? If one or the other, reflect on why that might be so.

Do you think that your own attachment history experience has influenced how you approach this part of the work?

Here are two possible situations to reflect on:

A. You notice that you tend to see the caregivers significantly longer than do other therapists. This might be an indication of the type of referrals you are getting. For example, if you receive a high number of referrals for caregivers in blocked care, the length of time in the parent-only work can be significantly longer. However, some additional possibilities to reflect on are:

   1. You have higher expectations than other therapists for the caregivers to meet their child's needs with fewer errors.
   2. You are slower than other therapists to address the caregivers' challenging behaviors or the possible roots of such behaviors in their attachment histories.
   3. You stress, more than other therapists, the importance in protecting the child from their caregiver's evaluative, misattuned, or possibly rejecting behaviors during the joint sessions.
   4. Any of these might suggest that you have unresolved issues

in your own attachment history (possibly a preoccupied attachment classification) that might lead you to be overly critical of the caregiver and/or overprotective of the child.

B. You notice that you begin the joint sessions sooner than other therapists. This, too, might be an indication of the type of referrals you are getting, such as if you have a high number of referrals of families at an early stage in their journey, before the child and the caregivers have developed blocked care. You might also have referrals of families in which the caregivers have already received parenting support and are already DDP-informed within their parenting. However, some additional possibilities to reflect on are:

1. You might be underestimating, relative to other therapists, the ability of the caregivers to be able to consistently provide safety for their child during the session.

2. You might be less sensitive than other therapists to negative effects on the child when the caregivers are being evaluative and judgmental.

3. Perhaps your own attachment history demonstrates a dismissive attachment classification that leads you toward minimizing the affective experiences of the traumatized child.

Even with good preparatory work with caregivers, it can be hard to judge the right time to bring a child into joint sessions. Once this joint work starts, you might realize it has been started too soon and the caregivers are not yet ready to support their child as needed. For example, this is clearly suggested when the caregivers' behaviors are critical and judgmental and they are unwilling or unable to follow the lead of the practitioner. In these situations, the therapist might need to go back to seeing the caregivers alone to provide them with further support, within which you can explore together their responses in the joint sessions. This would represent a major effort to repair the relationships among the caregiver, child, and therapist. Without this, the future success of the therapy could be jeopardized.

SESSIONS INVOLVING THE CAREGIVER, CHILD, AND THERAPIST

Once the therapist and caregivers have decided to begin sessions involving the child, they need to be ready for even more complexities in the sessions.

Yes, the child needs to be safe, and so do the caregivers, and so does the therapist. If any one of them is not safe and becomes defensive, there is a great risk that everyone will become defensive.

If the child becomes defensive, it is crucial that the therapist inhibit the tendency to join the child in defensiveness. When the therapist can remain open and engaged with the family, they can support the caregivers to not become defensive, then all the adults can remain open and engaged with the child. This helps the child become less defensive and to become more open and engaged.

During this complex interaction, the therapist's responsibility is to take the lead in ensuring that repair occurs when needed and all become safe again. The therapist does not passively observe escalating, defensive behaviors between the caregiver and child, but rather guides the interaction toward repair and the reestablishment of safe engagements.

Segments of the following session will demonstrate this active role of the therapist in maintaining a regulated, open, and engaged manner of relating with both the caregivers and the child to guide them away from a self-protected stance and toward an engagement that reflects joint safety.

TIME FOR REFLECTION

As you read this fictional example, reflect on the defensiveness of the parents.

- Can you think of reasons why they might have become defensive?
- Notice ways that the therapist helps the parents to reduce this defensiveness.
- Do you think that the therapist has been successful?
- Can you think of more that the therapist could do?

The following scenario represents parts of three sessions involving adoptive parents, Sue and Tim, and their 12-year-old adopted boy, Luke. An active boy with many interests, Luke likes to decide for himself how he will spend his day, and he does not like his parents directing or even guiding his behaviors. He wants to be left alone to do what he wants. With adolescence coming, his parents worry that he will become increasingly oppositional and distant from them.

Luke was adopted at five years old, after three years of significant neglect with his biological parents followed by two years during which he challenged foster parents, much like he does with Sue and Tim.

Luke's school life is characterized by fairly regular conflicts with his teachers and peers, but, because of his engaging personality, the conflicts never seem to get out of hand, and, for the most part, he is liked.

Sue and Tim had six sessions alone with their therapist, Ellen, before the joint sessions began. Ellen perceived them as motivated to learn the DDP interventions that she was suggesting.

The sessions were somewhat challenging for Tim, who had been raised by an authoritarian father who insisted on respect, which often meant compliance. He could, however, acknowledge that a more relationship-based form of discipline might have been just as effective in his learning "right" and "wrong" while creating a more relaxed and closer relationship with his parents.

Sue had willingly expressed a "good girl" attitude to please her parents, and she found herself naturally going along with what they wanted. At times, when Luke challenges her, she doubts herself—she must be doing something wrong—or she becomes angry with him for not appreciating the life that she and Tim are giving him.

During their sessions with Ellen, both Sue and Tim seemed eager to learn other approaches that might help their son to be happier and might bring them closer together.

Third joint session. A few days before the third session, Luke had come home late from a friend's house, and when his parents wanted to talk about it with him, he became angry. He went to his room and refused to talk. After first establishing a relaxed conversation with Luke, we join the session as they finish chatting about a recent trip he and his parents took to a historical museum that had a display involving ancient civilizations.

Ellen:	It sounds like it was a great exhibit of life that long ago. I'd love to see the book about it that you picked up there, Luke. Could you bring it with you next session?
Luke:	Sure, yeah, it was really cool.
Ellen:	Seems that all three of you enjoyed it a lot. Glad you were all able to go. It's a shame that you had a hard time a few days later, when you got home late and your parents were upset, and maybe you were too. What was that like for you, Luke?
Luke:	(*with some anger that Ellen knew about it*) I don't want to talk about it!

Tim: That's why we're here, Luke, to talk about the problems. Now answer her question.

Ellen: I know what you want, here, Tim, but my guess is that Luke doesn't want that. Would you let me and Luke work this out?

Tim: I'm just saying, if he wants us to solve our problems, he needs to be willing to talk with you when you ask him something.

Ellen: (*ensuring that her tone is relaxed and accepting, not critical*) I really see that this is important to you, but if Luke and I are to talk about this, we need to work it out together, the two of us. I don't want him to talk with me only because you tell him to. Are you OK with my saying this, Tim?

Tim: Yeah, I know, but . . . (*Ellen puts up her hand and Tim stops; she gives him a sympathetic smile.*)

Ellen: So, Luke, I can understand why you'd rather not talk about it. You were all upset, and why chance going there again? My hope is that I might help you all to have a better understanding of what was hard for each of you. Maybe I can help to find a way to work it out more easily the next time.

Luke: I guess, but I don't think it will help.

Ellen: Maybe it won't, Luke. But could you help me to understand what was hardest for you, when you came home late?

Luke: They treat me like a baby! Of course it would bother me.

The session continued quite well, as Luke showed his vulnerability about his belief that his parents don't have confidence in him, and his parents were able to express empathy for his experience.

Fifth joint session. Ellen spoke with Sue and Tim alone briefly before bringing in Luke. Sue seemed anxious, and Ellen asked if something was bothering her.

Sue:	This is hard to say, Ellen, but I'm worried that Luke is taking what you say as agreeing with him that he can do what he wants and has a right to get angry with us when we correct him.
Ellen:	Thanks for telling me that, Sue. I need to know how you see things, and of course you would be worried if you thought that I was undermining your authority with your son. I'm sorry if I said something that had that effect on him. Do you recall what I said?
Sue:	It's not so much what you said but how you talk with him about his anger and defiance. Like it doesn't really bother you. I thought that as well as helping him to understand why he does it, you would also make it clear that he shouldn't be angry at me like that.
Ellen:	Thanks for helping me to understand what's bothering you about his behavior. What about his anger bothers you the most—does he call you names or threaten you?
Sue:	No, he doesn't do that, but he raises his voice at me. I think you said that's not necessarily disrespect, but it just doesn't feel right that he yells at me.

Ellen: Are you saying that it's OK for him to be angry, but you want him to express it more quietly?

Sue: I guess that sounds silly. But why does it bother me so much when it doesn't seem to bother you at all.

Ellen: Oh, Sue, I can see how hard this is for you. You know that I see anger as a natural emotion that is experienced and expressed sometimes in all close relationships, but that's not your experience! It really bothers you! What bothers you the most about it?

Sue: It makes me feel that he is saying that I'm a poor mother. Maybe even that he regrets that I adopted him! And then I start to doubt! Maybe he's right! Maybe I am a poor mother!

Ellen: And how hard would those thoughts be! I know how important it is for you to be Luke's mother! You so much want to be his mother and to be the best mother he could have. And his anger causes you to doubt, to get discouraged, to think that maybe you're a failure as his mother! Oh, Sue, that must be so painful.

Sue: Do you think I'm a poor mother, Ellen?

Ellen: Just your being here and honestly facing your doubts causes me to be so impressed with you! You are facing your pain and doubts for your son! You are so committed to him! No, Sue, I don't think that you're a poor mother! But what is most important is what you think.

Sue: I never was quite right as a daughter. Even though I tried to be a "good girl." And now I don't feel quite right as a mother.

Ellen: Ah, Sue. I think your son's anger might be very hard, but it seems to be causing you to address self-doubts that you've had most of your life. His anger might well help you to become stronger; to become more confident; to discover who you are; and, maybe someday, to discover how fortunate Luke is that you are his mother.

Eighth joint session. Ellen was able to help Luke to explore the basis of his angry outburst at his father. His father had given him a chore to do, and Luke had yelled that the only reason his father wanted to adopt him was to get a servant to do the work around the house.

Tim: How can you say that? You have more chances to play, be with your friends, and just have fun than I ever had when I was your age!

Ellen: Tim, would you let Luke tell us more about his experience now? Luke, what are you saying? What does your place in your dad's life seem to be?

Luke: Like I said. My place in the family is to do what he tells me, to make his life easier! That's the only time he shows any interest in me.

Tim: That's not so!

Ellen: Tim, I know it's hard, but can we listen to what Luke is saying now? (*Tim nods.*) Tell me, Luke, what does that mean, if your dad seems to talk with you only when he wants something from you?

Luke: (*showing distress in his face and voice*) It means that I'm not that important to him! He's not proud of me, like a father should be proud of his son.

Ellen: If that's how it seems to you, Luke, that would be very hard . . . very lonely.

Tim: I am proud of you!

Ellen: Tim, I can see that this is hard for you to hear. What makes it hard?

Tim: I want so much to be a good dad, and it seems like Luke doesn't think I am. I want so much to have a better relationship with him than I had with my dad, and now it seems he's not proud of me.

Ellen: Thanks for your honesty, Tim, that must have been hard for you to say.

Tim: Thanks, but what am I supposed to say now?

Ellen: Just speak honestly, Tim, but speak about how his experience affects you. Remember I spoke with you about empathy. Express that now, just as long as it is what you are feeling.

Tim: I don't know how to.

Ellen:	If it would be true to say it, say, "Luke, I'm sad that you don't think that I'm proud of you. That would be hard and discouraging and lonely."
Tim:	I am sad for you, Luke, that you don't believe that I'm proud of you. Very sad, because it would be lonely, you wouldn't be able to trust me.
Luke:	Sometimes, I don't, dad.
Tim:	I am so proud to be your father, Luke. So proud. I have to find a better way to show you that, so you can believe me and trust me. (*Tim squeezes Luke's hand and Luke begins to cry. Tim moves closer to him, hugs him, and begins crying too.*)
Luke:	And I'm proud of you, dad, I really am.

The examples given in these segments of three sessions demonstrate that the therapist needs to be ready to assist the caregivers when they become defensive and focus on their own experience rather than expressing empathy for their child's experience. The therapist needs to address these behaviors with PACE, remaining open and engaged with the caregiver and without becoming critical and defensive.

During the joint sessions, the therapist tries to be aware of the psychological states of the child, the caregiver, and themselves, including whether or not the caregiver is aware of their own state and the state of their child. The therapist has three minds to focus on, the caregiver has two, and the child is receiving support and guidance to help them to focus on their own mind.

While the therapist needs to ensure that the caregiver is mindful of the safety of the child, there is no similar expectation that the child be mindful of their caregiver's safety. This remains so even when the child says, "I don't love you!" or "You don't love me!" or "You're mean!"

However, the therapist might consider addressing the child's statements if the child swears at the caregiver or calls the caregiver names. The intention of such statements may well be more than the expression of anger. They may represent the child's intention to hurt the caregiver or may simply be a lack of awareness that they are causing the caregiver pain. In either case, the therapist might address the child's statement in a manner similar to the following:

Therapist:	It's clear, John, that you are really angry with your father for not letting you go to town. I also notice that what you said is likely to have hurt your dad. Any idea why you expressed you anger in a way that would hurt him?
John:	He wasn't hurt!
Therapist:	I think he might have been, John, since most people would be hurt if someone they know swears at them or calls them names.
John:	He doesn't care!
Therapist:	What if you did hurt your dad, John? What if you did? Do you want to hurt your dad?
John:	No.
Therapist:	I'm glad, John. Letting him know you're angry over what he said is different from hurting him. You're angry that he decided you couldn't go to town. I'm glad you don't want

> him to be hurt though. Would you be willing to tell your dad that you are sorry if he felt hurt when you swore at him?

John: I didn't mean to hurt you, dad.

Dad: Thanks, son, I'm glad to know that.

John: But I am angry at you, dad, for not letting me go to town.

Dad: I know you are, son. I'm sad that it is bothering you so much. And I'm glad that you told me.

When you are engaged in joint sessions with the caregiver and child, your own family history can be activated in many ways.

1. The joint session may activate qualities in your past relationships with your parents.
2. The joint sessions may activate memories of your own childhood and your sense of self and relationships with your parents.
3. If you are a parent, the joint sessions may activate memories of your life as a parent and of your children, including your worries or conflicts regarding them.

Your family of origin is likely to have an impact on your experience of families you work with, which in turn may influence the narrative you have about your family of origin. While being intersubjectively present with the family in the joint sessions, your narratives involving your past and present experience of family can be active and influencing your perceptions, thoughts, and feelings. It is crucial, therefore, that you have resolved the experiences you had as a child and as a parent so that you can focus on the best interests of the family in therapy.

TIME FOR REFLECTION

You might consider brief reflections on your family of origin and your current family after DDP sessions to explore how your family history may have impacted your perceptions and the ways you engaged with the family in therapy with you.

If you notice any themes or patterns emerging, you might explore this more deeply with a trusted colleague or supervisor.

ENDING DDP INTERVENTIONS

DDP is a comprehensive, integrated, model of intervention developed to help children who are suffering from the pervasive features and consequences of developmental trauma. In deciding when DDP is no longer needed, the practitioner needs to consider many factors, beyond relief from specific symptoms. These factors include the range of therapeutic goals that the practitioner and family need to consider when deciding whether it is safe to cease the formal, ongoing sessions.

These factors include:

1. Consistent progress can be seen in the child's psychological functioning, including the child's affective regulation and expression, reflective functioning, attachment behaviors (including their ability to trust), and readiness and ability to engage in reciprocal relationships.
2. Relationships within the family are characterized by comfort and joy, along with conflict resolution and repair, while being consistently open and engaged with one another.
3. There is little sign of ongoing blocked care.

4. Parents are able to maintain an attitude of PACE, engage their child in the meaning of family behaviors, maintain "the two hands of parenting," routinely initiate relationship repair, and experience the child's strengths and vulnerabilities that are present under their behaviors.

5. Habitual shame is no longer present, with few signs of "the shield of shame."

6. Members of the family have developed individual and joint narratives that include a resolution of past developmental trauma and the development of coherent autobiographical narratives.

7. The experiential knowledge that the family has acquired in the therapy sessions has been integrated and internalized, and this is routinely expressed in their daily lives.

8. Members of the family are not perfect. Rather, they have the confidence and skills needed to address individual and joint challenges if they return or manifest for the first time.

While the practitioner is no longer physically present in their lives, the practitioner's psychological presence is still experienced as a source of guidance and support for both parent and child.

CONCLUSION

There might be a tendency to think that the nuts and bolts of DDP are somewhat soft and flexible. DDP is, after all, an experiential therapy involving relationships, narratives, affective states, and reciprocity. However, for DDP to provide the therapeutic space it is intended to, it needs to have firm and clear guidelines—nuts and bolts. These ensure safety for the child, especially, but also, and equally importantly, for the caregivers. The structure of DDP provides such safety.

Initially, the therapist meets with the parents alone. The parents are helped to understand the need for this before beginning joint sessions. The therapist also works hard to ensure that the parents do not experience the need for this part of the work as a judgment or them being blamed.

When the DDP therapist meets first with the caregivers, the therapist is creating an alliance based on providing the attitude of PACE, just as the therapist will later provide this experience for the child. This builds their trust in the therapist and helps them understand the attachment and trauma-based principles of DDP.

This work creates confidence that the parents can join the therapist in providing acceptance and empathy for their child. This guides the decision to begin the joint work with the child. The parents experience safety with the therapist and this helps them to follow the therapist's guidance within the joint sessions. This, in turn, ensures safety for the child.

Finally, attention is given to providing a safe and supportive ending to the work. The therapist works hard to provide this ending in a way that doesn't leave the child feeling a sense of loss or abandonment, resonant of past endings. Instead, the whole family leave confident that they will remain in the heart and mind of the therapist.

Yes, it is the nuts and bolts that enable the DDP therapist to provide safety for all. They relate to one another in an open and engaged manner that enables the family members to understand their current joint narrative, laden with fear and shame, while developing a new narrative of hope and joy.

Worksheet 5.1

 Reflective Exercise:
Responding to Defensive Caregivers

Here are some statements that caregivers may make during sessions. Think of nondefensive responses to these statements.

1. So, you're blaming me like everyone else does!

2. We're talking about my child's behavior, not my childhood! How I was raised has nothing to do with why I'm here!

3. My child simply has to learn to do what their told! My expectations are reasonable! Is that so hard? Can't you focus on that with the kid?

4. PACE might be fine for feeling good together! But what am I supposed to do in the middle of a conflict?

Reflections on Worksheet 5.1: Possible Responses

1. So, you're blaming me like everyone else does!

Response: That must be so hard to feel everyone blames you. I'm sorry that it seems that I'm blaming you too! I must have said it poorly. Let me say it differently, because I am definitely not blaming you.

2. We're talking about my child's behavior, not my childhood! How I was raised has nothing to do with why I'm here!

Response: I believe how we were raised does affect how we raise our kids. We are learning more about how this happens. If this is true then it will be really helpful for us to understand your strengths and vulnerabilities from your childhood. Will you explore this with me and see if it makes sense to you. I wonder if you will notice some changes in your parenting when you better understand the impact of your own childhood.

3. My child simply has to learn to do what their told! My expectations are reasonable! Is that so hard? Can't you focus on that with the kid?

Response: Your expectations do seem reasonable to me! So, we need to understand what's getting in the way of his cooperating with your directions. Maybe we can help him to tell us what is getting in the way.

4. PACE might be fine for feeling good together! But what am I supposed to do in the middle of a conflict?

Response: Thanks for being clear on your worries about PACE. Yes, we cannot avoid addressing the conflicts. PACE can be a helpful attitude during conflicts too. I guess I need to be clearer about how that works. Maybe we can take some examples and see how it would look.

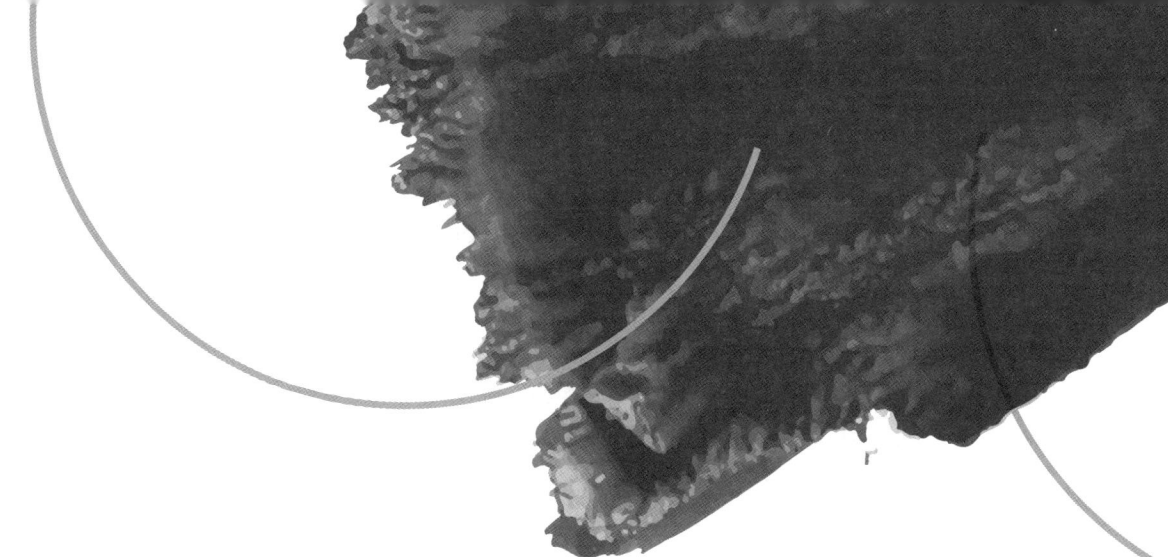

Chapter 6:
The Complex Therapeutic Alliance With Parents

> *All the while, the therapist is engaged with the parent in a manner similar to how the parent is—or will be—engaged with the child. As the parent comes to feel safe with the therapist, the parent begins to enter into reciprocal conversations that lead to developing stories. These include stories about parenting and the parent's own childhood, as well as general stories involving areas of pride and shame in the parent's life. From there, the therapist is able to get a sense of the parent's view of self and her narrative. With this foundation in hand, the therapist then begins to develop with the parent ways that they may—together—assist the child in resolving themes around the child's relationship with the parent. (Hughes et al., 2019, p. 112)*

REFRESHER

Within dyadic developmental psychotherapy, the relationship between therapist and parents is unique. The therapist supports the parents in their parenting while the parents support the therapist with the therapy. Parents need to feel trusted by and safe with the therapist. They need to know that they will be supported in their strengths and in their vulnerabilities. They need to trust that the therapist values being in a relationship with them.

As the therapist works with the parents, the parents are getting an embedded experience of the DDP model. The therapist holds the attitude of PACE, developing an affective–reflective dialogue; provides coregulation as needed; cocreates narratives; and offers repair during relationship ruptures. The parents experience radical acceptance from the therapist, experiencing first-hand the paradox that change emerges at its strongest and most spontaneous when they are being accepted for who they are and where they are at. The parents are helped to bring these same principles to their parenting.

An important part of this work involves the exploration of the parents' attachment history and how this has shaped them as parents. Through this exploration, the parents develop self-compassion that they can access at the trickiest times. This exploration also increases the parents' trust that the therapist understands and will support them if they become triggered during the child's therapy.

As we will explore in Chapter 7, the therapist needs to remain alert to signs of blocked care within the parent. Therapists are advised to support the parent to reduce this block before bringing the child into the work. Therapists also help parents understand blocked trust in their child. This understanding increases their compassion for their child as well as for themselves for how hard it is to take care of a child who resists or refuses care.

For the therapist–parent relationship to be strong, the therapist needs to watch for times when they feel defensive in response to the parent, which reduces their capacity to remain compassionate and have empathy for the parent. The therapist needs to notice signs of blocked care in themselves and seek support for themselves at these times.

In preparation for the child's therapy, the therapist guides the parents to be cotherapists. The parents remain parents while also assisting the therapist in providing the child with the therapeutic environment that they need to heal past traumas and to discover a healthier present.

ON BEING A PARENT IN A DDP SESSION WITH A CHILD

Witnessing one's child's therapy is a unique experience. Parents have ideas of what therapy is and what will happen, and these ideas can be different from the reality. Examples of some parents' ideas of therapy include: expecting the child to sit and talk; getting down to the "serious stuff"; and talking about behavior. These expectations can lead the parents to feel frustrated when they witness the therapist engaging the child in light "connect and chat" or apparently condoning the child's need for a mobile phone! The parent witnesses the child describing family life, often not putting them in a good light! Parents reflect on a range of experiences when participating in their child's therapy, ranging from the negative—feeling judged, blamed, exposed, uncertain, and confused—through to the more positive—feeling relieved, connected, and understanding more deeply.

TIME FOR REFLECTION

We invite you to imagine being a parent in your child's therapy session through the following scenario.

Please envision this scenario in a way that matches your and/or your clients' own cultural background, heritage, religious beliefs, sexuality, ability, and family composition.

If you are considering this as part of a study group, you might use the opportunity to experience being a parent through role play.

What feelings are evoked in you? Notice any doubts or uncertainties that arise. Do you feel surprised by anything? Are feelings toward the therapist evoked? Toward Jordan?

Fourteen-year-old Jordan lives with you, his parent(s), and a younger sibling. You (the parent) and Jordan arrive for a therapy session. Jordan is full of bravado. He boasts about his recent late night out with a group of sixteen- and seventeen-year-olds. He talks about hanging around the park and intimates that he joined them in drinking and perhaps more. He scoffs at your concerns for him, claiming that he knows how to keep himself safe. When you try to remind Jordan that he is too young to be out that late and that these peers are really not a good crowd to hang out with, Jordan tells you to "butt out, this is my session!" and adds, "anyway, you're one to talk. You were out late last weekend drinking with your friends. What sort of a role model are you?"

Jordan is firmly in control and will not be vulnerable by revealing that he did feel scared, especially when coerced into doing things he did not want to do, nor that his parents' drinking reminds him of how his birth parents were often drunk when he was little.

You watch as the therapist chats with him. The therapist does not pick up on your concerns, but focuses on Jordan's experience. What was it like feeling accepted by this group of peers? And then, more alarmingly, what was it like having parents out late and knowing they are drinking? For thirty minutes Jordan continues with his act, and it seems that the therapist is just going along with it.

Then to your surprise the atmosphere changes. The therapist has commented on how brave Jordan is and how clever he was to learn to take care of himself from such a young age. The therapist remarks on how sad he feels that Jordan needed to do this. Suddenly a much younger, more vulnerable Jordan emerges. You are astonished to hear how the peer group threatened and coerced Jordan into meeting them at the park and to bring along cans of lager from your cupboard. You didn't realize how much your social drinking bothers Jordan and how worried he is that you will return home drunk and beat him. You manage to respond with acceptance and empathy when invited by the therapist, but inside you are wondering how you did not know all this. Why does Jordan not talk to you about his worries?

We hope imagining this scenario highlights the importance of time spent with the parents before bringing the child into sessions. DDP practitioners often experience pressure to "get on with it," which often means "fixing" the child in some way. Commissioners and referrers do not always understand the process of therapy. Also, they are working under severe budget constraints. It is easy to rush the work because of these pressures. Imagining being the parent can reinforce the importance of building the alliance before embarking on dyadic work with parents and their child.

DEVELOPING AN ALLIANCE WITH PARENTS

Developing a therapeutic alliance with parents rests on a foundation of security, trust, and mutual respect. It develops out of our empathy for the struggles they are facing and our positive regard and unconditional acceptance of them. In this section we will explore what can make it hard to build this therapeutic alliance. But first, a little detour into the world of the nervous system and the importance of being open and engaged.

An understanding of the nervous system helps us to understand the importance of staying open and engaged in a relationship and the difficulties that can arise when the therapist or parent becomes defensive.

TIME FOR REFLECTION

Think back to the scenario with Jordan and his parent.

- What indicates that Jordan's nervous system was in a defensive state?
- How do we know when he moved into an open and engaged state, ready to interact with his therapist reciprocally?
- What might lead the parent into their own defensive state?
- What helped them to stay open and engaged, ready to engage with Jordan when needed?

We suspect you agree with us that the biggest indicator of a defensive nervous system was Jordan's need to control the session. Let's reflect through the lens of polyvagal theory (Porges, 2017), which we introduced in Chapter 2.

It is likely that Jordan had an active sympathetic nervous system, reacting to his neuroception of social danger ("I am going to be criticized, rejected, and probably abandoned"). This neuroception happens fast and beneath conscious awareness. Consequently, Jordan responds without knowing why. His fight response shows in his control, his bravado, his rudeness to his parents and most likely to the therapist too.

The therapist's open and engaged stance recognizes and accepts Jordan's complicated feelings of pride, shame, fear, and sadness. This provides enough safety for Jordan to move into social engagement. Now he can share his experience with curiosity and relief. His sympathetic nervous system, now blended with his ventral vagal state, mobilizes him for exploration rather than fight. It is possible that by the end of the session he will be open to receiving comfort from his parent. When his parasympathetic nervous system is blended with his ventral vagal state, he can immobilize in safety, providing rest, relaxation, and restoration.

Throughout the session, Jordan's parent needs to remain in an open and engaged state. This is threatened by listening to Jordan. What Jordan says elicits fears for the parent, a sense of failing as a parent and worries that the therapist might also criticize them. The parent's sympathetic nervous system might become activated, triggering a desire to express anger toward Jordan or the therapist. Alternatively, the parent's dorsal vagal system might become activated, triggering a desire to hide from the therapist.

We expect that you identified two things that helped the parent in this scenario to stay open and engaged: their own resilience as a parent with good reflective abilities, coupled with their trust and safety with the therapist. Their, likely, neuroception of danger is overridden by the cues of safety provided by the therapist. This allows their nervous system to stay in a ventral vagal state, and thus their capacity for reflection is optimized.

THE THERAPIST–PARENT RELATIONSHIP

As Stephen Porges (2017) reminds us, social engagement is a biological imperative. Our nervous systems are designed to respond to each other. When we stay open and engaged the other person will join us in this state. Of course, the reverse can also happen, when with someone who is defensive, we become defensive too. Understanding your own nervous system and how you can maintain social engagement is helpful when working with parents who are in defensive states.

It is not uncommon for parents to present defensively, especially when they first meet us or after a particularly challenging time. Sadly, parents often experience feeling judged and blamed, even when that was not the intention of the other. They arrive at our door because of difficulties and challenges, anticipating our judgement as well. To establish a therapeutic alliance, we need to hear the parents' worries, fears, and any sense of shame behind their defensive presentation. As they experience safety, their defenses will relax.

We continue with the example of Jordan: You meet with the parent following the joint session. They are frustrated because Jordan has continued to go out against his parents' wishes, meeting with the same group of friends. This has led them to doubt the effectiveness of the therapy session, becoming convinced that Jordan has just been taking them and the therapist for a ride. They arrive at the session feeling angry with you for allowing this to happen.

Parent:	He's exactly the same. He stayed out late three times this week, so much for feeling coerced by the other kids. He's gone straight back to them. And as for therapy I think it's just made it worse! You've just taken his side, talking about his hard life. He thinks this means he can do whatever he likes.
Therapist:	I'm sorry to hear that. It feels like I'm taking his side and that

this is making him even less open to respecting your boundaries or talking with you. No wonder you're frustrated.

Parent: Frustration doesn't go near it. I wonder if you really get how hard this is. He's putting himself at so much risk. This behavior has to stop, and I trusted you to help me. He just hoodwinked you into being nice to him. He wasn't opening up, just telling you what you wanted to hear. He said as much when we got back in the car.

TIME FOR REFLECTION

- How would you feel as the therapist in this scenario? Perhaps this parent often gets angry with you, blaming you when things aren't changing. You thought things had changed and that the parent had made some shifts, enough for you to feel confident to begin therapy with Jordan. You are now wondering if this has been a mistake.
- Notice how this feels in your body. What feelings and thoughts arise?
- Are you experiencing defensiveness? How does this impact how you feel about yourself and the parent?
- Do you notice your own feelings of blame and judgment, and where are these directed?

Times like this, we can easily doubt ourselves. "I'm no good at this. Why did I ever think I could be a therapist?"

Alternatively, we move into blaming the parents. It can be hard to like them and easy to feel frustrated that they are not following our guidance. We may wonder if they even like their child and may doubt that they can change.

When we move into noticing only weaknesses and not strengths in ourselves or in the parents, we are at risk of blocked care. This can be hard to spot in ourselves. We need trusted supervisors and colleagues to notice for us. They remind us to attend to our own self-care and help us to explore what is going on for us.

Building an alliance with parents begins with knowing ourselves. Why do we find some defensive parents easier to work with than others? Understanding our own attachment history will help us to understand our triggers. When we build self-compassion, we are more able to stay open and engaged, even in the most triggering of situations.

TIME FOR REFLECTION

Know your own triggers: We invite you to recall a situation when you felt defensive with a parent.

- Can you pinpoint what was activated in you?
- Are there any experiences from current or past relationships that feel familiar here?

Understanding what pushes your buttons can develop your self-compassion and allow you to remain flexible in the moment of being triggered.

If you are in a study group, you could ask your colleagues to role play the situation. Practice noticing when the trigger point arises, being compassionate to yourself, and maintaining an open and engaged stance.

WORKING WITH DEFENSIVE PARENTS

Now that you have done some self-exploration, it is time to reflect on ways of supporting the defensive parent. As we do in our DDP training, we have chosen to focus on parents who monologue. This can encompass several scenarios:

- the parent who is frustrated that you are talking with them rather than working with the child; they assume this is because you are blaming them for their child's challenging behaviors
- the parent who is angry because they feel let down by services, whether health, social care, or education
- the parent who is angry or frustrated with their child
- the parent who is feeling unsupported by their partner
- the parent who is certain there is something wrong with the child that needs diagnosing and does not feel listened to

We suspect you recognize some of these from your own experience and that you can add others to this list!

The difficulty comes when the parent feels so angry and frustrated that all they can do is vent this at you. Some venting is helpful. The difficulty arises when it doesn't stop, turning into a monologue, which can have a paralyzing effect on the therapist (see Table 6.1).

In these situations, the practitioner needs to shift the monologue to a dialogue. This opens up the intersubjective relationship, allowing a collaboration between parent and practitioner that at last feels helpful.

TABLE 6.1 MONOLOGUES AND DIALOGUES

Monologue	Dialogue
Nonintersubjective and nonreciprocal	Intersubjective, reciprocal
Venting at someone	Relating with someone
Lack of engagement; not conversational	Engaged in a conversation
Feels unsatisfactory for venter and listener	A satisfying conversation
Venter does not feel heard, and listener does not feel helpful	Offers a sense of being heard and helped
No cocreation of narrative; stuck in rigid and frustrating story	Cocreation allows a helpful change of perspective to emerge
Listener feels bored and sense of time not passing	Listener is interested and involved
Listener's mind drifts; they struggle to listen	Listener is focused and attentive

TIME FOR REFLECTION

Let's explore this through an imaginary monologue/dialogue.

Here is an example of a DDP practitioner and a grandmother talking together. As you read through this, notice at what point the grandmother moves from monologue to dialogue.

- What do you think helped this shift to happen?
- What were the benefits of the dialogue compared to the monologue?

If you are in a study group, have a go at some monologue role plays, perhaps based on this scenario. These can be fun to play around with as the "practitioner" tries to shift to a dialogue and the "parent" tries to resist. The competitive among you might test who can stay in monologue the longest, resisting the masterful pull to dialogue that your colleague is engaging!

Dilys is caring for her three young grandchildren. This family lives in a small community in Wales, U.K. The children's mother, Dilys's daughter Cerys, has been in and out of rehabilitation programs because of drug and alcohol problems. She has recently made some progress, and a decision has been made to return the children to her care. Dilys is very unhappy with this decision and is in conflict with the children's social worker.

Practitioner: Hello Dilys. Thanks for inviting me to your home so we can talk this through.

Dilys: (*with high energy and passion*) To be honest, I'm glad some-one's willing to listen to me. That social worker doesn't know what she's talking about. She's only 24 and has never brought up kids herself.

Practitioner: OK. OK. So you're telling me that . . .

Dilys: . . . basically, she just doesn't understand that my daughter is not fit to look after her children. She has no clue about them. OK, I get that she's made some progress because she's got off the alcohol. But you need to understand that this has been going on since she first went off the rails at fourteen. She has real problems. This is my daughter. I know her.

Practitioner: Yes, of course you do. Tell me, how old is Cerys now?

Dilys: She's 29, and I'm telling you she can't take care of those kids. She has been given so many chances.

Practitioner: (*moving forward to make eye contact with Dilys; with energy and animation to match Dilys's affect*) I hear you Dilys. So, over half her life she's had problems with . . .

Dilys: The social worker just won't listen to me. I'm her mother. I know her. She won't be able to do it. She'll look as if she's getting better, and then when everyone stops watching her it will all start again. We've seen it so many times. If those children go back, it will all happen again.

Practitioner: (*continuing with energy*) OK. Got it. OK. So, it's not the drinking so much because I heard she was reducing the drinking and she's on a program to help, but you're saying great, but it won't last and still she has to learn how to parent the children.

Dilys: (*still not looking at the practitioner and not fully hearing her*) She sucks everyone in. She's stopped drinking, well done for that, but as soon as those kids go back, she will start drinking again.

Practitioner: (*establishes eye contact again and says with urgency*) Dilys, I hear your worries. I really hear you. Stay with me here, OK? (*Dilys nods*) She seems to be doing better, but you don't trust it. I hear that you've been here before. It never seems to last, does it? How hard for you to witness this in your daughter.

Dilys: (*quieter and slower*) It's not going to last, I know, but the social worker just won't listen to me.

Practitioner: (*quieting and slowing*) Dilys, it must be so hard when the social worker doesn't listen to you. (*puts hand on shoulder*) I am hearing you, (*looks intently at Dilys*) OK? (*Dilys nods.*) Can you take a breath, and I will tell you what I'm thinking? (*Dilys nods*) I can see you're feeling really passionate about this.

Dilys: (*looking directly at the practitioner*) Of course I'm feeling passionate about it. They're my kids, and they're going to get hurt again. I can't stop it if they send them back to her.

Practitioner: (*with more energy again*) Yes, you love these kids. You've taken care of them for two years, and you've done well.

They're starting to improve in school. They're close to you. They sit and cuddle with you. Do they call you Nan?

Dilys: They call me Mom.

Practitioner: They call you Mom. You're doing so well. You're trying to give them a life, to help them to move on after the hard time they had. Right? And now you worry, because you care so much for them, that all the work you've done might be for nothing if they go back to their mom. I really hear how much you love these kids. And as we're talking about this, I'm thinking that this must be extra painful for you. I mean, you love your grandchildren, but we're talking about your daughter. Is this hard, sort of facing that you think your daughter isn't a very good mom and when . . .

Dilys: We did our best for her, but she wouldn't listen to us.

Practitioner: I'm sorry. I didn't mean to imply that you didn't do your best. I really apologize, I'm just saying that you and her, my guess is, right now you're not close.

Dilys: No, we don't speak.

Practitioner: (*quieter and slower*) For a mother and daughter that's very hard. So sad that you can't help her. When Cerys was the age of your granddaughter, when she was a little girl, were you close to her?

Dilys: Yes, she was great then. We used to do lots together. She would cuddle into me while I read to her. She liked to bake.

She went off the rails when she was a teenager. She decided she didn't want us anymore. I tried to take care of her, get her back on track. She just wouldn't listen. I did try.

Practitioner: I'm not blaming her or you. I'm just saying that closeness has gone.

Dilys: Yes, it's gone.

Practitioner: Yes, and there's a sadness in your heart. I bet you would love to be close to your daughter and your grandchildren. To feel safe knowing that your daughter will take care of them.

Dilys: And she can't do it. Everyone says give her a chance, that she's made good progress. I just don't see it.

Practitioner: My guess is you would want to give her a chance if it didn't hurt your grandchildren. I mean, you still love her, and she needs a chance, but if it's going to hurt your grandchildren, you're saying, wait a second, she had her chance. She's the adult. We're not going to hurt the kids anymore.

Dilys: Yes, we've got to protect them. Everyone is saying she's done really well, but they don't know her like I do.

We think you will agree that Dilys is now in a dialogue with the practitioner. Dilys feels heard and can feel some sadness about her loss of closeness with her daughter. They think together about how hard this is, living in a small community with everyone knowing their business, how exposed they both felt when things started to go wrong. Dilys can now think about how she and her daughter can both be supported to talk together. Maybe there is a way forward to help Cerys parent her children, supported by Dilys. Dilys is still uncertain about this, but she is willing to think about it.

Practitioner: My guess is this will take a while, Dilys. You and Cerys have had such hard times. You don't trust her, and she doesn't trust you. We need to do some work with the two of you because the children love you, and they love their mom. Part of them, I expect, wants to live with their mom. Part of them wants to live with you. They're really mixed up in a lot of ways. If we can help you and Cerys get along and have confidence in each other, this will help the children. If Cerys can learn that you will support her, then the children are going to feel less confused and less conflicted. They will have a mom and a grandma to care for them.

Dilys: Yes, that would be good. I could be a grandmother again. I'd like that.

MONOLOGUE TO DIALOGUE

Here are some techniques that help a therapist to shift from mono-logue to dialogue.

• Be more directive than usual. Actively interrupt the monologue. This means slowing the parent down and using an animated stance to engage them in the conversation. Communicate a sense of urgency to understand and be helpful. It is this urgency that requires you to interrupt, not that the parent has nothing to say or that you are being rude.

- Repeating yourself can help: "Wait a minute, wait a minute, I've just noticed something . . ."
- "Wow" statements can draw attention and help the parent to feel heard: "Wow! I notice you are really frustrated about this. I get it, I would be frustrated if . . ."
- Often a person monologuing is avoiding eye contact, looking just over your shoulder, for example. Leaning toward them and establishing eye-contact can slow a monologue down, giving you an opportunity to respond.
- Similarly, if it feels appropriate, a hand on a shoulder or knee can remind the parent that you are there to support them.
- Something as simple as asking someone to breathe can help them to shift: "Whoa, take a breath. I can hear how hard this has been."

Ultimately it is hard to resist someone who gets it and wants to support you. As monologue becomes dialogue, cocreation and joint understanding can begin.

EXPLORING ATTACHMENT HISTORY

When parenting traumatized children, trauma can seek out trauma. A parent holds their own unresolved difficulties, and this becomes triggered by the child's need for control. The child seeks for the parent's weak spots and pushes on them. Knowing their own history, the strengths and the vulnerabilities, can help a parent to manage these trigger situations and thus be able to respond to the needs of the child, however they are expressed.

TIME FOR REFLECTION

We invite you to reflect on how your own attachment history shows up in your current relationships. Are there times you find yourself reacting to others as if they are someone from your past? If you are a parent, can you recognize how your own attachment history has impacted your parenting and how this differs with different children?

It is not just our significant attachment relationship experiences that can impact our parenting. When exploring your attachment history, be alert for other equally impactful experiences, such as in the example below.

EXAMPLE ONE: IMPACT OF RELATIONAL EXPERIENCES

Psychiatrist Dan Siegel writes about a memory from his pediatric internship. This memory arose when he experienced feelings of panic, dread, and terror in response to his infant son crying inconsolably.

> I was with my infant son one day when he began to cry. I felt helpless to console him, and I began to have that strange panicky feeling of needing to flee. Then an image came to my mind, first as a sensation of fullness in my head. The panic began to feel centered, less widespread. Then I began to see something internally, which competed with what I was seeing externally. . . . I saw a child on an examining table, screaming, with a look of terror on his scrunched-up, reddened face. My pediatrics internship

partner was holding down his body. I had to not hear the child's screams. I had to not see his face. . . . He was burning up and we had to draw his blood to rule out an infection. . . . I opened my eyes. I was sweating. My hands were trembling. My six-month-old son was still crying. And so was I. (Siegel & Hartzell, 2003, pp. 18–19)

It is also important to look beyond our immediate parents' generation. The way of being we develop is rooted in the worlds of our ancestors. The experiences that they lived through are passed on, influencing our relationships, including our parenting. When these experiences are embedded in trauma (e.g., in racism and discrimination), this trauma is also passed on intergenerationally, ready to be enacted when conditions trigger it.

EXAMPLE TWO: IMPACT OF INTERGENERATIONAL RELATIONAL EXPERIENCES

Therapist Resmaa Menakem (2021) writes movingly about this in his book *My Grandmother's Hands*. He reflects on his grandmother's life on a plantation where she was routinely whipped by the overseers, how this impacted her use of "whuping" with Resmaa and his brother when they put themselves into physical or social danger, and the temptation he later had, that he chose to override, to "whup" his own son:

Unhealed trauma acts like a rock thrown into a pond. It causes ripples that move outward, affecting many other bodies over time. After months or years, unhealed trauma can appear to become part of someone's personality. Over even longer periods of time, as it is passed on and gets compounded through other bodies in a household, it can become a family norm. And if it gets transmitted and compounded through multiple families and generations, it can start to look like culture. (Menakem, 2021, p. 39)

Extending exploration of attachment history to encompass heritage and intergenerational experiences can be revealing both for our clients and ourselves.

REFLECTIONS FROM DAN

Dan recalls a story told to him by his father. When his father was in his last year of high school, the principal called him and his father (Dan's grandfather) into his office. He told Dan's grandfather that his son was very bright and should go to university and study to be an attorney. After listening quietly and respectfully, Dan's grandfather said, "Thank you, sir, but my son will be getting a job. We are not in the class of people that go to a university."

Years later, Dan's father told him that he always wondered what his life would have been like if his father had thought him of sufficient worth to go to university. When Dan applied to attend university, he felt gratitude that his father had told him the story. He realized that though his father had missed the opportunity to continue with his education, he fully supported Dan.

Despite this, Dan realized that some feelings of not being "of that class of people" had found their way into his mind. He recalls having haunting doubts that he had reached one step beyond the class—or place—that he was born for when he struggled with a particular test, when he was convinced that his dissertation held little value, and when his early efforts to have a manuscript accepted for publication ended in failure.

REFLECTIONS FROM KIM

Kim notices the impact of loss-of-belonging through displacement in her family history. Her Jewish ancestors were displaced from their country; her father was evacuated during World War II; her mother experienced a traumatic move from northern to southern England, leaving her family when Kim was just six weeks old; and her father's story of an illegitimate baby given up for adoption. This history has impacted her choice of career, much of which has focused on creating stability for families and children. She has had to work on a pervasive need for approval and an oversensitivity to thinking others are disappointed in her, which is linked to her need to belong.

Reflecting on family history and intergenerational impacts can promote resilience, strengthening us as people and as DDP practitioners. We can reflect on our family history with trusted supervisors or colleagues, within small study groups, or in affinity spaces with peers experiencing similar lived experiences. When we notice issues that feel unresolved, we might seek the support of a therapist.

TIME FOR REFLECTION

Reflect on your ancestors.

1. What do you know of their heritage, their lives, and any traumas they lived through? How did they experience the world wars? Do you know how they arrived in your country? Have they always lived here, or did they emigrate, arrive as refugees, or come to the country to help? Were they, for example, part of the Windrush generation, arriving in the U.K. from Caribbean countries to help fill post-war U.K. labor shortages? Were they enslaved or part of an Indigenous population, a first nation who experienced the trauma of colonization? Do you have an ancestor who suffered because of thalidomide or another disability? Maybe members of your family suffered oppression and discrimination because of their sexuality or religious beliefs. How did class status impact your ancestors?

2. Think about the intersection of these different experiences and the additional impact this might have.

3. How might these experiences still be alive within your family, impacting how you experience the world? What intergenerational trauma might you be holding in your body? How does this show up?

4. How might this impact you in your personal relationships and as a practitioner?

Within DDP interventions, attachment history exploration takes place as part of parenting support and as preparation for therapy sessions with the child. At the end of this chapter, we include an interview guide (Worksheet 6.1). This guide is introduced in DDP Level One training (see Figure 6.2 for a summary).

It explores a way to reflect on attachment history while keeping it grounded in the parenting of the current child. This embedded exploration helps to focus on the interviewee as a parent whose parenting is influenced by their own history. This leads to a better understanding of the parent, increasing empathy and compassion for them and building trust and respect. This understanding will be important for ensuring safety in the room when parents join their child's therapy sessions. The therapist will have a better idea when the parent is likely to feel triggered and thus be able to support them to respond to the child with empathy and acceptance.

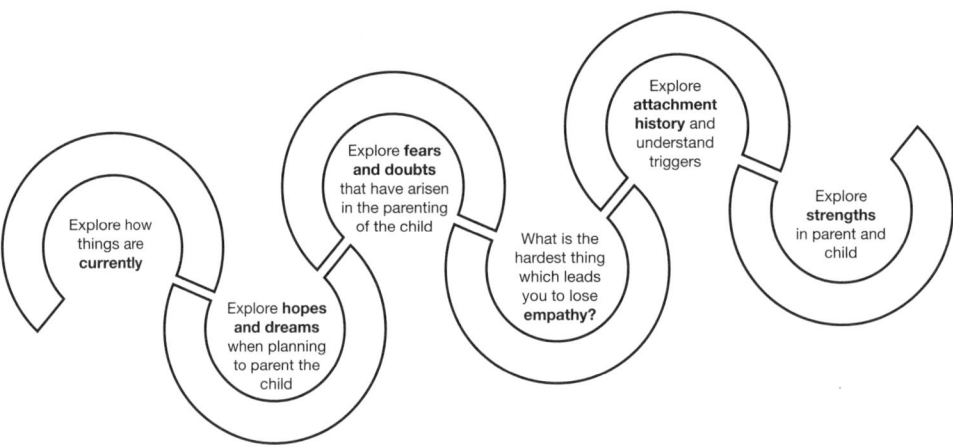

Figure 6.1 Exploring Attachment History Within the Context of Parenting

Notice that in this sequence, the DDP practitioner beins in the present. It is important for the parent to have an opportunity to share their immediate worries and frustrations without fear of judgement.

The practitioner then explores the hopes and dreams they had when planning to be a parent for this child. This gives the practitioner an opportunity to know the parent more fully, and the parent experiences being viewed as a good parent with positive motivations. Knowing that the practitioner sees them this way helps the parent to return to current fears and doubts with more vulnerability.

The practitioner then asks "the magic question": What is it about this child that is hardest for you, when are those times when it is difficult to maintain empathy for them? This is the question that guides the conversation into an exploration of attachment history.

As the parent describes their past relationships and considers how they were supported during times of separation, loss, or distress, the practitioner suggests links with their current experience of parenting the child and moments when the past triggers difficulties in the present.

The interview ends with the practitioner acknowledging the unique strengths that the parent demonstrates, and they both consider strengths of the child.

EXPLORING ATTACHMENT HISTORY: AN EXAMPLE

In the following example, we illustrate how a conversation might develop when following the interview guide just described.

Janice is a single parent of seven-year-old Maira, having fostered her since she was brought into care at age two. Janice wanted to adopt Maira, but it was decided that child services would search for a family who shared Maira's Pakistani-British racial identity rather than place her with Janice, who represents white culture. This search was unsuccessful, and Janice was appointed special guardian when Maira was four years old.

Janice requested a Pakistani-British DDP therapist for Maira, hoping that their shared heritage would be helpful. The therapist, Aleena, meets Janice to explore her attachment history as part of the DDP intervention.

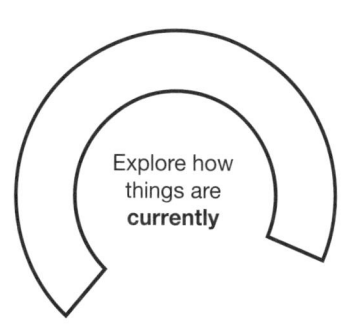

Explore how things are **currently**

The session begins with Janice describing the difficult week she has had with Maira.

School has been closed, and this has unsettled Maira, who has needed more support and attention as a result. "I have this angry little being following me around everywhere," describes Janice. "I just feel completely stifled by her."

We join the interview at this point.

Aleena:	That sounds overwhelming, Janice. Is she often angry?
Janice:	Yes, she is now. She was such a quiet toddler. It seemed to change the day I was told she could stay. I suppose I was naïve, thinking Maira would be grateful. Instead, she seems to hate me. She's so angry, although she won't let me out of her sight either. Very confusing.
Aleena:	Not what you were expecting at all! And hard to feel like second best because you weren't the first choice as her parent.
Janice:	Yes, I worry sometimes that the social worker was right. Maybe she needs two parents who reflect her heritage. Maybe that's why she's not happy with me. I'm hoping you can help me. You understand Pakistani culture. You could help me get it right. I don't want her to lose part of herself.
Aleena:	Yes, it's so important to help her retain her heritage. I'm glad you're thinking about this. You're not a Pakistani mother and never can be. This will be painful for Maira as she grows up. Accepting this means you can support Maira with the complex feelings she's likely to have. I'm happy to talk about this, but for now let's focus on

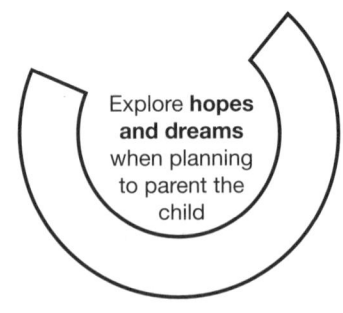

Explore **hopes and dreams** when planning to parent the child

you. I can hear the doubts here. Can we take a step back? I wonder what you were expecting. What were your hopes and dreams when you decided to be Maira's parent?

Janice: Well, I wanted her to have a stable family. There were a lot of different family members caring for her in those first two years. I suspect her mother had undiagnosed depression. As a mental health nurse myself, I know marginalized people don't always get good support. Instead of being treated for depression, I think she just got blamed for her parenting. Maira was handed from one relative to another before coming into care with me. I couldn't help Maira's mom, but I wanted Maira to have the best possible chance of a happy life. I grew up with a mother with depression; it's not easy. I want Maira to be free of all that.

Aleena: So, your big hope and dream was to give Maira a life that is stable and happy.

Janice: Yeah, I guess. I want Maira to go out into the world and be who she wants to be. I want her to be accepted and for her to accept herself. She's not living with her birth family, that is part of who she is. That's tough by itself. The loss of her birth mother, the instability she experienced, they will all have an impact on her. She's also living in a white family. What does that mean for her Pakistani heritage? It's important to me that she can embrace this.

Aleena: So, you have your hopes for Maira, but lots of doubts too. She isn't the little girl you imagined she would be. She isn't happy, and you worry that you aren't the right parent for her. You worry you could get in the way of her being comfortable with herself, both in terms of being in a special guardianship and in embracing her heritage. Big doubts and fears.

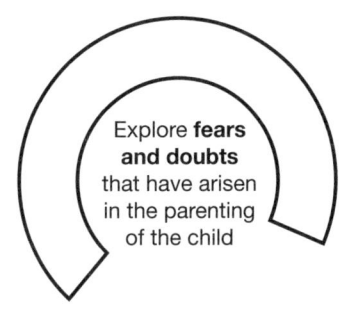

Explore **fears and doubts** that have arisen in the parenting of the child

Janice: I do worry about her . . . that she can't be happy. I try to be there for her, but it's hard when she's never satisfied. I feel like I can't get it right.

Aleena: I can see how hard you try, and with no one to support you. I imagine that makes it even harder.

Janice: Well, that was my choice. Maybe you think that I shouldn't have taken on the special guardianship, that a single mom isn't what Maira needs.

Aleena: Janice, I'm sorry. I didn't mean to imply that you shouldn't be parenting alone. I was just thinking how hard this must be, having no one you can turn to when it's feeling tough. Someone to share your doubts with, you know.

Janice: I'm not good at turning to people. I get on with it. That's what I've always done. You can't wait for others to help you; you have to find your own way in life.

TIME FOR REFLECTION

While exploring the parenting of Maira, some attachment themes have emerged. Reflect on these. How might you move into exploring attachment history?

Aleena: I'm assuming that's how you've always been, someone who tries and deals with things on your own. I'm wondering, what's the most challenging thing about parenting Maira? What do you find hardest?

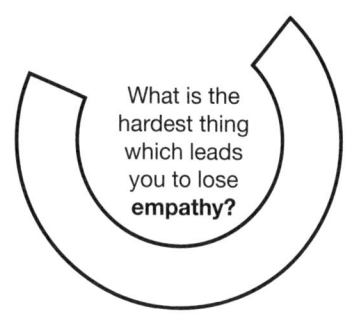

What is the hardest thing which leads you to lose **empathy?**

You know, those times when it is really hard to have empathy for her.

Janice: Well, I try not to get annoyed. Before I had Maira I just kind of did what I wanted. But when you've got somebody there and they're constantly wanting your attention, they're talking to you all the time and you're trying to get everything done. That's the thing I have the most problems with, not giving her enough attention.

Aleena: It's the constant need for attention that she expresses. Well, I can see how that can be hugely frustrating and emotionally draining. I'm just wondering, for you, what's especially hard about that?

Janice: I don't know. I think because I know I should just stop and listen to her. So that's my failing, I suppose, in that sometimes I don't do that.

TIME FOR REFLECTION

The therapist has asked the magic question: What is the trigger point for Janice when she loses empathy for Maira? Reflect on Janice's answer. How would you respond to this? What attachment themes might you follow?

Aleena: I suppose my reflection back to you is that you put a lot of pressure on yourself to get things right. And when someone needs that much attention, you can't possibly get it right all the time.

Janice: No. Some days it feels like I get nothing right!

Aleena: I bet, and there's no way you can respond to everything. So, I'm wondering if this triggers anxiety in you because there's a part of you that wants to be there and responding to her every single time. That's what 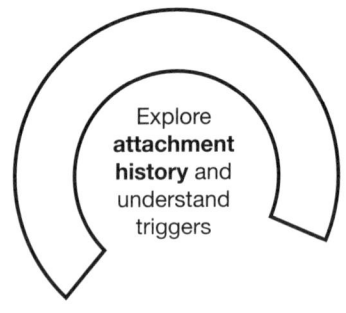 you feel she needs? So, the next question is: Where does that drive to get things right come from? I imagine this isn't just about Maira. Do you recognize this in yourself generally?

Explore **attachment history** and understand triggers

Janice: Oh yes, I'm always trying to please people, and I always worry that they're not happy with me.

Aleena: So, who has been hardest to satisfy in your life, to get it right for?

Janice: Oh, that will be my parents. I think maybe you've guessed that. (*both laugh*)

Aleena: So, tell me about your parents.

Janice: Um, my mom, well, she had depression, I think I mentioned. And we, my brother and I, always had to do the chores for her, be quiet when she was in bed, you know, that sort of thing. Of course, as children we didn't always remember, then our dad would be cross with us. He was never satisfied with us!

Aleena: So, you could never be good enough for him?

Janice: I remember. . . . It was when I cut my head open. It would have been a Saturday night. My parents used to meet their friends at the pub. We were too young to be left at home, so they took us with them. We had to play in the pub garden. Well, on this day, we were trying to get conkers [horse chestnuts] down from a tree. I picked up this brick and threw it. I clearly forgot about gravity. (*laughs*) Anyway, it landed on my head; there was blood everywhere. Dad was furious. He had to take me to the hospital to get stitches. All he could think about was his beer that he'd left.

Aleena:	And your mom?
Janice:	I don't remember. Dad always dealt with things.
Aleena:	You don't remember her holding you, comforting you?
Janice:	I don't remember. She must have been there.
Aleena:	Oh, Janice, that's sad. You must have been scared, and no one comforted you.
Janice:	I was just a nuisance, ruining their evening.
Aleena:	How hard, a hurting little girl and no one to comfort her. So, we started off thinking, what did you find hard parenting Maira? One of the things is trying to constantly meet her need for your attention. And there are a couple of things around this that I'm thinking about. One is: the way you got your dad's approval was being self-reliant, someone he could depend on. When that happens in the absence of nurture, comfort, it becomes "I have to do this in order to get that." Do you see what I mean? It just feels to me like it's left you with a lot of pressure to get things right and to be the perfect mom.
Janice:	Well, yes, that kind of makes sense. I've never thought of it like this before.
Aleena:	The second thing is: Maira's neediness was something you learned not to show when you were little. Maira has a very

different style from you when you were a child. I expect her mother's illness and experiencing so many caregivers in her first two years have left her with an intense need to be noticed and cared for. She won't stop seeking this, fearful that if she is soothed by you, your emotional availability will disappear, just as it so often did when she was little. She is very attention-needing, you were very capable and self-reliant, her ambivalent attachment style contrasts with your avoidant one. Maira needs to keep signaling her need for you, while her inability to feel soothed by you triggers your feeling not good enough. That must be difficult for you. You don't recognize her in yourself. Do you see what I mean?

Janice: Yes, I think so.

Aleena: She's different from you. How do you respond to that? It's hard because part of you must be feeling, "If only this kid would not show this stuff," because that's your style. And then another part of you is wanting to let her be the child she needs to be, perhaps because you weren't able to be. When you needed attention, needed comfort, you didn't get it. You couldn't live up to all the expectations on you as a child, and you worry that you're still not doing it as a mother. Can you see the pressure you put on yourself because of your own childhood experiences? Does that makes sense?

TIME FOR REFLECTION

When exploring attachment history, memories from childhood often arise. These might be memories that have not been thought of for a long time and are only just now seeming significant.

- Have you experienced this when exploring your own attachment history?
- Think about how exploring your story with someone who is safe and interested in you can lead to making connections that have not been thought of before.
- How did this impact you as a practitioner?

In the Janice example, we will imagine some of the complexities that arise from the intersection of experiencing loss and separation from one's birth family as well as from one's racial identity and heritage. This will help the mother and social worker to identify areas that they can work on together. The exploration of attachment history blends with the work they will continue to do together.

Janice: Yeah, my dad was very critical. You always had to live up to his expectations, and honestly, it was as if my mom wasn't in the house half the time. Mind you, they could both be critical. I hated listening to them talk about other people, always putting them down. I think that's something that's stuck with me too. We had these neighbors who moved in next door, a Pakistani family. I haven't thought about this for years. It just came to my mind as you were talking. My parents didn't like them. I wonder, maybe it was the Irish thing. My grandmother came from Ireland as a 16-year-old, you know, with my father as a child. Her family had cut her off. She ran away to avoid the nuns. They'd have taken the baby away. I was close to my gran until she died. She told me about it. But with my parents, we never talked about it, never acknowledged our Irish heritage. I think my dad was a bit ashamed. My parents were so "English." I think maybe that's why they felt they needed to put people down. With the family next door, it was about "look at us. we're better because we're English." I don't know if this is making sense. There was a little girl my age. I wasn't supposed to talk to her. We used to play together at the bottom of the garden, through a hole in the fence. She never understood why she couldn't come around or why I didn't talk to her at school. I feel bad about that. Maybe that's why I wanted to parent Maira—maybe it was to make up for that, and maybe a way of showing my father.

Aleena: It's complex, isn't it? I can see you putting a lot of things together that are making sense of your struggles with Maira. You had such a lot to be managing as a child, a depressed mom, an exacting father, and pressure to be a certain way that also meant denying parts of yourself; your Irish part, for example. Then experiencing racism while trying to find your own values. All these things come together, making you the mother you are.

Janice: You know, it's hard to tell you this, but when Maira is at her worst, I look at her and think, "What will become of you? you won't amount to anything." I don't say it to her, but the thought is there. Then I feel bad for thinking it. It's just what my parents used to say about the family next door. I wonder, maybe I wanted to keep Maira to show them. Show them they're wrong. Then I find myself thinking it too. I'm just like them!

Aleena: I can see how hard you are on yourself, Janice. We get lots of pressures on us from our childhood, some conscious and some less so. We bring our parent's values with us, and some we try to get away from.

Janice: Yes, but my motive to keep Maira, was it for the right reasons? I don't want the reason to be to get back at my parents or from a sense of pity for her—a white savior thing! She's just a kid, and no matter her race or being unable to live within her birth family, she deserves all the best in life.

Aleena: You are thoughtful about this. I think, at the end of the day, that's what counts. I can see you have a lot of influences on you from your childhood. We all do. It's what we do next that counts. I can understand that when Maira is angry, demanding, and expressing her need of you, it's hard to manage. In some ways you see your own needs that weren't met. You never learned how to express them, and it's hard to know how to help Maira when this wasn't modeled for you. And your motivations to parent her, yes, perhaps they are mixed up with a rejection of your parents' racism and your treatment of your childhood friend. Exploring those motives is important. If you don't do that work, you may end up putting a lot of pressure on Maira to be the child you want her to be.

Janice: You mean, Maira being happy and embracing her identity would make me feel better, would make amends for how I treated my friend, and would show I had rejected my parent's racism. But I didn't even know those motives were influencing me until just now.

Aleena: That's why this exploration is so important. Making what is unconscious, conscious will help reduce the pressure on Maira. You will be better able to focus on what she needs and not be driven only by what you unconsciously need.

Janice: Wow, this is making my head spin! I am thinking about the struggles that Maira is having. I know she is experiencing racism at school. I'm just not sure how to talk to her about it. I also see her rejecting her Pakistani heritage, and it breaks my heart. Like with the dolls, she was choosing a family of dolls for her doll's house. I wanted her to choose the ethnically similar family. She told me they were ugly, and she wanted the white family. I just got frustrated with her. Was it because my need for her to be happy in her identity is more about proving something about me? I need to focus on what she needs, don't I? I have brought her into my white family. It must be so confusing for her. How do I help her to be in touch with and proud of her Pakistani roots while she's also absorbing my values and culture as her white mother? There are so many ways I could get this wrong!

Aleena: What I see is a mom who is really strong for her daughter, willing to keep on trying even though it feels like she's getting

Explore **strengths** in parent and child

it wrong, a mom who is asking important questions about how to support her daughter's complex identity. That's what Maira needs, and she knows she needs you. She keeps on demanding even though she's anxious that she doesn't deserve you.

And you want Maira to achieve, to be successful. In a strange way it's like reclaiming your Irish heritage and amending for the past. She needs you to believe in her, but even more, I think she needs you to believe in yourself, take the pressure off yourself. As you work through this, you will be able to leave the past behind and focus on Maira's needs in the present.

Janice: You have given me a lot to think about. I do want Maira to get what she needs from me, and I feel very poorly equipped sometimes. We've had plenty of training about trauma, but not about racism. How can I talk to Maira about what she's experiencing? I think this is a talk I've been avoiding.

Aleena: Sadly, racism is a reality for her, and this is a talk that needs to happen. We also need to talk with the school, to make sure she is getting the right support there. The racism Maira experiences is a racial trauma, and it will impact the way Maira is relating to you. We know that often children who experience racial trauma will display aggression, experience more vigilance and suspicion, and may have a shortened sense of the future. It won't be just losses that lead to her being angry and needing attention, although it is, of course, important not to lose sight of this; her experience of losing one family and being moved into another is also a big part of the trauma she has experienced.

Janice: This feels complicated. I have to help heal the trauma wounds from Maira's early family experience and loss, some of which echoes my experience of having a depressed mother and a lack of emotional availability from my parents. I always lived with my birth family, but I can see some influences here that could make caring for Maira complicated. I also have to help her with racial trauma. I can see some possible connections here with her mother's illness and what she has experienced.

Aleena: Yes, and this trauma is ongoing for Maira, and you can't always protect her from it. It can happen anytime she leaves your house. Maira is also internalizing racism—picking up societal values around the superiority of white over Black and brown—evidenced by her rejection of the doll figures for her doll's house. Then she experiences racism from white people; the same skin tone as you, her mother. Can you see how confusing and troubling this is? When Maira looks at your face, she sees someone who loves and cares for her *and* she sees the white face of her racist attacker. Along with the loss of her birth mother, this makes it hard for her to know how to trust you and to believe in your love for her. Helping her with her identity is going to be a complicated process.

Janice: Wow, this is a lot to take in. I'm beginning to see what an even bigger commitment I have taken on in parenting Maira.

Aleena: It is a lot. You have got strengths from your childhood: Your self-reliance, ability to go it alone. Your commitment to helping Maira get the best from life. These can be vulnerabilities too, the need to get things right, the pressure to see Maira being happy and able to achieve. I admire your strength to find your own values in life and to be willing to face the impact of your childhood experience. Your mother's depression and your father's critical stance have been a part of what made you the person you are and will impact your parenting. Making sense of this will build your resilience.

Janice: Yes, and Maira is strong too. I guess she's terrified that she's going to be left again, but she's hanging in there. Maybe my expectations—that she be happy, that she embrace her identity; that she achieve—maybe she feels like she's failing me. Maybe that's why she gets so angry with me. Her anger is a strength too, letting me know that she is struggling. It's time for me to reduce my expectations and focus on what she needs.

Aleena: Yes, and I'm here to help you. We can do this together.

TIME FOR REFLECTION

As you reflect on this interview:

1. Notice how current parenting and attachment history exploration are woven together. What helps to maintain the focus on parenting within this exploration?
2. Think about Janice's experience of parenting Maira. What do you think will be the hotspots, those times when she gets emotionally overwhelmed in Maira's therapy sessions? How might these also impact her parenting?
3. Notice how the conversation develops. Do you see Janice being more vulnerable as she discloses issues regarding rac-

ism and family history in response to memories that arise? What helps her to trust Aleena with this very personal experience? How does this change her thoughts about herself and her daughter?

4. What areas of work, within therapy and outside of it, might Aleena and Maira identify with?

5. Reflect, too, on being this therapist. How might this interview help the therapist to support this mother? What might it be like to be a Pakistani-British therapist supporting a white British mother? What might be triggering for the therapist? What supervision might she seek?

DEVELOPING PARENTAL COMPASSION

As the interview with Janice illustrates, parenting children who find it hard to trust is challenging. Jon Baylin describes how this can lead to chronic ambivalence toward the child (Baylin, 2015[4]). There is a natural tension between the parents' loving intentions, their desire to give the child a better life, and their disappointment and sense of failure when the child doesn't trust them or their parenting.

Children in states of blocked trust read these ambiguous signals as negative and threatening, thus reinforcing the mistrust they are holding.

Within DDP interventions, we need to help the parent to find compassion for themselves and for their child, especially when discouragement and a sense of failure are strong. Sessions like the one we have just explored can help parent(s) and therapist to find this compassion and to work through the ambivalence.

---

4   A brief paper written for the DDP Network Library by Jonathan Baylin, PhD, July 2015.

TIME FOR REFLECTION

Reflect on the dialogue with Janice.

- What ambivalence does Janice reveal in her parenting of Maira?
- Do you think the therapist's compassion for Janice will have increased from this work?
- Are there things that could threaten this compassion?
- Can you identify ways in which Janice's compassion for Maira is increasing as she explores her own history?

BRINGING PARENTS INTO SESSIONS WITH THE CHILD

By the time you begin parent–child sessions, you will know the parents well. They will feel safe with you, experience you as trusting them to support the work with the child. You are ready to plan for bringing the child into sessions.

In preparation for this work, the therapist:

- explains how the sessions are likely to unfold, what to expect of the therapist, and what the therapist will expect of them.
- plans with the parents how to manage tricky moments (e.g., what they will do if their child dysregulates or infringes important boundaries; which rules will continue to be observed, such as no hitting, and which will be relaxed—swearing is likely to be tolerated in sessions, especially when it emerges authentically as a way to express intense emotion).
- discusses how to manage times when the parent experiences frustration or anger toward them and how to indicate that they urgently need to have a conversation that would not be appropriate in front of the child.

- explores what signals parents can use to indicate that they are struggling and will not be able to respond with empathy.
- provides the parents with opportunities to experience aspects of the DDP intervention that might feel strange and unusual, such as the therapist talking for the child or the parent being invited to respond to the story they have witnessed unfolding between therapist and child.
- decide when parent-only sessions will be interspersed with the parent–child sessions. The therapist will create ongoing opportunities for checking in with the parents and to explore what is happening both at home and within the therapy sessions.

The alliance between therapist and parent will be important when tricky moments arise in the therapy. The parent needs to be open to the guidance of the therapist so that safety for the child can be maintained.

REFLECTIVE EXERCISE: RESPONDING TO PARENTS

At the end of the chapter, Worksheet 6.2 provides an opportunity to explore responses you might make to a parent during child and parent sessions. How can you guide the parent toward maintaining safety for the child?

CONCLUSION

Dyadic developmental psychotherapy is a unique family intervention involving parents alone and parents and children together. While the therapeutic focus is always on the children, within the DDP model there is recognition that this needs to be done in collaboration with the parents. The therapeutic alliance between parent and therapist is a critical part of successful interventions.

Worksheet 6.1

Moving into Attachment History: A Guide[5]

1. Explore symptoms reported in child
Symptoms are the motivation for the parent coming; don't minimize them. Explore how parents make sense of the symptoms. Find out what they have tried.

Help parents to know that you "get it." Listen to their anger and frustration so that they are and feel heard and their experience is not being minimized or judged.

2. Explore hopes and dreams
Acknowledge that parents did not expect things to turn out this way. Explore the hopes and dreams they held before the child arrived.

Usually, parents are motivated by good things. As you explore these good motivations, parents' trust that you see them as good people grows.

3. Explore doubts and fears
When did the parents start to think their dreams were not going to come true? This isn't the child they thought they would be parenting. For example, parents may acknowledge fears that they are a bad parent, that they should not parent, that this is the wrong placement for the child. This discussion will likely reveal feelings of grief, loss, resentment, and shame.

Accept and empathize with feelings of discouragement. This allows a reexploration of symptoms, now with sadness and vulnerability. This builds trust and feelings of safety.

---

5 Adapted from *DDP Level One Training Book* © 2019, DDPI.

4. What in the child is the hardest thing for them to have empathy for?

This is the "magic" question, and it connects to their own attachment and relationship history. By approaching history this way, the exploration is embedded in the context of their current parenting.

Help parents to experience you as curious and nonjudgmental about their experiences and how their experiences are linked to their parenting.

5. Explore attachment history

Help the parents understand the feelings they have in response to the child that are linked to this history. Understand their triggers.

Ask parents to recall actual events, such as how did they calm or comfort themselves as a child when they became upset, ill, or separated? Reflect on how this experience impacts their parenting.

6. Explore strengths of parent and child

This is something to build on, even if it starts very small. Build on the strengths seen in the parent and see strengths in the child. This process increases acceptance and commitment. It can lead to feelings of pride and joy. Successes will increase, and failures will decrease. Guilt will occur without shame. Any continuing difficulties of the child can then be met with PACE, not parental shame and resentment.

This moves the discussion into a more hopeful dialogue. It helps the parent understand the difficult impact the child can have on them and helps them to develop new and realistic hopes and goals.

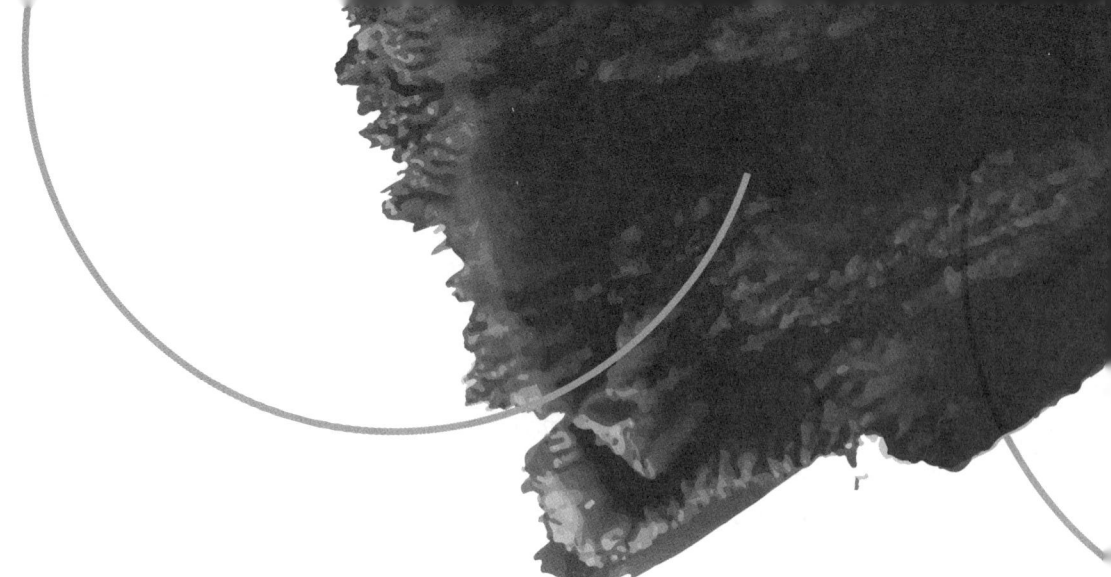

Chapter 7:
Parenting Children with Developmental Trauma

Dyadic developmental parenting is an important part of helping children to recover and heal from developmental traumas. This relies on parents using both hands of parenting to connect emotionally alongside empathy-led "correction" through behavioral support. PACE is the central attitude to build these connections so that children can experience safety where they previously experienced threat and trust where they have only learned mistrust. (Hughes et al., 2019, p. 152)

REFRESHER

Dyadic developmental parenting (DDP-informed parenting) is an approach to raising children that is informed by DDP principles. Children recovering from developmental trauma need to live in environments where they can experience safety and security; where they learn to trust in unconditional love and support; and where they believe in their own goodness because their parents see this goodness in them, even during the hardest of times.

DDP interventions involve supporting parents to provide these healing environments. The children do not believe in the safety and comfort parents offer. They do not believe that the parents' authority has good intentions, and they do not trust in their own lovability.

The children learn to miscue their attachment needs:

"I will act as if I don't need comfort when I am emotionally troubled."

"I will act as if I don't need you to explore with me when I am feeling emotionally safe."

The children resist invitations to join intersubjectively:

"I will not allow you to influence me, to hold my mind in your mind."

These children learn to stay in control. Parents' care, comfort, authority, and interest in the child's experiences threaten this sense of control.

Optimal parenting is provided by the authoritative parent offering "two hands of parenting." They provide the child with warmth, nurturing, and fun alongside supervision, discipline, and boundaries.

DDP-informed parenting is no different. There are, however, additional elements within each hand; elements that all children can benefit from but that are essential for the child with developmental trauma (Figure 7.1).

Within the attitude of PACE, the first hand also offers the child safety and security, even when these are resisted and rejected.

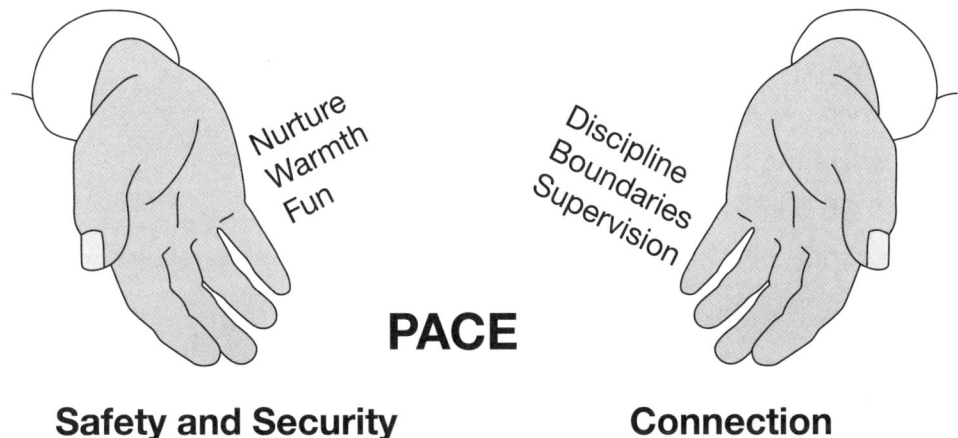

Figure 7.1 Two Hands of Parenting

The second hand pays extra attention to emotional connection. This lets the child know that they are loved, that they will not be abandoned, and that parents will support them with any discipline or boundaries that are needed. The parent maintains their parental presence even when the child is rejecting, hostile, violent, and abusive. Only in this way will the child learn that they are loved no matter what and that this time, hurt and abandonment will not follow.

You can learn more about DDP-informed parenting in the books listed in the list of resources.

SUPPORTING PARENTS TO PARENT WITH PACE

 TIME FOR REFLECTION

Spend a moment reflecting on your work with a parent that you found particularly challenging. This is a reflection about feeling rather than thinking. If you notice yourself trying to understand or make sense of why you find this parent difficult or wondering what you could do differently, gently put these wonderings to the side.

Focus on the experience of being with this parent and notice:

- the feelings it creates in you
- what is happening in your body
- where the energy sits within you
- any thoughts, images, sensations that arise
- any hurt or angry parts of yourself that appear, and gently soothe them

Now direct your thoughts back to the parent and notice how you are feeling about this parent.

- Any feelings of frustration or irritation?
- Any sense of hopelessness or inadequacy?
- Any feelings of empathy, acceptance, and curiosity?
- Any feelings of enjoyment of the parent?

At the end of this exercise, you might want to jot down any thoughts you are left with, things you would like to discuss in supervision, things you want to be curious about when you are with the parent next.

Kim sits with an adoptive mother, Gem. Gem is parenting two boys, who present a range of challenges. Gem is struggling with the children's need of her alongside their continuous rejection. She and Kim have explored how this triggers memories from her own upbringing and the parenting she has received. They have spent time reflecting on Gem's hopes and dreams and grieving for the family she thought she would have. They have gone through the children's early history, exposure to drugs and alcohol and witness to domestic violence and physical abuse. They have thought about the impact of this experience and why the children struggle to feel safe even after seven years living in their adoptive home. Gem attended the Nurturing Attachments Group, spending a year with a group of adopters exploring DDP-informed ways of parenting the children. And yet, Gem is here again, still experiencing the same frustrations, still struggling with the hurt of parenting these children, still feeling the sense of failure that these boys are not the happy, loving children she imagined and that she does not feel like the calm, caring mother she thought she would be.

Kim wonders what more she can do to help Gem. As Gem talks of her frustration with the boys, Kim reminds herself of the hurt this mother is experiencing. She reflects on the years she has been supporting Gem and soothes herself around the sense of failure that this brings up in her. She moves away from her need to fix and instead sits with Gem in her despair. She is fully present, accepting the sense of disappointment and failure that Gem is experiencing; being curious about the emotional experience of this, deepening her empathy for this person who has always struggled to feel good enough, as a daughter and as a mother, and finding moments of playfulness as they enjoy being together.

A part of Kim wonders, "Is this enough? Gem has driven an hour to see her. Will she be frustrated that there are no answers, no new things to explore?" At the end of the session Gem stands up to leave. She stands taller and looks lighter than when she arrived. She smiles at Kim. "Thank you," she says, "I think I can accept them more now." Kim invites her to phone when she needs another session.

This was an important experience for Kim. She learned that acceptance was what Gem needed most at that time. Kim needed to trust in acceptance, otherwise she would have moved into focusing on finding solutions for Gem. Gem would likely have experienced that as dismissive and minimizing of her experience, and she likely would have continued to feel alone and unsupported in her difficult experience of parenting the children. She would not have experienced Kim's belief that she was a good parent, doing the best she could and wanting to love her children. Gem would likely have left with stronger feelings of not being good enough.

As DDP practitioners, we do provide instruction on what PACE is. This information is a necessary part of helping parents bring PACE to their parenting. To develop PACE as a way of being, however, takes more than education. Parents need to experience PACE for themselves. The DDP practitioner provides a predictable presence, conveyed with the attitude of PACE. This helps the parent to feel connected to the therapist, trusting that whatever they share will be acceptable. DDP-informed parenting support provides the parent with the experience that we hope they will begin to provide for their child.

To provide this experience, practitioners also benefit from experiencing PACE from others.

TIME FOR REFLECTION

Reflect on times you had supervision with a focus on your work with a parent.

1. When and how did this supervision feel helpful? When did it leave you feeling energized, with a renewed motivation for working with the parent?
2. When did this supervision feel less helpful? What got in the way of this being supportive?

Reflect on times you had supervision with a focus on you, when you explored together what you brought to the work and how the work impacted on you.

3. When and how did this supervision feel helpful?
   - If your supervisor was empathic to the struggles you were experiencing and curious about the emotional experience of the work, did you feel understood and supported; accepted, not evaluated?
   - What was your experience of this supervision?
   - How did it impact your work with the parent?
4. When did this supervision feel less helpful?
   - Are there ways in which you didn't feel heard?
   - Were you left with feelings of frustration, doubt, uncertainty?
   - What was your experience of this supervision?
   - How did it impact your work with the parent?
5. Finally, reflect on how you let your supervisor know what you need from supervision.

A. Are you clear about this yourself?

B. Do you feel confident directing your supervisor to what you need?

If you currently supervise others, you might do this same reflection as supervisor rather than supervisee.

Just as with supervision, when we provide parenting support, we need to make decisions about how we provide this support. As we will explore later, DDP-informed support represents a slowing down. We let the parents know that we are interested in their experience. We judge when the parent is ready to think about the child and about their parenting. Parents, just like all of us, are not always good at signaling what they need in the moment. We figure this out with them, fine tuning what they need as they respond to our interventions.

TIME FOR REFLECTION

Notice how the practitioner adjusts their focus with the parent in the following dialogue about her son's troubling behavior:

Parent: He's been rifling through my underwear drawer again. He doesn't even try to hide it. I walk into my bedroom and the drawer is pulled open. When I call him on it, he just says sorry, as if that makes it alright.

Practitioner: Oh, I'm sorry to hear that. He hasn't done that for a while now, has he? Do you think he's feeling extra

	insecure at the moment? I wonder if something is stressing him.
Parent:	Nothing more than usual, I don't think. He just seems to enjoy making me feel uncomfortable.
Practitioner:	What about the underwear you bought him to wear, is he still using these?
Parent:	I've tried everything you suggest. It doesn't seem to make any difference. I just want him to stop!
Practitioner:	I apologize, this is so hard for you. I think I was too focused on your son and forgot what a horrible thing this is to experience. It's such a violating feeling when someone is doing something so intimate in this way. I know we've thought about this before, but shall we spend some time thinking about you in this? How would that feel?
Parent:	Yes, that would be helpful. I can really feel this building up in me.

As the parents experience our PACEful attitude, they are getting an embodied sense of DDP-informed parenting. Alongside PACE, the DDP practitioner models the other DDP principles.

- They develop AR dialogues with the parent, discovering and exploring the story of their experience.
- Emotion is coregulated as narrative is cocreated.
- They attend to the verbal and nonverbal communications and are alert for relationship ruptures, ensuring that these are repaired in a way that demonstrates that they value the relationship.
- The practitioner combines the PACE attitude with education, guidance, coaching, and exploration.

- Sometimes this also involves holding a boundary with the parent. Just as we want the parent to do with the child, we offer PACE and emotional connection while gently but clearly outlining our thinking about what is not acceptable.

For example:

"I can see how helpless you are feeling. Whatever you do doesn't make a difference. I worry that your understandable frustration is leading you to communicate in a way that isn't helping your child. Telling them that they will only be able to stay if they stop hitting you is likely to increase their insecurity, leading to even more violence toward you. I understand you need to let them know that violence isn't acceptable. Are you willing to explore with me some different ways of communicating this?"

As we model DDP in our interactions, we are strengthening the parents' capacity to bring a DDP-informed approach into their parenting.

Our aim is to stay in an open and engaged state, just as we do in work with the child. This means accepting, without evaluating, the emotional experience of the parent. What they think, feel, wish, believe is not right nor wrong; it just is. This acceptance is especially important when we wish to help a parent to change their practice. Without this acceptance, defensiveness is likely to be high and that can trigger us to respond defensively. Most conflict arises because of the assumptions we make about another person's motives.

For example, a support worker judges a parent for locking their foster son in his bedroom when he was being violent. The support worker assumes that the parent got frustrated with the son and locked the door in anger. The foster carer assumes that the support worker is looking for reasons to end the placement and is finding fault with everything they do. Neither of them will be able to think about alternatives to locking the child in his room when they are busy defending themselves against the assumptions of the other.

REFLECTIVE EXERCISE:
ACCEPTANCE OR EVALUATION?

Reflect on the brief scenarios below. Do you think that the practitioner is becoming defensive, leading to evaluation, or staying open and engaged, leading to acceptance?

1. **Parent:** How will my son ever learn not to steal if there are no consequences? You just want me to be soft on him because you feel sorry for him.

   Practitioner: It's not about feeling sorry for him, I just think there are more natural consequences that you can support him with. It feels like you want to punish him more than you want to teach him. Can we think together about more helpful consequences than removing his computer privileges?

2. **Parent:** I feel you criticize every judgment I make. I don't think it's helpful for my son to have contact with his father just now. That's why I didn't take him.

   Practitioner: I apologize that it feels like I'm criticizing you. I have to help you make good decisions though. You can't make decisions about contact even if you do believe he'll be happier as a consequence.

3. **Parent:** I just don't feel supported by you. You're never there when I call. I needed to talk with you last night after they took the overdose. I didn't need the duty worker telling me what to do.

   Practitioner: I can only imagine how hard it was finding out that they'd taken all those tablets. I'm sorry I wasn't on call last night.

> Can we go through what happened? After that I would like to think about why you're not feeling supported by me at the moment.

Notice that in the first two responses, the practitioner is holding some assumptions about the parent's motivations. Curiosity is lacking. This will increase defensiveness and the likelihood of conflict. In the third, despite the unjust criticism, the practitioner remains open to wondering why this parent is not feeling supported by them. The practitioner may have some assumptions in mind. The focus, however, is on exploring what happened. This may give the practitioner some clues as to the parent's emotional state, which can help with a curious exploration of the parent's beliefs. The parent will experience the practitioner as interested in them and their experience, reducing feelings of defensiveness and increasing feelings of being supported.

BARRIERS TO DDP-INFORMED PARENTING

There are a number of reasons why parents might struggle to implement guidance for parenting their children in a DDP-informed way. At these times, it is important that DDP practitioners slow down and seek to understand these difficulties rather than offering more guidance. With this understanding the practitioner can ensure that they are providing the support that the parents need.

BLOCKED TRUST AND BLOCKED CARE

Children who have experienced developmental trauma often enter states of blocked trust (Baylin & Hughes, 2016). This means responding to damaging caregiving environments by blocking the pain of rejection and the capacity for delight. The child has found a way to survive in a world that holds no comfort or joy (Figure 7.2). Blocked trust moves with the child, making it difficult for them to discover that comfort and joy are now available.

The challenges the child is presenting, especially the difficulties the child has in entering reciprocal, intersubjective interactions with the parent, are experienced as hurtful and rejecting. The parent does not feel loved by the

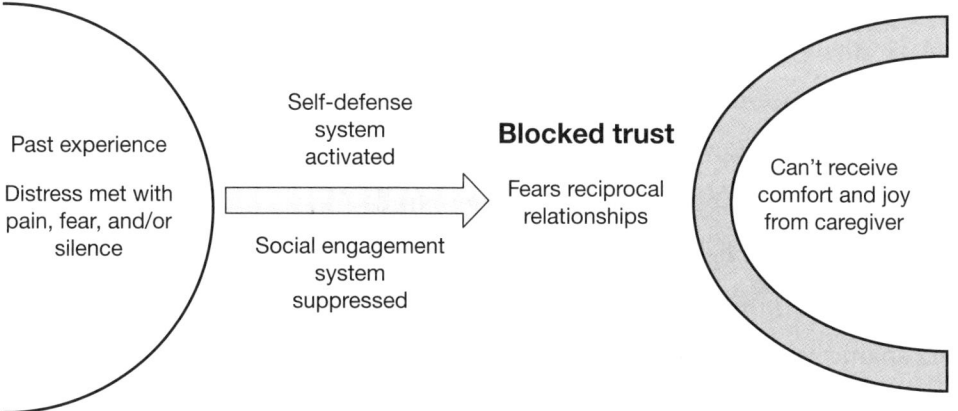

Figure 7.2 Blocked Trust

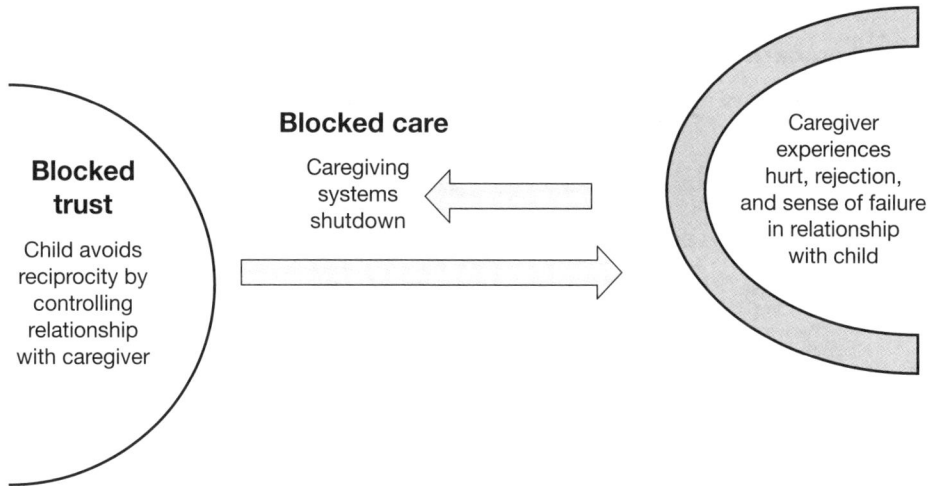

Figure 7.3 Blocked Care in Response to
Blocked Trust

child, and their love for their child is threatened as a consequence. Most of the
caregiving systems within their nervous system start to shut down, and joy in
parenting is lost (Figure 7.3). This state of blocked care can reduce the ability

to mentalize at a time when we hope to strengthen the reflective capacity of the parent.

When blocked care is present or emerging, the DDP practitioner needs to spend more time with the parent, providing support and offering the reciprocal relationship that they are struggling to find with their child (see Table 7.1).

The parent is helped by knowing that blocked care is a biological process that emerges from certain relational experiences. This reduces feelings of failure and shame and helps them to be more open to the practitioner's care and support. Being cared for by a friend, colleague, or family member helps the parent care for the child who is rejecting.

TABLE 7.1 IMPACT OF SUPPORTIVE RELATIONSHIPS ON BLOCKED CARE

Blocked care shuts down care-giving systems	Supportive relationships reduce blocked care and increase PACE
Depletion of oxytocin leads to a drive to avoid the child.	Drive to approach the child increases.
Depletion of dopamine leads to experiencing the connection with the child as unrewarding.	Increase in sense of reward from caring for child. Joy in relationship rediscovered (playfulness).
Mentalization decreases, affecting child reading, as understanding decreases.	Mentalization increases, leading to improved understanding of child (curiosity) and increase in acceptance and empathy.
Memories of past relationship stress is activated, impacting meaning making.	Meaning is made based on an understanding of the child rather than on past experience.

TIME FOR REFLECTION

We all have times when we feel the touch of blocked care. It might be when parenting children, caring for elderly relatives, or working in a caring profession.

Think back to your own experience of this, however fleeting. Quietly sit and move into the memory of what that felt like.

- Notice what feelings, worries, beliefs, or hopelessness you experienced.
- Notice how you felt about the caring role you were in.

Now move yourself forward in time as you emerged from blocked care.

- How have the feelings, worries, beliefs, or hopelessness changed?
- If you moved from "I can't do this anymore" to "I can do this," what did that feel like?

Finally, reflect on what helped you to move out of blocked care.

- What did you do?
- How did others help you?

DEFENSIVE STATES

Parents may have strong defenses in place, often in response to feelings of discouragement and failure and a need to conceal this vulnerability. It is easy to join them in defensiveness. This gives us distance from the emotionally overwhelming experience of the parent but reduces our support. As psychologist and Catholic priest Henri Nouwen said: "It is no secret that many of our suggestions, advice, admonitions, and good words are often offered in order to keep distance rather than allow closeness" (Nouwen, 2017, p. 196).

TIME FOR REFLECTION

Below is a list of common defenses that parents present. Reflect on each one and notice your response to it.

1. **Let's think about how services have let me down.**

   The parent becomes preoccupied and angry about the services they are or are not receiving.

2. **Let's talk about the child.**

   If we wonder about the parents' experiences, they skillfully—and often unconsciously—move us back to thinking about the child.

3. **Let's solve the problems.**

   Both parent and practitioner become preoccupied with finding answers to immediate problems that the child is presenting.

4. **Help me to feel better.**

   The parent expresses some fears about failing, about not being good enough, but then backs away from thinking about this experience.

If you are in a study group, you might explore these through role play, which may provide you with an embodied experience of these scenarios.

- Do you find yourself being pulled into the distraction?
- Do you want to reassure or offer solutions?
- Do you feel you want to defend or explain something?

- In what ways are these keeping you away from your immediate goal of exploring and offering PACE for the parent's experience?
- There are times when it is helpful to focus on the parent's concern. Reflect on how you can distinguish between a helpful discussion and a defensive distraction.

In Scenario one, we might feel frustrated, too, and have sympathy for the parent. We might feel an urge to defend our colleagues. Either way, we become distracted from exploring the parent's experiences. Services can and do let parents down, including, at times, our own services. It is helpful to hear and understand the parent's experience with acceptance for their anger and frustration. We might think about how we can advocate for the family, ensuring that services are provided helpfully.

In Scenario two, we often already have some understanding about the child and what might help them, so we are keen to communicate this. We can easily be pulled into this focus. If we instead slow down the parent, helping them to reflect on their own experience first, we can guide them to make helpful reflections about the child. For example, the practitioner might ask:

"What's that like when your child . . ."

"Why do you think your child . . ."

"When your child says that, does it remind you of other times when someone . . ."

The parent moves into an open, rather than defensive, state and the exploration becomes more helpful as a consequence.

Going along with Scenario three can help us to feel like we are doing something useful, and it distracts from the feelings of discouragement that problems are not going away. Often, the solutions we offer are ones that the parent is very capable of finding for themselves. If those solutions were helpful, they would already be doing it. We know we have missed a step in supporting the parent when attempts to offer solutions are met with resistance:

> *"I've tried that."*

> *"Yes but . . ."*

> *"That isn't going to work because . . ."*

When parent and practitioner are ready to focus on ideas for supporting particular challenges, the discussion will feel more collaborative and joint problem-solving will occur.

In Scenario four, we move into offering reassurance instead of acceptance and curiosity as we, again, back away from exploration. This can happen when sitting with our discomfort feels hard. Our motivation is to make the parent feel better rather than to communicate acceptance and empathy for their experience. This shuts down curious exploration. When we can sit with uncomfortable feelings, the parent may feel safe enough to express their vulnerability and to feel supported. The parent is then able to hear how we experience them differently. We offer affirmations rather than reassurance, shifting their own experience of themselves:

"I see how much parenting this child makes you feel like a failure. I am not surprised, when it confirms so much of what you heard from your own father as a child. I see so much strength in you; you keep on being there for them despite the hurt you are feeling. I do hope one day you will be able to see this strength too."

SAFEGUARDING CONCERNS

One of the most challenging times in parent support is in dealing with concerns about risk:

- A parent might disclose hitting their child.
- A child might make an allegation against a parent.
- A concerning report comes in from the child's school.
- A parent describes a moment of parenting that you feel is dangerous, physically or emotionally.
- A parent tells you that they are feeling suicidal.

We all have a duty of care at these times. We need to talk to the parent, and we must report our concerns to the relevant people. We know that this may trigger a process that is extremely stressful for the family.

At these times, practitioners may feel that they need to put DDP to one side; that it will distract from the necessary safeguarding procedures. They are concerned that there is no time to slow down: action must be taken.

Respectfully, we disagree. Of course, if the child is in immediate danger, then action will take precedence. However, barring this, slowing down is needed. If we do not, we are in danger of triggering defensive responses from the parents and throughout the network. In such situations, there are no winners, and risk to the child will increase, either from within the family or by being removed from it.

Actions are needed. This might be, at most extreme, removing a child; it might be increasing family support or providing educational opportunities for the parents. We might need to involve mental health services. Any action is most likely to be helpful, or managed with the least harm, when we are working with the parents, all of us in an open and engaged state.

- Slowing down, maintaining an attitude of PACE, and cocreating the narrative of what has happened while offering coregulation to an, often, distressed parent will help to avoid defensive responses.

- We hold on to our assumption that these are good people, doing the best they can, and that they want to love and care for their child.

- As we communicate these assumptions in our willingness to listen and to understand, the parents feel our support and become able to reflect with us on how this situation arose.

- Our risk assessment will be informed by this understanding.

- Sometimes, often in states of fear and shame, the parents are angry with us. This can feel hurtful. We are the ones believing in the parent and trying to support them; now we feel under attack.

- We need to take care of ourselves, plan on who we will reach out to for support.

- We can then focus our empathy and acceptance onto the parent as we remember that these are parents in pain and fear.

- If possible, we can then collaboratively decide on next steps.

- We are honest about who we must tell and the timescales within which this will be done.

- We plan together how we will do this and what the parents will do in the interim:
    - Can we meet jointly with the child's social worker?
    - Does one parent need to leave the family home for a time?
    - Will the parent attend the mental health appointment, and who will support them? Who will talk to the child, and how will the child be talked to?
    - Does the school need to be informed?
    - Who will be able to support the parents and the child through what may be a long and challenging process, full of uncertainty?

REFLECTIVE EXERCISE: DDP AND SAFEGUARDING

You may explore how the DDP principles can inform safeguarding using Worksheet 7.1 at the end of the chapter.

SUPPORTING PARENTS IN CONFLICT

When we meet parents in conflict, it can be difficult to maintain the focus on parenting the children as we get caught up in the couple dynamics.

Let's imagine a part of a session with parenting couple Erin and Cassidy. They are a cisgendered, lesbian couple. They have adopted two siblings, Kai, a boy, and Abigail, a girl, ages six and seven, respectively.

Esther is a social worker who has supported Erin and Cassidy since before the children moved in. She has recently begun the DDP practicum to guide her work with parents. Esther is cisgendered, bisexual, and a single parent of an adolescent son. She does not discuss this with Erin and Cassidy because of her concerns about holding appropriate boundaries. In her previous training, self-disclosure was discouraged.

Erin is a lawyer. She describes her family as very focused on achievement. Her father's style is on the authoritarian side, respect for parents is highly valued. After their initial worries that being so open as a lesbian would affect her career, Erin's parents have always supported her and Cassidy, including their wish to adopt. Erin has a behavioral approach to her parenting and finds it difficult when her children do not respect her.

Cassidy, a part-time teacher, had a challenging childhood with parents who could be emotionally neglectful and harsh. They didn't speak to Cassidy for two years when they found out she was a lesbian. They are now more accepting, something Cassidy feels has happened since they adopted Kai and Abigail. Her father, however, still holds rigid and critical views. For example, he is vocal in his belief that Kai needs a father figure and will undermine Cassidy's and Erin's parenting in front of Kai. Cassidy has recently attended a DDP-informed parenting group and is enthusiastic about the value of PACE. She struggles to apply boundaries within her parenting, worried that this will lead to the children feeling emotionally abandoned by her.

The parents have arrived at this session concerned about Kai and his developing defiance to their authority. They are in conflict about how to manage this.

TIME FOR REFLECTION

Reflect on how you might support these parents.

- What themes might you explore as you talk with them?
- Think about the intersection of heritage, experience of being parented, and sexuality. You might consider this scenario with parents of different heritage, sexuality, and gender. How might these intersect and impact the conversation?
- Think also about how these interact with the parents' attachment histories.

How might these reflections influence your intervention?

Now consider this imaginary dialogue:

Erin: I just feel that Kai needs some good discipline. He is rude and defiant and is horrible to Abigail. He needs to learn some respect. Without respect, I don't know what his future will bring. How can he be successful in his career if he doesn't know how to respect his boss? How will he be successful in relationships?

Cassidy: But Kai is so little, and he's experienced so much. He just needs to feel in control, it helps him to feel safe, that's what we learned in the course. If we can support him to feel loved, I think the respect will come.

Erin: Cassidy, you are so soft with him. He just walks all over you. I don't see how that can be good for him.

TIME FOR REFLECTION

How are you going to help Erin and Cassidy?

First, notice what feelings are aroused in you by each of these parents.

- Do you feel more affinity with one of the parents?
- Do you think the gender of the parents makes a difference in how you experience their approach to parenting?
- Do you think that this is impacted by stereotypes we might hold about mothers' and fathers' approaches to parenting?

How might this impact your support of them? Now consider how you might move forward.

If you are in a study group, you might explore different interventions you could make at this point and see how they are responded to. There are no right or wrong answers.

The following is one way of moving forward:

Esther: It sounds like Kai is challenging both of you right now. You've always been so clear and together in the parenting of your children. Am I right that you're not feeling very together just now? (*Both parents nod.*) I can see you both have strong and important values. Can we all take a breath, slow down, and see if we can think about this together.

Erin: I must admit, I'm feeling a bit outnumbered right now. I know that Cassidy got a lot from your course, and I can see some benefits. I just don't see how that will help if she can't provide boundaries.

Cassidy: But you're all boundaries, Erin. How will Kai feel understood if you don't stop and listen? And look at how my dad is with Kai. It must be confusing him. After the children have visited my parents, Kai is so rude to us. I think he is muddled and needs support from us.

Esther: OK, OK. I can see you both have strong feelings. Erin, I'm sorry if you're feeling outnumbered. It can be hard when one partner attends a course and the other doesn't. I want you to know I respect your motivation to help both Abigail and Kai. I want us to find a way forward that helps you both feel authentic to your values and that brings you together in your parenting. Can we begin there? You're both so committed to these children. I can see how much you want to get it right for them, to give them the future that you dream for them. I see you very together in this. (*Erin and Cassidy look at each other and nod.*) Erin, tell me about your dreams.

Erin: I want both of the children to grow up to be strong, able to achieve in whatever they choose to do. My family helped me to do that. My father could be a bit scary at times, but he instilled respect in me. My grandparents too. That was so important.

Esther: Yes, I hear that. Respect is an important value for you in parenting successfully. Cassidy, how does it feel hearing Erin?

Cassidy: I'm not sure I learned respect in my family. You just had to fend for yourself. That's what I don't want for the children. But I hear Erin. I can see the value in respecting your parents. I'm just not sure you can punish a child into respecting you. It certainly didn't happen with my father! If I'm honest, I worry that in the end he'll turn Kai against us.

Esther: That sounds like a big worry, Cassidy, and hard to experience your father as not believing in you and what you can offer, Kai. I know you had a difficult time being accepted when you came out to him. I imagine it is very disturbing to experience the impact of his views on Kai. So, what are your dreams for the children?

Cassidy: I want them to be happy. I want them to feel loved. Of course, I want them to do well, to achieve, have a career. I just don't think that would be enough.

Esther: I know how hard it was to feel loved in your family. You work so hard to make sure that your children experience the love that you struggled to find. Erin, how does it feel hearing Cassidy?

Erin: I always felt loved in my family, it was never in doubt. Maybe I take love for granted. Of course, I want the children to feel loved. I just don't think it's enough on its own. We fought so hard to be allowed to parent them as lesbian adoptive parents. If we don't get this right, everyone who criticized us will be thinking, "we told you so," especially your father, Cassidy. I worry about his influence on Kai as well.

Esther: I know you had a hard time being accepted as adopters. It felt like you had to jump through a lot of hoops, didn't it? And you're still having to cope with judgements, even abuse, from others. I understand the pressure you are experiencing to prove yourselves as parents. I know this isn't easy.

Erin: I know we can do it. Even so, we need to be thoughtful about what the children need and how we provide it.

Cassidy: Well on that we can agree. We're very different parents, Erin. I think we each bring something to the parenting. We just need to ensure we're doing this together.

Esther: I really appreciate how you are listening to each other. And I so admire the values and the thoughtfulness you are bringing to your parenting. Learning to respect and to feel loved are important, as are ensuring the children get all their needs met. Between you, the children are going to thrive. Raising the children as a lesbian couple is going to bring extra challenges. Please don't stop telling me about these. Can we work together to bring your parenting in line with each other while still holding on to your values?

Erin: I would like that. I don't want to be hard on Kai. I'm just not sure how this PACE stuff will teach him how to behave. I can see he's feeling more secure since Cassidy did the course, but there don't seem to be any boundaries. I don't think it will help if he can just do what he likes.

Cassidy: You are right, Erin. I don't think I'm too good at boundaries. I just worry Kai won't feel loved. He does behave better with you. I just want you to see his fears. He's so frightened we'll get rid of him, and I do wonder if my father is contributing to this.

Esther: So, we need to find a way forward that helps Kai to feel loved and wanted while also giving him some boundaries that will help him to feel safe and to learn respect for you as his parents. It sounds like we're all on the same page.

TIME FOR REFLECTION

We invite you to reflect on how this conversation has gone.

- Do you think the parents are both ready to explore DDP-informed parenting together?
- Will Esther be able to take the conversation forward without either parent feeling undermined?
- What obstacles can you see that might need to be navigated?
- How would you continue to explore Cassidy's worries about her father and Kai?

A parenting session will often focus on the child who is being experienced as most challenging in the moment.

- How will you ensure that Abigail's needs are not overlooked as you continue supporting these parents?

DDP is a model that encourages the therapist in the use of self, drawing upon their own experiences, feelings, and personality to enhance the interventions. Therefore within DDP there is a different view of thoughtful self-disclosure than in some other models.

- If you were Esther's DDP supervisor, how might you help Esther to reflect on what she might feel comfortable sharing about herself?
- What are the pros and cons of Esther telling these parents she is bisexual and is raising an adolescent boy?

PSYCHOLOGICAL, PARENTAL, AND SOCIETAL INFLUENCES ON PARENTING

In this example, a helpful understanding of Erin's and Cassidy's parenting can be gained from taking a psychological perspective; that is, considering how their parenting is influenced by their own experience of being parented. Erin's family is high achieving and behaviorally focused. Love is plentiful but so is good behavior. This may have influenced Erin to be a parent who focuses more on behavior than the inner life of her children. Cassidy experienced parental neglect, where self-reliance was the only option. Cassidy may have developed to be a parent who avoids conflict so that her children don't experience her as harsh and indifferent, like her parents.

We might also consider the wider cultural impacts on Erin and Cassidy. Erin's parenting fits with a sociocentric society, more typically seen in non-Western countries. Interdependence is valued, leading to parenting that values children assuming responsibility, showing obedience and fitting in with the social group. Cassidy, although impacted by neglect, seems to have values and needs that fit with a Western, individualistic society, where independence and self-reliance are valued and children are encouraged to follow their own path.

These formulations are neither right nor wrong, but each offer themes that the DDP practitioner can explore with the parents, cocreating a unique story about them as parents and the many influences on them.

There are layers of influence on all of us as we grow and develop. The DDP practitioner can hold these different layers in mind both for their clients and for themselves. Exploring psychological, parental, and societal influences can enrich how we adapt our practice to the needs of the family.

TIME FOR REFLECTION

At the end of this chapter is a summary table of differences between sociocentric and individualistic societies (Worksheet 7.2).

1. Which of these societies most closely matches the society that you grew up within?
2. How might parenting approaches reflect these different societies?
3. Think about the ways DDP practitioners might need to adjust their interventions to align with the different worldviews reflected in these different societies.

SLOWING DOWN IN PARENTING SUPPORT

If we are going to help parents to adopt a DDP-informed approach, we need to slow down during our parent support interventions. Parenting-support-in-the-moment is based on a parenting in the moment model developed by Kim (Golding, 2017a, p. 188). You will see that this models less immediate focus on problem-solving and advice giving than other approaches to parenting support. (See summary in Figure 7.4 and Worksheet 7.3 at the end of the chapter.)

This process of parenting support starts by exploring the parent's experience before helping the parent to understand and connect emotionally with the experience of the child. This precedes deciding how to provide behavior support. The focus is on making sense of the behavior and how it has been triggered by the child's underlying experience. This often involves reflecting on the child's past, as well as current, experience. The parent, having experienced this process with regard to their own past experience, is likely to understand the relevance of this for their child and thus will be comfortable engaging with this exploration. This will then increase understanding and empathy toward the child.

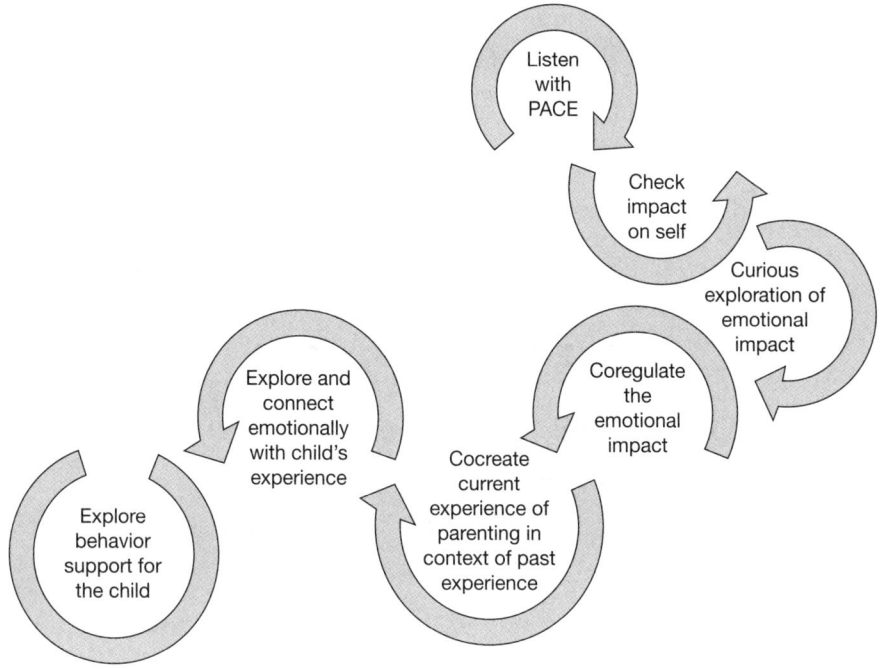

Figure 7.4 Summary of DDP-Informed
Parenting Support

Still, the parent needs to manage the day-to-day impact of the child's behavior and to support the child to develop prosocial behaviors. The usual starting point for parent support interventions has been reached via a longer, richer route. This often shifts the parent from a coercive style of managing behavior to a collaborative support style that maintains emotional connection. The child is supported to manage natural consequences and to repair relationships. The parent will also become more alert to times when consequences aren't needed; times when the child will benefit from more regulatory support or closer supervision.

CARING FOR THE CAREGIVER—EXAMPLE:[6]

This dialogue provides an example of a conversation between a parent and DDP practitioner. The whole session is likely to take around one and a half hours, thus this provides just a glimpse of the process.

TIME FOR REFLECTION

As you read through this example, reflect on what feels different from more traditional parent support.

Notice how the sequence in the parenting-support-in-the-moment model is followed.

What defenses do you think Monica is experiencing?

What empathy does she discover for herself and for her son?

Monica is an adopter, meeting with the practitioner for a support session. Monica and her partner, Zack, are parenting two boys, aged nine and 10 years. The older boy, Aaron, is causing them most challenge with his generally oppositional behavior: lying, stealing, and resisting their nurturing. This session focuses on him.

Practitioner: Hi Monica, you're looking tired. Tough week?

Monica: Oh, you know, same old, same old. Aaron is up to his usual tricks.

Practitioner: It's a bit unrelenting, isn't it? How are you feeling this week?

---

6   This example appears in the DDP Level One training supplementary materials for trainers, p. 15 © 2020, DDPI.

Monica: Well, it's just he never changes, whatever we do. He stole again this week. I was stupid, I left my purse out. The twenty quid went of course. Will I never learn?

Practitioner: That sounds frustrating. It's tough when you can't put your purse down without thinking about it.

Monica: I think something is going on at school. He won't talk about it of course, but I've a feeling he's struggling with his friends again. Not surprising, he's so bossy with them. They'll only take so much.

Practitioner: And then he won't talk to you either. I guess that's hurtful.

Monica: Well, we've tried rewards. he seems happy to earn points, but as soon as he gets the reward, it is back to usual. Punishments don't work either. We took his iPad away. He didn't seem to care. Nothing seems to work. I just feel out of ideas.

Practitioner: So, he's lying and stealing; friendships are tricky; and whatever you do, nothing seems to work. On top of that, he doesn't want to talk to you. It must be hard to feel you are making any difference.

Monica: Yes, as I said, same old. There are glimpses of a lovely boy underneath, but honestly, it's hard to see this most of the time.

Practitioner: Monica, I want to slow you down a bit. You know what I'm like! (*Monica laughs.*) I've noticed that whenever I ask about how you are feeling you talk about Aaron. Is it hard to think about you in this?

Monica: (*laughing*) I'm doing it again aren't I? I know you will stop me though. It's just so hard to think about. Painful as well, I guess. Go on, do your worst.

Practitioner: Aaron is tough; he's resisting all the good parenting you have to offer. It's hard to have good moments with him. I'm guessing that has to hurt.

Monica: He's a lovely lad. I can see that. And he's had a tough time . . .

Practitioner: (*touching Monica on the arm*) But it has to hurt. Let's think about you now.

Monica: (*thoughtfully*) Well, yes. It does hurt. (*tears come to her eyes*) It's so hard!

Practitioner: I can see your tears. So hard. What do you think is the hardest thing about parenting Aaron?

Monica: (*brushing tears away*) I don't know. I just see what he could be, I guess.

Practitioner: And you aren't able to help him be this child, are you? How does that feel?

Monica: (*more animated*) Pretty useless. He just doesn't respond to anything.

Practitioner: (*also animated*) Yes, he makes it so hard for you. (*quieting*) And does that make you feel like a failure.

Monica: (*tears come again*) Yes, that's it. I just feel like I'm letting him down. I'm failing him because nothing ever changes. I dread to think where he'll end up—prison like his birth father, I guess.

Practitioner: Such a big fear, and I'm guessing you would think it was your fault?

Monica: Well, yes. I said I would take him on. What's the point of adopting him if we can't make a difference?

Practitioner: That sounds like a big worry. What's it all for if you can't make a difference? I would like to stay with these feelings for a bit longer if it's OK with you. (*Monica nods.*) I am wondering if, perhaps guessing that, Aaron isn't the first person who has made you feel like a failure.

Monica: (*thinking hard*) Well, I've been lucky. Zack is great; we have a great relationship. My birth kids have done well. I have lots to feel good about.

Practitioner: What about before you married, anyone then? (*tears spring to Monica's eyes*) I'm guessing you have felt like this before.

Monica: I had an aunt. We were very close, but she died. I was about ten. She lived a couple of streets away. I visited her every day on my way home from school. As she got sicker, I would cook her stuff, try to get her to eat. Then one day my Mom met me from school and told me she was in the hospital. I never saw her again. They wouldn't let me visit.

Practitioner: Oh, Monica, how sad. So, you never got to say goodbye?

Monica: She was only 18. Everyone said how clever she was, all the great things she should have done in life. For the longest time, I thought it was my fault. If only I could have gotten her to eat, maybe she would have got better. Last year, not long before she died, my Mom told me what was wrong with my aunt—cancer. I hadn't known.

Practitioner: So, for all those years, you thought that you hadn't looked after her well enough. What a big burden to have carried all that time.

Monica: I didn't think about it as I got older. I got on with my life. Met Zack, had the kids; but yes, I guess somewhere it was still there, nagging away.

Practitioner: As I'm listening to you, I'm thinking about your feelings about Aaron. They're making a lot of sense to me now. Those big fears about failing him. I'm guessing they're even bigger for you because of what happened with your aunt. I wonder if somewhere deep inside you have a sense that you have to get things right with Aaron, because it feels like you didn't with your aunt?

Monica: Well, I don't worry that Aaron might die, but when you say it like that it makes some sense. I haven't really thought about my aunt for years, but she has always been there in the background. I do worry about Aaron's future, and maybe it's more important to me because my aunt lost her future. It kind of makes sense, but I'm still not getting anywhere with Aaron. I'm not sure how this will help with that.

Practitioner: I wonder if it's extra hard when Aaron doesn't respond because it's taking you back to the past. It's hard to wonder what is going on for Aaron when you're becoming preoccupied with the sense of failure you feel. You may not have understood what was being triggered for you, but the feelings are very real.

Monica: It's strange, I feel a bit lighter somehow, like maybe there is some hope. How odd, we've hardly even talked about Aaron, and nothing has changed there. I've been so desperate to stop all his behaviors, maybe I've lost sight of something.

Practitioner: Any sense of what?

Monica: Well, why does he need to steal, for a start, and what makes it so hard for him to talk to me?

Practitioner: Those are great questions. I can see you're really trying to understand Aaron. What does he do with the money he steals? That seems a good place to start. He buys lots of sweets, doesn't he?

Monica: Yes, and then he tries to buy his friends with it. Of course, it links to how he's feeling doesn't it? He doesn't believe people will like him for who he is. Maybe that's why he doesn't want to talk to me as well.

Practitioner: I wonder how you could let Aaron know that you get this. Like, when he's stolen, or fallen out with friends. Do you think you could help him to know you understand how bad he's feeling?

Monica: Yes, I could. But I've just focused on what he's done wrong, or what he could do differently. I don't think I've ever told him I understand how hard all this is for him. I can certainly do that.

Practitioner: You might need to be a bit patient. I think this will feel a bit strange to him. Give him time, and if you feel a bit despairing let me know, we can think about it together.

Monica: Yes, you're right, I can imagine being impatient to see change, but I understand that better now. What should I do when he steals though? I can't just let him get away with it.

Practitioner: No, of course not, but you might be surprised how Aaron feels when he starts to tolerate your acceptance. You might find he's feeling pretty bad about it.

Monica: And then I punish him, just making him feel worse. But I've tried rewards as well. Wouldn't that make him feel better?

Practitioner: Rewards can be tricky. They can lead to feeling more pressure to get things right. Then when he messes up, he'll just feel like he's letting you down, more evidence that he's the bad kid he fears he is.

Monica: Well, if I can't punish and I can't reward, what is left?

Practitioner: I do think he'll be helped with consequences, but they need to help him to feel better about himself, such as consequences that help him repair the relationships. In fact, if you can think about this with him, once he's feeling understood, he'll probably have all sorts of ideas about what he can do. You can figure it out together.

Monica: That feels good, and it feels more focused on him. I see that now. I've just been trying to get him to stop stealing, kind of to make me feel better, so I can see some progress. When there isn't any progress, I just want to pile on the punishments, make him behave. Now I see that it needs to be more about him, doesn't it?

Practitioner: Your motivations are really good, but yes, I don't think you will be able to punish him into being good.

Monica: Thank you, I really think this might be a way forward, but I mustn't rush it. I need you to help me take it one step at a time.

Practitioner: Sure, we can figure this out together too. You're still going to have plenty of strong feelings evoked by Aaron and his behaviors. It's one step at a time for all of us, isn't it?

CONCLUSION

DDP-informed parenting interventions represent a slowing down during support. The practitioner emotionally connects with the parent's experience before focusing on the child's emotional world. This then informs behavior support.

Worksheet 7.1

 Reflective Exercise:
DDP and Safeguarding

In the first circle list the DDP principles and in the second circle the tasks needed to follow the safeguarding process. Now reflect on how you would bring these two circles together so that the safeguarding tasks are accomplished using the DDP principles.

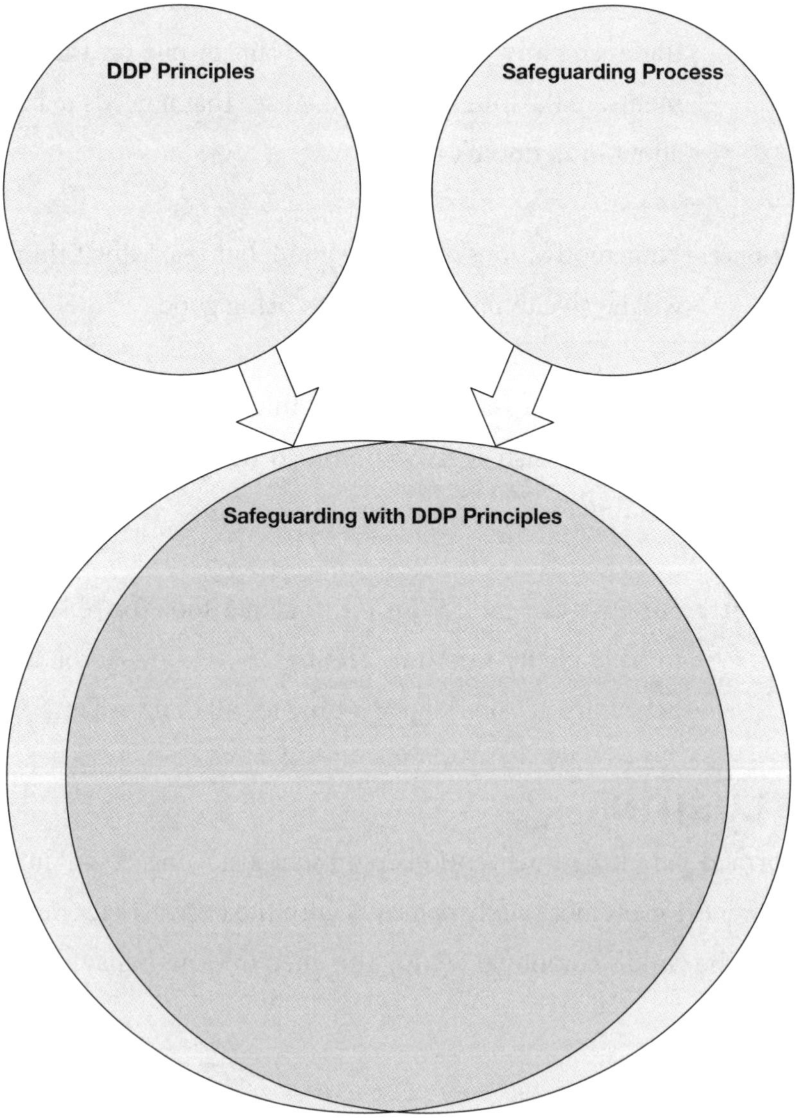

DDP Principles

Safeguarding Process

Safeguarding with DDP Principles

Reflections on Worksheet 7.1: Possible Responses

DDP Principles

Safe
Relational
Open and engaged
PACE
AR dialogue
Cocreate via storytelling
Coregulate
Relationship repair

Safeguarding Process

Act within legal framework
Investigate and interview
Assess risk
Partnership across agencies
Share information
Record
Decide on future actions
Monitor and review

Safeguarding with DDP Principles

Safe: Take immediate action within legal framework to ensure safety of everyone involved.

Relational: Clear boundaries conveyed nonjudgementally; maintain dignity of those involved.

Self-regulate to remain open and engaged within all relationships involved.

Stay curoius and support emotional experience of the other through coregulation.

PACE: Listen with acceptance and empathy while being clear about the issues of concern.

Communicate clearly and PACEfully with family and professionals involved.

AR dialogue: Remain supportive of affective experience while gaining and giving information needed.

Cocreate via storytelling: Listen to everyone's narrative, build a shared story of issues, potential solutions, and actions.

Relationship repair: Attend to ruptures and offer repair.

Worksheet 7.2

Differences Between Individualistic and Sociocentric Societies

This table presents generalizations, which inevitably miss the complexity of the individuals described, of two broad cultural categories. There are many differences between and within cultures that need to be considered when working with families.

(Sources: Keller, 2022; Lancy, 2017; Harwood et al., 1995)

Individualistic	Sociocentric
Independence, self-reliance, and autonomy are valued; children encouraged to follow their own path	Interdependence and relatedness are valued; children encouraged to be responsible and obedient to fit in with the social group
Nuclear family households	Large extended-family households
Primary attachment figure supported by secondary attachment figures	Multiple caregivers, including peers and siblings
Sensitivity expressed by responding to distress signaled by infant through crying; parent reacts to explicit signals from infant	Sensitivity expressed by anticipating needs and minimizing expressions of distress in infant; parents engage in high level of emotional closeness to anticipate child's needs

Individualistic	Sociocentric
Security of child through balance between autonomy and relatedness	Security of child through learning proper, contextually appropriate demeanor
Competence equated to children's ability to explore, self-express, and regulate affect	Autonomy, self-expression, and affect regulation are important only to supporting social cohesion and connectedness
Dyadic parent–child communication	Complex polyadic networks (several communication partners at the same time)
Emotion viewed as force that can enhance the self or hinder its completion	Emotion viewed as leading to behaviors that can strengthen or threaten the well-being of others
Children have high status: granted personal space; have access to toys; and learn through teaching	Children have low status: live in communal space; play with found objects, such as tools and utensils; and learn through observation
Focus on children's agency and mental states, preferences, wishes, and needs	Focus on social context, moral obligations, and respect

Individualistic	Sociocentric
Autonomy is linked to self-maximization; goals for children are unique and expressive	Autonomy is linked to independence without the guidance of parents; goals for children are that they belong and maintain harmony

Worksheet 7.3

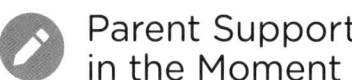

Parent Support in the Moment

1. Listen with PACE: Connect and explore how things currently are

Curiously explore the parent's immediate experience of parenting the child. Hear the worries and frustration the parent is holding. Provide time for the parent to offload and feel heard. Accept expressions of anger, frustration, or despair about the support being offered.

2. Impact on self: Check response to parent

Check in with yourself: Am I regulated; can I stay open and engaged? Am I becoming irritated, angry, defensive? Do I feel pressure to fix? Can I be compassionate to myself while staying open to understanding the parent's experience?

3. Curious exploration

Explore the emotional impact the child is having on the parent. Notice feelings of pain, hopelessness, and failure. Meet any defensive responses with PACE.

4. Coregulate the emotional impact of this exploration

Acceptance and empathy provide coregulation of experiences, such as shame, anger, fear, and despair, that are evoked by this exploration.

5. Cocreate: Explore the current experience of parenting in the context of past relationship experience

Identify "hot spots"—points of greatest vulnerability. Explore whether the parent has felt like this before. Notice when past experience is impacting the present. This includes attachment history. Discover the stories together. New meanings of current feelings and behavior in relation to child are cocreated.

6. Explore the child's experience and connect emotionally with this

Curiously explore child's current presentation and understand this in relation to past and current experiences. Help the parent to connect emotionally with the child's experience. Cocreate new meanings of the child's behavior, and increasing feelings of empathy.

7. Explore behavior support for the child

Think together about how to emotionally connect with the child, how to offer connection even when it is being rejected, and how to build on this connection to support the child's behavior. This includes exploring discipline, consequences, structure, and supervision.

IN CONVERSATION FOUR

Tena koutou katoa.

I greet you all with a traditional welcome.

Ko Murimotu toku maunga.

*Murimotu is the name of the mountain that connects me back to the land
that I am a descendant of.*

Ko Aotea toku waka.

Aotea is the name of the ancestral canoe.

Ko Whangaehu toku awa.

*Whangaehu is the name of the sacred river used by my ancestors to
nourish and heal.*

Ko te Ati Haunui a Paparangi toku iwi.

Te Atihaunui a Paparangi is the name of my tribe.

Ko Ngati Rangi toku hapu.

Ngati Rangi is the name of my subtribe.

Ko Lorraine Wiersma toku ingoa.

My name is Lorraine Wiersma.

Ko Ella raua ko A. F. toku tamahine.

Ella and A. F. are my daughters.

No reira, tena koutou, tena koutou, tena tatou katoa.

Greetings again. Now we are all one.

Kim met with Lorraine to talk about her experience participating in the Nurturing Attachments and Foundations for Attachment groupwork programs, delivered by Sally and Rob in New Zealand.

Kim:	Hello Lorraine, thank you for meeting with me. I'm looking forward to hearing about your experience of participating in the groupwork programs. Can you tell me a little bit about yourself?
Lorraine:	I am 62, both my parents have passed, and I am daughter number five in a family of eight children, two boys and six girls. I have two children, one of whom I have fostered for nearly five years, I'll call her A.F. I stumbled into fostering; I was supporting a friend to find her birth parents and sitting in on the social worker interview. We got to talking and sharing and I mentioned that I worked in the disability sector and that I had an 18-year-old daughter, Ella, who has cerebral palsy with high, complex health and communication needs. They asked if I had thought about fostering and invited me to an information evening. I've got to say, it wasn't something that had appealed to me, not ever; but I got to thinking over the next few days, "What happens to

kids who come into care already carrying diagnostic labels that are attached to their behaviors, thinking, processing, and learning? Kids who use wheelchairs or have high medical needs?" I thought about the complexity of caring for children with so many layers of need. What would Ella's life be like if she was in care? That thought alone got me to the info night, where I agreed to go through the training to become a foster carer with the proviso that children with disabilities would be my priority. As it turned out, the social workers had a child in mind for me, a very vulnerable child who had been bounced around the system for all of her six years. She was a little bitty thing, nonverbal, with a lot of attachment, trauma, and abuse issues. We lost our hearts to her immediately. It's been four years, four really hard, life-changing years, during which this child has given me opportunities to be the best I can be and has shown me sides of myself that I never knew existed. She has brought such joy to our household, a spark of wildness that Ella really enjoys; it's a totally different dynamic from just being Ella, her Dad, and I. Ella has the opportunity to be a big sister and A.F. is able to have the role of the little sister.

Kim: And is your foster daughter from an Indigenous background as well?

Lorraine: A.F. *whakapapas* [traces her genes] back to Samoa. Historically, here in New Zealand there hasn't been a lot of matching up of cultures within the foster care system. I *whakapapa* to Māori and Dutch bloodlines. This was not empathetic to a Samoan child. I have to outsource, if you like, [to meet] those needs to give her that cultural sense of belonging; for example, her language, her history, her being around people that look like her.

Kim: Yes, I see. And thinking about you engaging in the groupwork, what was the cultural mix in the groups you participated in?

Lorraine: There was a South African woman, myself, being Māori, and the rest were New Zealand European. As we made our way through the course, I realized that there were actually many non-Māori caring for Māori children. I found that really challenging. The carers would talk about the children in their care doing or saying certain things that I, being able to see through a Māori lens, could relate to but they thought these things were "weird," one carer actually said that. They would strongly discourage the children doing or saying these things because they saw it as strange.

Kim: Can you give me an example?

Lorraine: Well, the children would call the female adults in the house "*whaea.*" It means aunty, even though they're not related. It's meant as a term of respect. This particular carer, who has three Māori children in his care, was kind of making fun of it within the group, saying "You won't believe it, they call everyone "aunty" and they're not even related!" I said, "Yes, that's what we do," and he said, "Well we don't."

Kim: Really insensitive.

Lorraine: There are a lot of New Zealanders who feel we should all be one. The "one" being New Zealand European. Their traditions, family etiquette, politics, values, etc. They want to wipe out any history these children have with their families because of their belief that they are bad, that they are related to gangs and will never overcome their dysfunctions. I think some carers want to scrub the children's memories of their birth families and start again.

Kim: That is very distressing. I can imagine that made being a part of the group quite challenging for you. I'm also wondering about your experience of the program itself. What fit, what didn't fit, how could it fit better? I wrote that program through my own lens of being white and British. I know Sally and Rob gave some thought to how that would best be applied to the Māori community, but I expect there is a lot that we could have done differently.

Lorraine: When Sally first approached me to talk with you, I thought, did it make a difference that I was Māori? I know that the course resonated with me right from the start. It challenged me to reflect on my parenting skills, where I got them from, how I was raised, the impact all the pivotal people had on me as I grew; I found it fascinating! The fact that we weren't just reading endless facts out of books, that it was so personal, made it easy to connect to. Often, a lot of our group time was spent supporting each other as we unpacked issues from our own childhoods or an experience we were having with a child in our care [that] was triggering us. There was some really intense learning at times, but Sally and Rob held a safe space for us all. Fostering is hard, and sharing those stories with each other, especially the ones where we felt like we couldn't do it anymore, was very affirming. I think being able to be vulnerable in the group and cry over a perceived failure or even over a massive shift in your learning was a huge part of the learning for many of us. Māori generally don't have a problem showing emotion and, again, Sally and Rob holding that space for us to do that was very important. I have quotes and passages from the course notes stuck up all over my house, but especially outside A.F.'s door, to remind me to not go charging in there, to take a breath, to reset.

Kim: So, the whole idea of slowing down in your parenting, which is a big part of the program.

Lorraine: For sure, it still amazes me what a difference it makes when I just sit beside her and she sees me calming myself. Sometimes she giggles at me, but if she's really angry, I can see her at least stop escalating. I'm almost like a distraction. Then I'll say something like: "Do we need some more calming time? I think I'm good now, you?" She usually says: "I not finished angry." Then I'll ask her what we should do next. Have chocolate is often the response. I've used and gotten some great results using some of the less confrontational deescalating techniques with different systems as well, like with the school principal. I've "wondered" why the behavior plan wasn't adhered to in an instance where A.F. was suspended. The old me would have just been raging at the injustice of it all and been thought of as out of control.

Kim: I was thinking, as you were talking, about the whole idea of community and healing within your community and how important that is to First Nations people. I think we Western people lack this. We can be insular. It sounds like Rob and Sally were able to create a sense of community for the group so that you could come together, whether for healing or increasing your self-awareness, and then link that back to parenting and how you parent children.

Lorraine: Absolutely! Self-awareness is key. So many aha moments for me throughout the course, usually around things my parents did and now why I do them or did do them. It's interesting to notice that when I get stressed, I revert to punitive measures. Once I calm down, I think it through from a PACE perspective and I'm able to be kind to myself and also do some relationship mending with A.F. So many things in the world have changed, so it's great to be able to parent in a way that is relevant now and will be well into the future as well. This way of parenting comes from a totally different place, so unlike my parent's style of parenting, which wasn't bad, but it was fairly heavy on rules, and with eight kids, there wasn't a lot of time for any individuality. I don't think it works for children now.

Kim: And was it important that Sally and Rob understood Indigenous culture?

Lorraine: Certainly, it was important that they had a broad lens around the effects of colonization and a general idea around why Māori [are] represent[ed] so highly in the foster system. I feel it would have been very unsafe for me otherwise. They were able to cool things down when they got a bit heated without making anyone feel like they were in the wrong. A couple of years ago over here, the authorities were removing babies straight out of the maternity ward from young Māori mothers. Some people in the group believed this was the right thing to do. Rob dealt with that by talking about the incorrect processes, not systems blaming as such, which I thought was very diplomatic.

Kim: That's so important, isn't it? That the facilitators were able to be sensitive to that and manage it in a way that maintained safety.

Lorraine: Yes, particularly when these people have Māori children in their care and have to build a relationship with their families.

Kim: I was thinking about the risk of you feeling so isolated in that group, as the only Māori carer there.

Lorraine: Well, I guess I might have felt like that if Rob and Sally hadn't been as good at their job as they were! I felt well supported, never unsafe.

Kim: Yes, the importance of the facilitators. That is key, isn't it?

Lorraine: I did wonder, during the group sessions, what a Māori facilitator for Māori families would feel like. I'm not sure that would be a good idea either. How would the non- Māori foster carers feel if Rob and Sally were Māori? I wonder if they would have engaged in the same way. Colonization can be hugely triggering for Māori, that would be another layer they would have to deal with.

Kim:	I guess it would, again, depend on that person and their openness to non-Indigenous as well as to Indigenous cultures. A Māori facilitator might well do that really skillfully, or might not, just like a non-Indigenous facilitator.
Lorraine:	Yes, perhaps.
Kim:	And your foster daughter and her disability? It sounds like you found the group helpful through that lens as well.
Lorraine:	It was really helpful because we discussed a lot about nonverbal behaviors. Her speech is limited. I have to be really mindful and not jump to conclusions. I learnt to let scenarios roll out and not make any judgements around them. I learned to recognize the signs that her anxiety was rising. She asks me: "This my home? You my Mom? Ella my sister? Hector my Dad?" I found that talking about her role within our family regularly throughout the day settles her. "Can you get your sisters blanket?"; "I wonder what Dads bringing home for dinner?"; "The littlest sister gets to choose first"; "Come here my bubba." The importance of speaking about her role, the importance of it is huge. All these conversations build up a story around who she is in our family.
Kim:	It gives her a sense of belonging. And as I'm listening to you, I'm thinking about her limited ability to communicate. You hold curiosity for her. You need to do that without making assumptions, but you have to make some guesses because she can't speak everything she thinks and feels.

Lorraine: Yes, we'll put out some sentences, not judgements, open ended sentences: "Do you think?" or "maybe . . ." Usually it's around what she perceived as an attack on her that she has responded to prematurely and aggressively. Later on, if we reacted curiously instead of punitively, she would come and be open to a chat and be curious back. Often she says: "Mom, I not know."

Kim: Within her limitations, you help her to be curious. Within DPP, we call that wondering from a not-knowing stance. You are tentative, so that she is free to express her comfort or discomfort with your ideas.

Lorraine: Yes, that works for me because I don't want to put ideas into her head about why she feels what she feels. This way of being also helps me connect and work through things with the birth mom as well. As a foster parent, I was told lots of things about A.F. and her birth mom—things that weren't true. They were judgements that could have been cleared up if at least one social worker, along a long line of social workers, had worked with more playfulness, acceptance, curiosity, and empathy. There is a saying in Māoridom: "What is the most important thing? It is people, it is people, it is people." PACE helps us connect and get to the heart of each other.

Kim: That's beautiful. So, anything else that you feel is important?

Lorraine: I did think about the risk of recolonization by taking the ideas of the program on board. If it doesn't come from our history, if it doesn't come from our knowledge, is it recolonizing [me] or even the children in my care? The course felt right for me, like in an intuitive way. It felt like personal growth, which then impacts my family, which then spreads out to my community.

Kim: I'm interested in exploring concern about recolonization. I'm thinking about choice and freedom. Cultures will grow and develop, and you as a Māori carer might embrace some parenting ideas that are non-Māori, but you have a choice about that. It has to fit. I guess, colonization is about them being inflicted on you and taking away your own heritage.

Lorraine: That's true, but I liken cultural identity and the impact on the life of someone who has had that identity taken from them to an amputated limb that has been reattached even if the limb works through systematically reprograming it, it will never be the same. Its journey has taken a different turn. There is no going back but moving forward. I am mindful of what my parents and my grandparents went through, and so I question, and I seek the best of both worlds, often finding common ground. Sir Mason Durie and his model of well-being, 'te whare tapa wha' likens us to the four posts of a house. All four posts—spiritual, emotional, physical, and family—must be cared for to support Maori health.. If all of these posts aren't solid and looked after, the whole house is going to fall down. I also saw these teachings in the PACE course.

Kim: That is so interesting. I have developed the house model of parenting. There's a nice link there. Thinking about the four posts, I just wonder if there is enough around the spirituality post within the program. That is something that we could learn about from Māori thinking.

Lorraine: I have observed that for some people, religion is a manifestation of their spiritual self. For me it's about my whole self being seen; all the experiences in my life have made me into who I am in this moment; I am more than just my physical body. As a Māori person, my belief is that I am related to the earth, that I come from the earth, that I will return to the earth. *Ko Murimotu te maunga, Murimotu* is the name of the mountain that connects me back to the land that I am a descendant of.

Kim: That's a beautiful point on which to end. Thank you so much; it has been lovely talking to you and learning from your experience.

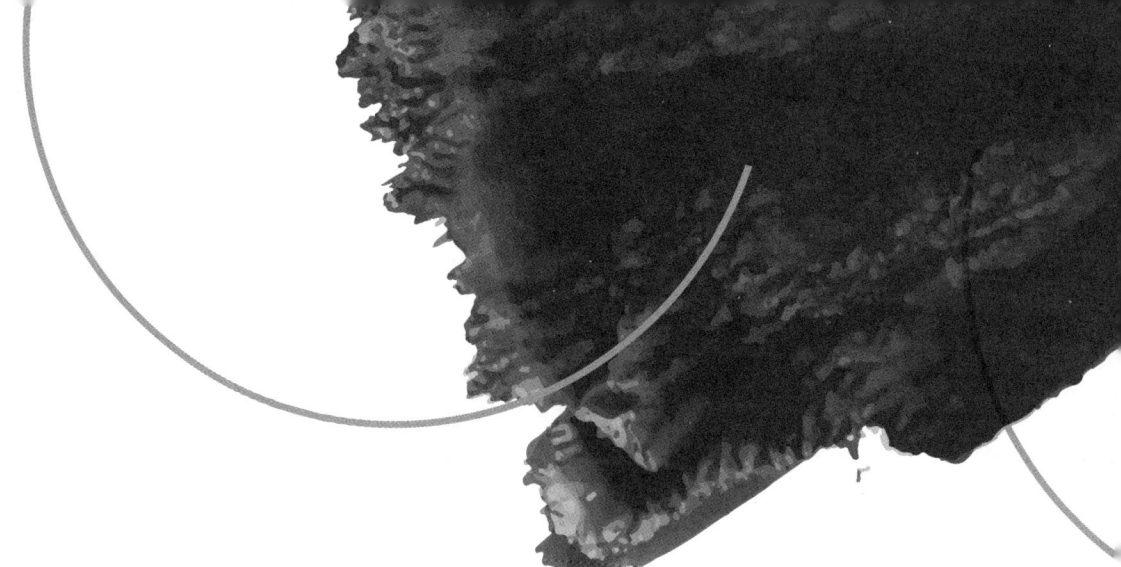

Chapter 8:
Providing Safe Settings: Dyadic Developmental Practice

Children who have experienced developmental trauma and disrupted attachments, whether or not therapy is provided, often require a range of services in social care, child mental health, education, and residential care. The delivery of these services, fully integrated with the principles and interventions of dyadic developmental psychotherapy (DDP)—attachment focused, trauma informed, developmental, and systemic is known as dyadic developmental practice. (Hughes et al., 2019, p. 153)

REFRESHER

Dyadic developmental practice expands the focus of DDP interventions beyond the child and family to also encompass communities, networks, schools, and organizations. Psychotherapy with the child is supported by DDP-informed parenting. Further support arises when DDP also informs the teams and systems surrounding the child and family. Interventions at all these levels need to consider the interconnections of identity with the early experiences of developmental trauma, separation, and loss.

In the practice model (Figure 8.1), we attend to the importance of understanding developmental trauma within context. This means reflecting on the impact of developmental trauma as it interconnects with the experience, culture, and identity of the child, family, and the practitioners offering the support. A simple diagram does not capture the complexity of meaning and uniqueness behind the words and labels and would therefore be in danger of being reductionist. However, we wanted to highlight the importance of understanding developmental trauma within a wider context, which impacts all of us. This includes the intersection of developmental trauma with the experience, sometimes traumatic, of growing up in a marginalized group. This includes differences because of gender, sexuality, class, race, religion, neurodiversity, or physical or mental disability. Knowing ourselves and those we are supporting is an important part of dyadic developmental practice.

To work with a child and family successfully, it is important that we understand *context*. We are interested in learning about the *culture, identity*, and *experience* that impacts them, as described below. This also includes the family history and background, education, professional training, family composition, and lifestyle of the individual. Each individual has their own world, journey, and story. To varying degrees, they experience a sense of belonging or not belonging and varying levels of stability or instability. Traumas, complex traumas (e.g., war, pandemic), and developmental traumas also contribute to this context.

- Culture is the family and community we grow up within. This encompasses the characteristics and knowledge of a group of people, including customs, values, social behavior, religious beliefs, cuisine, music, and arts.
- Identity encompasses those influences that have informed the development of the individual, including race, sexuality, sexual orientation, gender, religion, class, language, physical and mental health, neurodiversity, ability, and disability.

- This all influences the experience of the individual throughout their lifetime.

Understanding these experiences will be an important part of DDP interventions. This is where identity and culture intersect, and we need to be aware of the power and influence an individual holds alongside the degree of marginalization that they experience. This applies equally to us and to the practitioners and families we are working with.

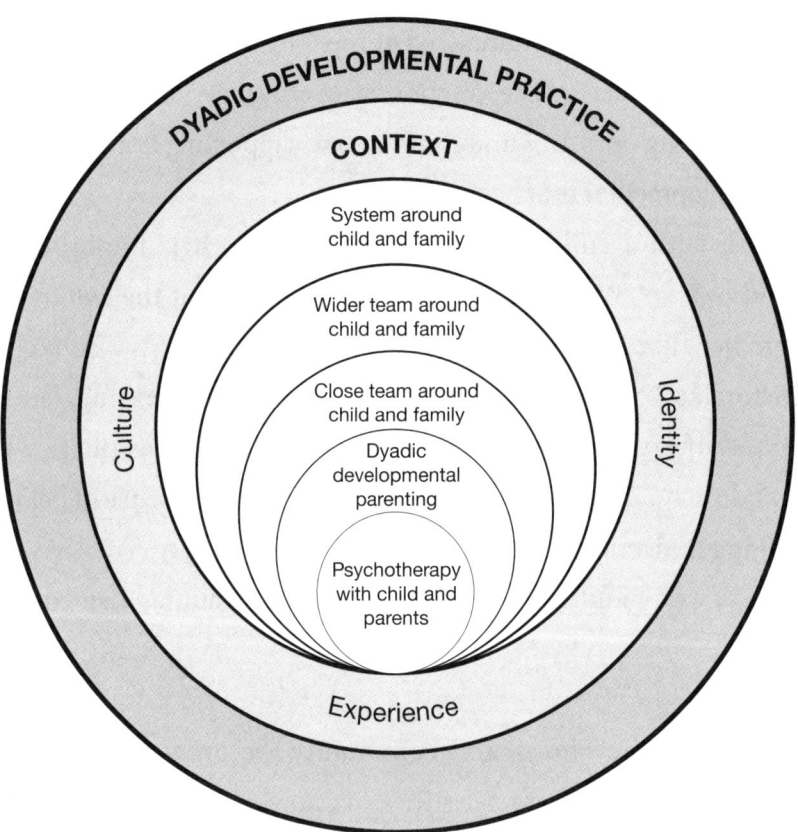

Figure 8.1 Dyadic Developmental Practice Model

Through the expansion of DDP into a practice model, children and families can receive help, support, and a range of services, all informed by a relational, attachment-focused approach. This approach understands and attempts to mitigate the impact of developmental trauma.

When people come into connection, as in DDP interventions, the context, culture, identity, and experience of all those coming together interconnect. The DDP practitioner has a responsibility to consider these interconnections, including their own, and use them to inform the interventions being provided.

When DDP-informed thinking and support are present throughout services, the support is more likely to be joined up and therefore more cohesive If the child can go to school in an environment that facilitates DDP practice, they are more likely to have their trauma needs understood and thus to feel safe and secure enough to learn.

Trauma impacts the child, the family, and the practitioners working with them. This commonly leads to the spread of defensive responding through the environments around the traumatized child.

For example, trauma encourages splitting; individuals within the network find it hard to hold on to or integrate opposing or contradictory thoughts, feelings, and beliefs. This means that self and others are seen as either good or bad. This splitting process spills through the network, producing high levels of shame. Individuals within the network then experience a sense of failure. They defend against this by seeking a source of failure elsewhere, which can increase the conflict.

- Teachers wonder about parental practice.
- Parents blame therapists.
- Social workers are seen as not intervening quickly enough or as intervening too quickly.
- The psychiatrist is seen as withholding treatment.

In these situations, the system becomes reactive rather than reflective, and disconnected rather than integrated.

Within DDP practice, all members of the network are held in mind. From an open and engaged stance, the DDP practitioner provides support, space, and time for reflection. This can be done through consultation with networks, organizations, and staff teams, through training, and via individual or group support.

Dyadic developmental practice relies on the DDP principles. These principles help the practitioner to offer coregulation as needed and to form connections with others through the attitude of PACE. Relationship ruptures are quickly repaired, while the AR conversations allow perspectives to be understood both at the cognitive and the emotional level. As individual narratives are shared, joint narratives can emerge, bringing a new perspective onto what can often feel like a stuck situation. A way forward that holds in mind the child's emotional world, often glimpsed through the behaviors being displayed, is then agreed upon.

In this chapter, we will explore dyadic developmental practice via consultation and school support. If you would like to learn more about DDP practice, there are a range of books that explore this in more depth named in the list of resources.

BRINGING NETWORKS OF PRACTITIONERS TOGETHER THROUGH CONSULTATION

Children who have experienced developmental trauma can have a range of comprehensive difficulties. These may be psychological, neurodevelopmental, or a combination of both. This can lead to a large number of services from within social care, health, and education as well as the private sector being involved with the family. Networks of practitioners are working to meet the needs of the children with varying amounts of connection between them. Collaborative work with the parents can be variable and the understanding of the child's difficulties can differ depending on the particular lens each practitioner is looking through. For example:

- A social worker may be focused on ensuring the child is living in a stable environment and managing contact with birth family.

- A teacher may be concerned about the child's attendance and engagement with the curriculum.

- A psychologist might be seeking to understand any mental health challenges in terms of the impact of past and current experience.

- A psychiatrist might be seeking a diagnosis and treatment for suspected ADHD.

- A play therapist might offer therapy to mitigate some of the impact of trauma.

The contact with all these professionals can be myriad and confusing for the parents, leaving them feeling frustrated, with a sense that their voice is not important.

Within this network of parents and practitioners, there is a wide range of knowledge and understanding about the child and about the child's experience. Individual narratives about the child can lead to useful support but pulling in different directions. Imagine the power of these stories when they are joined up. Consultation can facilitate a coordinated narrative that takes account of individual perspectives woven together to produce an integrated support plan for the child and family.

Developmentally traumatized children project powerful emotions onto those parenting and supporting them, and these emotions can become unconsciously transmitted throughout the network, organizing the way individual members respond (Sprince, 2002, 2005). Consultation can be open to this emotional layer, providing space to identify and contain the emotions. This can deepen understanding of the child's experience within the network, leading to consistent and more effective action (Dent & Golding, 2006).

To achieve this level of reflection the network needs a space that is not constrained by the agenda of statutory meetings. This reflective space brings people together to find a shared vision of the child and a way forward. While differing views are likely held, the DDP practitioner searches for common threads that can bring everyone together, leading to a coherent, shared plan for a way forward with short-, medium- and long-term goals.

With sufficient time, each individual within the network has a voice and, much as in a choir, bringing voices together can lead to the emergence of something magical. The network comes to a shared understanding and a shared vision of the way forward (Figure 8.2.).

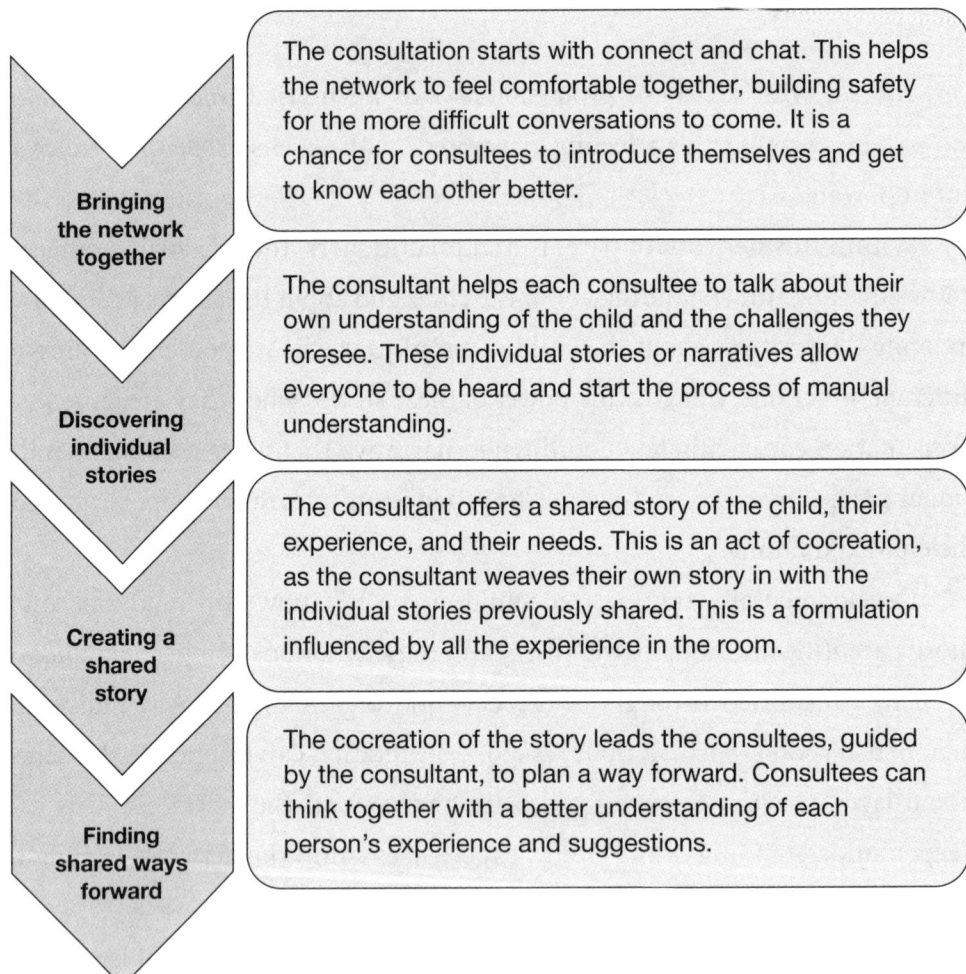

Figure 8.2 The Process of Consultation

REFLECTIVE EXERCISE 8.1: DDP PRINCIPLES WITHIN CONSULTATION

Consultation is a powerful tool for the DDP practitioner working with a network of parents and practitioners from a range of agencies. Worksheet 8.1, at the end of the chapter, provides an opportunity to explore consultation alongside a consideration of the core DDP influences and principles.

CONSULTATION—AN EXAMPLE

The focus of this consultation is twelve-year-old Mac. He has a younger sister, Ivy. The children are of Black African heritage. The children are in foster care while their mother is in the hospital for severe anxiety and depression. Mac was assigned female at birth and is now requesting boys' clothes and to be called "Mac" rather than his given name. Moira, Mac's foster carer, is keen to support him. She asks everyone at the consultation to respect this. At school, Mac is described as settled with friends and making academic progress. At home, Mac is struggling to settle and can be prone to dysregulated outbursts. He is spending a lot of time in his bedroom on his computer.

BRINGING THE NETWORK TOGETHER

Ann, the consultant, and the consultees sit around a table while drinks are distributed. This is the first time they have all met together as a network, and this is an opportunity to connect and chat. Ann introduces herself and then asks each of them to say a little bit about themselves (Figure 8.3).

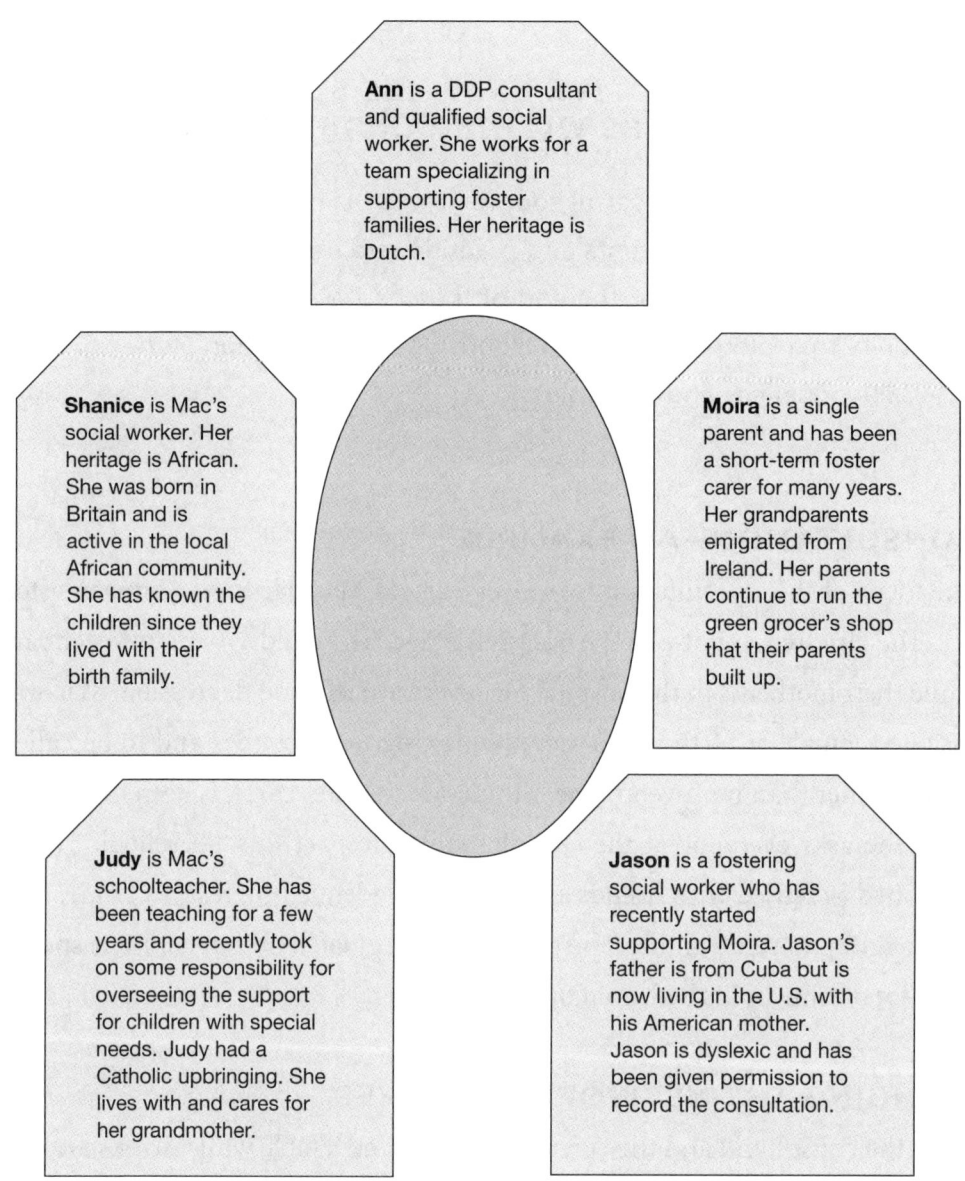

Figure 8.3 The Introductions

DISCOVERING INDIVIDUAL STORIES

Beginning with Moira, Ann invites each consultee to talk about their concerns and hopes for the consultation. Here are the individual stories that emerge:

Foster carer, Moira, is finding Mac's dysregulated outbursts increasingly difficult to manage. She has enrolled the children into after-school activities to reduce Mac's screen time and to ensure they get a range of experiences. She expresses concern that Mac is not understood in school. She feels he is "under the radar" and needs more support than he is getting. He does have friends, but the friendships rarely last, and she worries that he is struggling with reading. Moira notes that Mac rarely talks about his family and that he doesn't complain about foster care, although he frequently asks when his mom will be better. She was pleased when Mac confided his wish to be recognized as a boy and has been supporting him. Family contact is coming up, and Moira wonders whether this should be delayed while they help Mac to explore the permutations of life as a boy and help to prepare his mother and extended family for this new development in Mac's life.

Fostering social worker, Jason, is working hard to get to know Moira and the children. He is concerned that Moira views the answer to Mac's difficulties as lying solely in helping him with his identity. While this is important, Jason wonders if the impact of Mac's mother's illness and living in foster care is being missed. He would also like to see the number of after school activities reduced. Jason notes that Moira is a single carer and that the network is dominated by female practitioners. Jason wonders if he might be a helpful role model for Mac. Jason lets the network know that he is part of the LGBTQIA+ community and has experience supporting young people transitioning. Jason offers to spend time with Mac, if the network agrees. He knows of a service for young trans people and wonders if counseling might help Mac to talk about his identity, his family, and his experience of foster care.

Child's social worker, Shanice, views Mac as a resilient child who is always compliant and well-behaved when she sees him. She worries that counseling would be pathologizing Mac and would prefer him to be supported within his Black African community. She also acknowledges that gender identity adds another dimension and that not everyone within the community would accept his desire to transition. She notices the behavioral issues are at home and not school and would prefer to see Moira get more support with her parenting rather than begin counseling for Mac. She would like school to keep an eye out for bullying, worrying that Mac is already singled out for his African heritage and that the change in his clothing and name could potentially make him more of a target. She is keen for family contact to go ahead and wants to ensure that Mac is prepared for this.

School teacher, Judy, is uncertain why she has been invited to the meeting, as Mac is doing well at school. Mac is a quiet child. He has friends and is making progress academically. She acknowledges that his reading age is a little behind, but they have implemented remedial support for this. She also reports that the other children have responded well to Mac's change in name and appearance, and she is not aware of any bullying. They are a diverse school that ensures that multiracial topics are an integral part of the curriculum.

TIME FOR REFLECTION

We invite you to imagine that you are the DDP consultant. If you are in a study group, you might role play the delivery of these stories.

1. How did you respond to the stories presented in this overview?
   - Are there aspects of this consultation that you anticipate finding difficult?
   - Is there anything you might want to avoid or that you might feel sensitive about?
   - How do you think this will impact on you as the consultant?
2. Notice what you might bring to this consultation in terms of your own values, beliefs, heritage, gender, sexuality, class, and identity.

- Reflect on where this could be helpful and/or limiting.
- How will you hold this in mind while attending to the consultees?

3. Reflect on the challenge of holding each person's experience as having equal value and of facilitating discussion and exploration without judgment.

4. Focus on your response to these consultees and their individual stories.

- Who do you warm to in the room?
- Who puts you on edge?
- As you imagine this, notice what is happening within your body. Where you are experiencing tension, for example?
- Notice any thoughts, assumptions, or worries that emerge.
- Notice what might make it hard for you to stay open and engaged.
- Are there any themes you might be reluctant to explore?
- How will you take care of yourself while running this consultation?

5. Next, reflect on the stories that are being shared.

- What themes are emerging on a reflective and an affective level?
- How might you respond to these themes to lead the consultees into discussion?
- Do you foresee any obstacles?
- Who might need more PACE from you to be open and engaged?
- Where might ruptures occur?

6. Now think about your narrative about Mac.

- What story do you bring to the consultation, based on your preparatory work for the consultation?

- Notice if this might be impacted by your own attachment history, identity, and life experience.
7. Finally, what do you add to your own story about Mac when you hear the stories shared in the consultation? Think about the shared story that could emerge from this consultation.

CREATING A SHARED STORY (NARRATIVE)

Here is a possible shared story that incorporates Ann's story and the themes that emerged from the consultees.

Ann starts by voicing her thoughts about Mac as an emerging adolescent with many of the typical pressures of his age group. He also has experienced developmental trauma through the impact of his mother's illness and his subsequent move into foster care. She acknowledges the complexity of holding this experience in mind while also focusing on current needs, such as supporting Mac in school as a child at risk of experiencing racism and bullying. She notes that the school, while supporting a diverse population, remains predominantly white and with limited experience of children transitioning gender.

As Ann is pulling this story together, she is also holding in mind, without sharing with the network, her own experiences (Figure 8.4).

Whilst Ann is noticing her private reflections which she will raise in supervision, she continues to be curious with the network. She voices her curiosity about the impact of Mac's early experiences. She notes the challenges for Mac of moving into foster care, along with his worries about his mother. She invites the network to wonder how he expresses these worries and any associated distress. Ann suggests that this experience has impacted Mac's development. For example, is Mac less emotionally mature than his peers? And if so, what impact is this having on his peer relationships? She questions what defenses have developed to

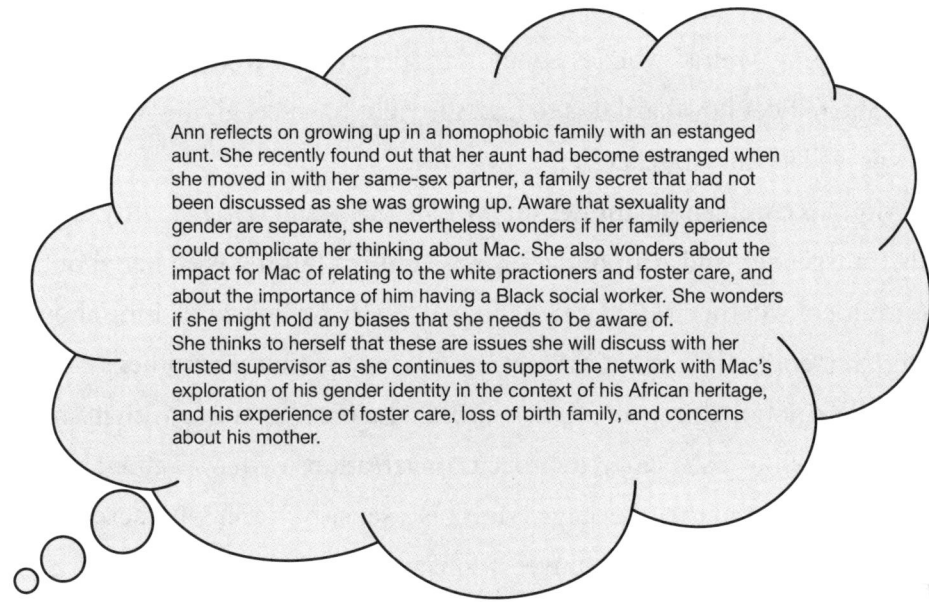

Figure 8.4 Ann's Self-Reflections

help Mac cope in a world that previous experience suggests could be emotionally unsafe. Is Mac's compliance, at school and with the social worker, one way he has learned to manage not feeling safe?

Shanice's reflection about Mac's resilience is acknowledged, alongside Moira's concerns about his isolation and difficulties engaging in activities. Ann observes how resilience helps Mac participate in school, engage with studies, and mix with peers. She talks about the cumulative stress of his coping strategies and considers the possibility that, when he is in the relative safety of his foster home, this stress is released through dysregulated outbursts. If Mac could speak about his distress, she imagines him saying: "I am trying to be good, Moira, but it is so hard. I don't want to be naughty. I miss my mom, and I don't want to have to go and live somewhere else until she is better." In response to this, Moira remembers times that Mac has described himself as naughty and thinks he does worry about moving again.

Ann reflects on Jason's concerns around after-school activities while acknowledging Moira's worries about Mac spending time isolated on his computer. She notices how hard it is to find the right balance, giving Mac opportunities as well as time to relax in his own way.

Moira is commended for her support for Mac's emerging identity as potentially transgender, and Ann notices Mac's comfort talking with her about this. She wonders whether Moira might find it easier to talk with him about his emerging identity than about his mother. Caring for another mother's child can have a big emotional impact., Ann reminds the team of the sensitivity needed for Moira, a white foster carer, to broach conversations with Mac about his Black African mother and their heritage. Moira is a sensitive carer who deserves support for what could be tricky conversations with Mac.

Ann points out the intersection of African and gender identity and wonders how comfortable Mac is talking with Moira about any racism or gender discrimination that he experiences. Ann affirms Moira's willingness to support Mac across these intersections and reflects on the range of experience within the network and how helpful this could be to Moira as she has these conversations with Mac.

Ann thanks Judy for attending and providing another valuable perspective about Mac. She also acknowledges the supports that school has put in place for Mac.

Picking up on the support Mac needs as a child of African heritage, Ann affirms the school's efforts to provide a multicultural environment, introducing the children to a range of cultures within their education. She also notices that children can be influenced by a range of things, in and out of school, that can lead to racism. Acknowledging the white space that they are inhabiting within the consultation, she invites Shanice to reflect on her concerns. Jason's knowledge of supporting transitioning adolescents is also explored to inform the network.

FINDING SHARED WAYS FORWARD

Bringing all this together, Ann reflects with the group on how much there is to consider when supporting Mac as a foster child with a mother in hospital. She notes that Mac is an emerging adolescent, trying to figure out his identity in terms of both gender and heritage. Ann invites discussion and reflection while moving the network toward potential plans for moving forward.

The group discusses the tension between counseling, community, and parenting support. They consider whether there is any community support that might be helpful for Mac to help him understand his ethnic heritage and whether there is potential for this to be supplemented with counseling. Jason's offer to be a role model is acknowledged with gratitude.

All this is followed by a discussion about family contact and how to support it. Ann wonders aloud if there is anyone Mac trusts in school who might work with Moira to gently explore his feelings about his mom being in the hospital and having to live in foster care.

Ann gives voice to the complexity of parenting Mac, affirming Moira's commitment to Mac and the positive way she has handled the challenges of parenting a child who is dealing with so much in terms of his gender identity and heritage while also having a mother in hospital and living in foster care. Moira engages in the discussion, sharing what parenting support she might find helpful. The group notes Moira's concerns about peer difficulties and they decide that she and the school will think together about how to support him to develop more lasting friendships. Judy enquires about additional support and/or training they could access to think further about children in foster care and the impact of their prior experience.

The consultation ends with a decision to meet again in two months.

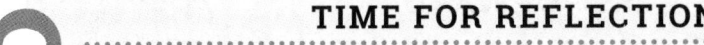

TIME FOR REFLECTION

Reviewing this example, think back to reflective exercise 8.1 and reflect on how DDP principles could enhance the consultation.

1. What principles did you see being drawn upon within this example consultation?
2. Were any opportunities missed?
3. In what ways did or did these principles not enhance the consultation?

DEVELOPING DDP PRACTICE IN SCHOOLS

TIME FOR REFLECTION

We invite you to drop down into a memory of being in a school, either as a student or more recently as a practitioner. It is a large school, and lessons are under way. You are here for a meeting with the headteacher.

Imagine walking along the corridors.

• What can you see, hear, feel, and smell?
• How easy is it to navigate your way through the corridors to find the room you need?

As you are walking along, a loud bell signals the end of the lesson.

- Notice what happens in your body as the bell rings and students pour out of the different classrooms.
- What has been added to the sensory stimulation you were already experiencing?
- How easy is it to know where you are and where you need to go among the sea of students and educators moving around the school?
- How does your body react when you hear an adult close by shouting at the students not to run? When you hear doors slamming? When you feel a cold draft of air as a nearby door opens to the outside?

And then calm descends as everyone arrives where they need to be. You find the right room, go in, and sit down.

- How ready are you for this meeting?
- How easy is it to assemble your thoughts; to attend to what is being said?

Schools have a range of obstacles to accommodating children who have experienced developmental trauma. The number of students, the size of the school, the levels of sensory stimulation, and the range of adults and peers to interact with make it difficult for the hypervigilant child to feel safe. The main aim of a school is to teach a curriculum to children in chronologically aged peer groups. Learning develops out of a drive to curiously explore the subject matter, a drive that disappears under feelings of threat.

Additionally, children who have experienced developmental trauma will have nervous systems that have developed a heightened sensitivity to potential threat. This defensive state does not provide the conditions for emotional growth, rest, and restoration, which enable emotional maturity (Porges, 2017).

This condition can increase a child's difficulty relating to peers. The behaviors of children with trauma can be challenging, and they may exhibit poor responses to traditional behavior management. Alternatively, they may be overly compliant or withdrawn.

When education staff understand the emotional needs of their students as much as their learning needs, they will be better able to coregulate their students and to discern whether behavioral support may also be needed.

As when bringing a DDP model into any organization, training is a starting point. but the DDP model is unlikely to make the difference hoped for without ongoing support, such as staff supervision, to embed it into educational practices. It can be helpful to have DDP champions in the school who can help keep ideas and new practices alive. DDP champions across a network of schools can support each other in study groups. There also needs to be buy-in from the leadership team, who can "model the model" and support the staff to develop in the agreed upon direction.

DDP practitioners enter school environments, often with no teaching experience themselves, ready to help the education staff develop a DDP approach within their school.

- Some of the staff they meet will be eager for this development and ready to try another way of doing things.
- Others will be willing to listen but are understandably cautious about adding more to an already full working life.
- Others will be skeptical, not wanting to see their way of doing things overturned, and perhaps have a sense that this new approach is soft and fluffy.

The practitioner needs to draw on all their DDP knowledge and skills to talk with the whole range of staff and to find a way forward that can be embraced by all.

REFLECTIVE EXERCISE: RESPONDING PACEFULLY TO CHALLENGING COMMENTS FROM EDUCATION PRACTITIONERS

Worksheet 8.2, at the end of the chapter, provides an opportunity to explore responding to members of a school staff group. Though you may receive many positive comments from them, some may be more challenging. We invite you to reflect on how you might respond.

All the comments in the above exercise have been said to us at one time or another. We have also encountered many lightbulb moments when educators realized the need for a different way and/or have experienced a powerful moment of success with a student. Supporting schools to embed DDP within their functioning is an up and down process.

REFLECTIVE EXERCISE 8.3: SUPPORTING SCHOOL STAFF

Worksheet 8.3 provides an opportunity to explore supporting a school staff group. Within this exercise, we symbolize this up and down process as a game of snakes and ladders.

One theme that frequently arises when supporting education teams to embed DDP principles within their schools is the use of boundaries.

- Some educators view DDP as being too soft and worry about the loss of boundaries that they think this implies. They adopt an authoritarian approach.

- Others like the nurturing approach and view the attitude of PACE as supportive but worry that applying boundaries will interfere with this. They can be too permissive in their approach.

A challenge for the DDP practitioner is to help these teams be authoritative in their approach, understanding how boundaries can be applied within a DDP model, which also provides emotional connection (Figure 8.5). This can allay anxieties on both sides.

REFLECTIVE EXERCISE 8.4: PROVIDING BOUNDARIES IN SCHOOL

In Worksheet 8.4 at the end of the chapter, there is an opportunity to explore how boundaries are traditionally applied in schools and how this can be adapted within a DDP model.

CONCLUSION

Within this chapter, we have explored dyadic developmental practice as a model for providing support beyond parent–child psychotherapy and parenting support. Using the examples of consultation support to networks and working with educators, we have explored how the DDP principles are used and modeled across a wide range of ways of working. Within this, we have considered the importance of inclusivity and antidiscriminatory practice. DDP encourages collaborative working, which facilitates the sharing of lived experience and knowledge to enhance understanding for everyone.

DDP practitioners have a responsibility to understand themselves, including any experiences of marginalization they have encountered, to ensure that these are not unconsciously played out within these interventions.

Dyadic developmental practice facilitates the application of DDP principles

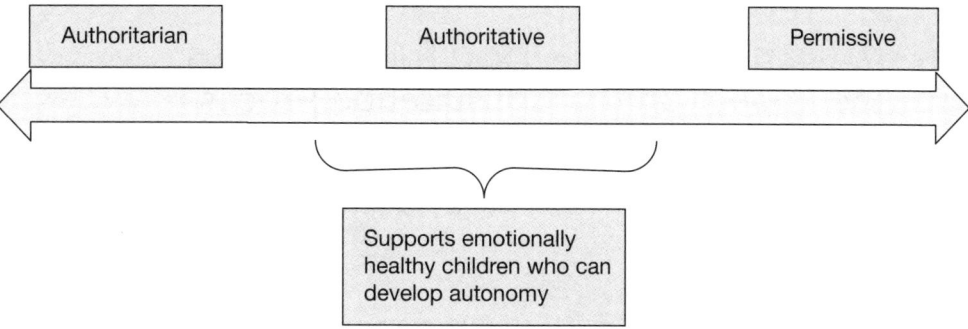

Figure 8.5 Authoritarian—Authoritative— Permissive Continuum

to the services, networks, and systems the child and family are living within, encouraging cohesive and joined-up support. This provides opportunities for healing from the impact of developmental trauma and its intersection with other trauma and forms of oppression the child and family may have experienced.

Worksheet 8.1

 Reflective Exercise: DDP Principles and the Impact on the Consultation Process

Consider each of the DDP influences and principles in the table below and how they could be used within the consultation process.

DDP Principle	Influence on consultation process
Attachment-informed	
Intersubjective	
Open and engaged with attitude of PACE	
Coregulation of emotion	
Cocreation using AR dialogue developed through storytelling	
Talking for and about	
Follow-lead-follow	
Relationship repair	

Reflections on Worksheet 8.1:
Possible Responses

DDP Principle	Influence on consultation process
Attachment-informed	The DDP consultant keeps the attachment needs of the child in mind, noticing examples of these needs being miscued and helping the network reflect on how this impacts the child in different settings. This reduces mistrust that can stem from different perceptions of the child. For example, a child appearing settled in school and more distressed at home may be viewed as the child displaying attachment needs differently rather than as the parents not managing or parenting correctly at home. This can strengthen the parents as primary attachment figures for the child and help parents feel more supported by the child's teachers, who are secondary attachment figures.
Intersubjective	Facilitating intersubjective connections between consultees increases reciprocity, allowing mutual sharing of concerns, perspectives, and ways forward. Safety is created through the collaboration that emerges as individual network members reduce their own, possibly rigid, views and become more flexible to the views of others.

DDP Principle	Influence on consultation process
Open and engaged with attitude of PACE	Individual network members may arrive at a consultation feeling defensive and with strong feelings about the child, their role, and what they want from the meeting. Conflict and tension can be high. As the DDP consultant maintains an open and engaged state, meeting the conflicts and tensions with PACE, each member will become more open and engaged to the process so that concerns can be openly shared and discussed. Defensive responses decline, and shared thinking emerges.
Coregulation of emotion	As affect emerges, the DDP consultant is on hand to coregulate emotional expression with a PACEful attitude, respect, and understanding for the perspective of the network member. The consultant will also notice, with self-compassion, any dysregulated affect in themself. Consultants need to remain regulated in many diverse situations and with a wide range of individuals.

DDP Principle	Influence on consultation process
Cocreation using AR dialogue developed through storytelling	The DDP consultant slows down the process of the consultation, ensuring that problem-solving isn't premature and that no one's concerns are dismissed or minimized. The dialogue they facilitate allows consultees to feel heard while all reflect on the child at the heart of the consultation. In this way, meanings become cocreated rather than individually held, and a rich and shared story that can touch and change the experience of those involved emerges. The consultant holds the emerging story and tells it back to the network in a storytelling, rather than lecturing, style of communication.
Talking for and about	Each consultee has an opportunity to witness and to be witnessed as the story emerges. The consultant talks *with* participants, *about* them, and sometimes *for* them to allow this witnessing to unfold. In similar fashion, the child, although not present, is held in mind as the network talks about them. Talking for the child can give the absent child a powerful voice.
Follow-lead-follow	The consultant seeks to balance being nondirective and directive, following themes that emerge within the discussion and leading consultees to a deeper understanding at affective and reflective levels.

DDP Principle	Influence on consultation process
Relationship repair	The consultant maintains connection with the consultees, but inevitably there will be ruptures in these relationships. The consultant notices discomfort, which may be expressed verbally and/or nonverbally, and takes responsibility for ensuring that a repair occurs. The consultant also needs to be able to accept that sometimes it is they who have made the relational mistake. The DDP consultant avoids going into shame about this because that would likely lead to them blaming the consultees.

Worksheet 8.2

 Reflective Exercise: Responding PACEfully to Challenging Comments From Education Practitioners

Think about how you can respond PACEfully and helpfully to the following challenging comments.

That's all very well, but I have 30 pupils in my class to attend to. I can't just focus on X.

I have a lesson to deliver; there is no time to ensure that X is regulated.

Where is the discipline in this? These children need to understand what is expected of them.

_____

_____

_____

_____

The school inspectors are not interested in how we reduce anxiety; they want to see learning outcomes.

_____

_____

_____

_____

I can't treat X differently. The other children would want to know why they can't have this privilege as well.

_____

_____

_____

_____

There is no room in this school to create a safe space for X. Your ideas are just unrealistic.

_____

_____

_____

_____

I have tried giving X no consequences, and his behavior is just getting worse.

_____

_____

_____

_____

We have so much that we need to do in school, I don't see how I can create reflective time for my staff.

_____

_____

_____

_____

This pupil needs to know what we expect. Give me a term, and I will tame her.

_____

_____

_____

_____

 ## Reflections on Worksheet 8.2: Possible Responses

Comment: _That's all very well, but I have 30 pupils in my class to attend to. I can't just focus on X._

Response: Of course not. I imagine it is very challenging to include a pupil with X's needs when you also have to care for and educate 29 other pupils. You must be exhausted by the end of the day. I can see your commitment to all your pupils. Would you be willing to think with me about the possible consequence of expecting X to be able to manage the teaching practices that the other pupils are thriving with?

Comment: _I have a lesson to deliver; there is no time to ensure that X is regulated._

Response: Time is a big pressure, isn't it? Here I am giving you another thing to think about. I wonder, have you noticed how the children who are best able to regulate are also the ones who learn most easily? Can you see benefits to increasing the regulation abilities of all your pupils? If so would you work with me to see if there is a way to build this into the lesson plan?

Comment: _Where is the discipline in this? These children need to understand what is expected of them._

Response: Yes, discipline is so important in raising and educating children. Their future ability to fit in and thrive within society is in your hands. I am thinking what a responsibility you have. I do think discipline is a part of the approach I am suggesting, but perhaps coming to it in a different way. Would you be willing to explore this possibility with me?

Comment: *The school inspectors are not interested in how we reduce anxiety; they want to see learning outcomes.*

Response: I heard that a school inspection is happening soon. I guess you are feeling anxious about this. Maybe we can think about some ways that might help you with your anxiety too (*smiling and both laugh*). It is hard to be at your best when you are anxious isn't it? I think this is a difficult time for me to be giving you more things to think about.

Comment: *I can't treat X differently. The other children would want to know why they can't have this privilege as well.*

Response: Yes, it is more complex when you have a classroom of children to consider. We all want fairness for our children. Sometimes children think that fairness is the same as treating everyone the same. I guess my ideas are feeling unmanageable to you, especially when you need to help the children to understand the differences as well. Can we think together about how to create a classroom culture that builds the value that fairness is ensuring that everyone gets what they need?

Comment: *There is no room in this school to create a safe space for X. Your ideas are just unrealistic.*

Response: I can see that space is at a premium in this small school. I am sorry I have given you unrealistic ideas to consider. I think we both agree that building safety is important for X, when they come into school already feeling unsafe. Can we get creative together and figure out some things that are possible?

Comment: *I have tried giving X no consequences, and his behavior is just getting worse.*

Response: I really have to apologize to you. I can see that I have explained my ideas very poorly. Consequences are important. You must be feeling very frustrated with me just now. Let me have another go at explaining that consequences work best when provided while staying connected with the child.

Comment: *We have so much that we need to do in school, I don't see how I can create reflective time for my staff.*

Response: The pressures on a headteacher, especially in a school of this size, are immense. I can see that staff well-being is important to you and that you don't want to burden them with more things to fit in. I am also thinking about how hard it is for you to fit this into your busy schedule. I am grateful that you have set aside some time to reflect with me today. Shall we start there, noticing how reflective space does and doesn't help?

Comment: *This pupil needs to know what we expect. Give me a term, and I will tame her.*

Response: Wow, that is a strong word. I think I may be jumping to conclusions about what you mean here. Can I take a step back and have you help me understand what "taming" means to you? Perhaps when I have a better understanding of this, we can think together about what would help this pupil.

Worksheet 8.3

 ## Reflective Exercise: Supporting School Staff

Here is a game of snakes and ladders to use to explore ways you (a DDP practitioner) might support a school staff group. This game provides a series of scenarios with questions to reflect on.

We encourage you to print the board and play the game!

Land on 2. You have had a good training session with the staff group. It feels like there is momentum to build on. Reflect on how you might start to embed the training. **Move up ladder to 21.**

Land on 8. At a supervision group, several of the staff report positive moments with a pupil with developmental trauma. Reflect on how you might affirm this progress without discouraging other staff members. **Move up ladder to 30.**

Land on 14. A pupil has been excluded for three days because they became dysregulated during a class. How can you help the staff group think about managing dysregulation without resorting to exclusions? **Move down snake to 4.**

Land on 16. The staff group is open to thinking about how to help an excluded child come back into school in a nonshaming way. How might you support them in doing this? **Move up ladder to 37.**

Land on 27. A parent of a pupil with poor attendance has agreed to attend a parent support group. How can you help the staff support this parent, who is experiencing anxiety and depression? **Move up ladder to 69.**

Land on 28. A parent attended the first parenting support group but left early, feeling that they were being blamed for their child's difficulties. How might you help a staff member to reach out to the parent and repair the relationship? **Move down snake to 10.**

Land on 34. A new behavioral policy has been written that focuses on the use of consequences but lacks attention to providing regulation support for pupils. How might you help the staff develop this behavior management policy into a behavior and regulation support policy? **Move down snake to 18.**

Land on 41. A staff member has cleared out a quiet area to make into a safe space for a pupil to go to when they are feeling stressed. Reflect on how to make this space feel safe and on how to help the pupil use it. **Move up ladder to 62.**

Land on 43. The school inspection is due, and staff are getting anxious. They have stopped using some of the ideas you have been guiding them to use and they keep canceling your visits to the school. How can you help the staff face this inspection, feeling confident in the new approaches that they have introduced? **Move down snake to 1.**

Land on 45. The school inspectors have visited, and they commended the school for their innovative approach to helping their pupils with trauma. How can you build on the momentum of this positive experience for the staff? **Move up ladder to 55.**

Land on 51. It has been a challenging term, with a lot of staff illness because of a nasty virus that has been going around. It is nearing the end of term and your last "reflective space" group meeting of the year. All the staff are getting very tired. Plan whether and how you would use this session with the staff. **Move down snake to 31.**

Land on 63. A gay member of the staff is persistently experiencing homophobic comments from a group of older pupils. Understandably, they are struggling to maintain an attitude of PACE. How will you work with the school to support this staff member? **Move down snake to 38.**

Land on 65. A staff member has asked for help to figure out why a particular pupil is triggering them. How might you help this staff member? **Move up ladder to 97.**

Land on 73. The headteacher has returned from training full of ideas for helping their pupils with emotional troubles. They ask you to help them embed the

DDP ideas you have been sharing with the school. How might you work with the ideas the headteacher has taken on board, weaving DDP into them? **Move up ladder to 94.**

Land on 77. One of the key DDP champions in the school is taking time off because of stress. How will you work with the senior leadership team on a stress reduction program for their staff? **Move down snake to 26.**

Land on 83. A staff member feels discouraged. It seems to them that all attempts to bring a PACE attitude into the school are being sabotaged by the leadership team. Most recently, they have been told that they cannot attend a DDP training that they registered for. How can you support the staff member to respond to these educators with PACE? **Move down snake to 59.**

Land on 93. A pupil has been experiencing peers touching their afro-textured hair even when they have asked them not to. The teacher dealing with this has suggested to the pupil that they have their hair straightened. How will you PACEfully support this teacher to understand that this is racist hair discrimination, and how will you explore with them how they can support this pupil to feel safe from racist abuse in school? **Move down snake to 66.**

Land on 95. The teacher training days have been planned for the year. There is no space for the follow-up training you have planned. How will you think with the leadership team about training priorities for the school without dismissing the importance of their priorities? **Move down snake to 53.**

Land on 100. Well done. The school has been nominated for a reward for their innovative practices and has invited you to join them at the award ceremony.

Worksheet 8.4

 Reflective Exercise:
Providing Boundaries in School

1. Think about how boundaries are traditionally set in schools.
2. Explore ways that boundaries informed by the DDP model can be provided.
3. Reflect on each of the examples you have given, and consider how these might be communicated to the child.

See how many examples you can come up with, using multiple copies of this sheet.

Traditional Boundary Setting	Boundaries the DDP Way
How boundary is applied:	How boundary is adapted:
Adults assume child feels safe and secure enough to manage the boundaries.	Adults attend to building safety and security for the child to help them manage the boundaries.
"Callum, I want you to turn around and face me. I can't teach the back of your head while you are busy watching the door."	*"Callum, you seem especially worried about who might be coming into our classroom today. Would it help you to sit closer to me? You can't attend to the lesson while you are watching the door."*
How boundary is applied:	How boundary is adapted:

Reflections on Worksheet 8.4: Possible Responses

Traditional Boundary Setting	Boundaries the DDP Way
Boundaries are in place to manage the pupil's behavior. Punishments are used as a consequence to enforce the boundary. *"That is the third time today I have seen you running in the corridor. You will report for detention next break."*	Boundaries are in place to support the pupil with their behavior. The pupil is supported with consequences to manage the boundary. *"Jasmine, you are running in the corridors again. Help me understand why you need to run. Then we can figure out how to help you remember to walk. In the meantime, I would like you to apologise to April, who you bumped into in your haste. Let me know if you need help to do this."*

Traditional Boundary Setting	**Boundaries the DDP Way**
Adult controls the boundary and provides coercive consequences to reduce the behavior and to get child to respect the boundary ("to" rather than "with" the child). *"There is no swearing in our school. You will be in isolation for the rest of the day."*	Adult decides on the boundary while supporting the child to manage their emotional response to it. This leads to collaborative consequences with the adult and child figuring this out together ("with" rather than "to" the child). *"Justin, you're so angry with Jack right now. I think it is hard for you to respect the no swearing rule. You need to find another way of letting Jack know how you feel. I will help you figure this out. Meanwhile, let's think together about the consequence for swearing in front of the younger pupils. How do you think you can make amends to them?"*

Traditional Boundary Setting	Boundaries the DDP Way
Adult provides conditional support based on the child observing the boundaries.	Adult unconditionally supports the child while helping them to manage the boundary.
"I am not prepared to listen to you until you are ready to follow our school rules."	*"I can see following our school rules is difficult for you. I am here to support you with this struggle. The rules have to be followed. Let's figure out together what will make this easier for you."*
All children, regardless of ability or capacity, have to manage the same boundaries. "One size fits all."	Understand the individual needs of the child. Fairness is not treating all children the same but giving each child what they need.
To whole class: "I want you all to sit still on your chairs, face forward, and concentrate."	*To whole class: "Let's see if we can support each other to concentrate in class. Some of you will need help to sit on your chairs, others will need things to fidget with. Let's figure out what you each need and then we will be the best class at concentrating."*

Traditional Boundary Setting	Boundaries the DDP Way
Expectation of obedience without question. Adults provide external locus of control (behavior is managed by adults, external to the child). Adults set the boundaries and ensure compliance through consequences. *"You will look at me when I am talking to you, and you will do as you are told."*	Help the child to understand the boundary, and support their emotional response to it with an attitude of PACE. Adults help child to develop an internal locus of control (learn to regulate their own behavior and to seek support when needed). Adults support child with boundaries, providing scaffolding support as needed and allowing the child to develop self-regulation. *"I can see it is hard to follow my instructions today. I wonder what you are finding hard. Let's see if I can help you with this, and we can find out what will help you to do what I am asking."*

Traditional Boundary Setting	Boundaries the DDP Way
Judgmental. Often the child is labeled as naughty. *"Your behavior is not acceptable. I will not have this naughtiness in my classroom."*	Nonjudgmental and supportive, conveyed through tone of voice and emotional connection with the child. Child is viewed as struggling emotionally. *"I can see you are finding it hard in school today. I'm guessing you're not comfortable behaving this way. How can I help?"*

Shaming. The child experiences themselves as bad.
   Public display: child is shamed in front of peers (e.g., use of zone boards, where a child's name is moved up or down the board depending upon their behavior).
 	
"If you can't behave, I don't want you in my classroom. Your name will stay at the bottom of the board."
	Child is supported to understand the consequences of their behavior and to experience guilt (not shame) and remorse. Adult supports child to make amends (including relational repair as needed).
	   Peers experience each other as emotionally and behaviorally supported when struggling.
	
	"I can see you are having trouble sharing today. Can you help me understand what the problem is? I will support you with that. Now Alice does not have time to finish her drawing. What do you think you can do to help Alice to know you are sorry and to help her catch up?"

Traditional Boundary Setting	Boundaries the DDP Way
Isolating the child. The child is moved away from the adult when the child cannot manage a boundary. *"You are not using the gym equipment appropriately, so that is the end of the lesson for you. You will sit here by yourself and do some work."*	Adult remains present while supporting the child to manage the boundary. If the child cannot tolerate the adult's presence, the adult remains available while respecting the child's need for distance. *"I can see you are struggling to use the gym equipment today. Sarah [teaching assistant] is going to help you. She can talk you through what you have to do. If you prefer, she will remain close by, and you can call her when you need help."*

Traditional Boundary Setting	Boundaries the DDP Way
Focus on behavior without curiosity.	Adult slows down and understands before acting. The extra time taken leads to a quicker and healthier resolution to the behavioral difficulty.
Boundaries have to be put in place under time pressures. Adults may feel that they don't have time to be curious.	This means having curiosity about what is underneath the behavior. This allows the child to experience PACE for the emotional experience that has triggered the behavior.
"You have been late for school every morning so far this week. Maybe a detention will help you get to school on time tomorrow."	*"You have been late for school every morning so far this week. Is something going on at home that is making it hard to get out on time? That does sound hard. Maybe we can sit down with Mom and see what can be done to help you."*

Traditional Boundary Setting	Boundaries the DDP Way
Boundaries are set and held rigidly. This is kept separate from child's emotional needs.	Boundaries are clear with flexibility to allow the child the support they need to manage the boundary. Emotional regulation is provided when needed, before or instead of a behavioral consequence.
"I know you have problems at home. However, you are in school now and the rules have to be followed."	*"You have so many difficult feelings just now. Things are hard for you at home. I think you need some quiet time in the book corner. I will help you catch up with math tomorrow. Do you want Sarah to sit with you for a while?"*

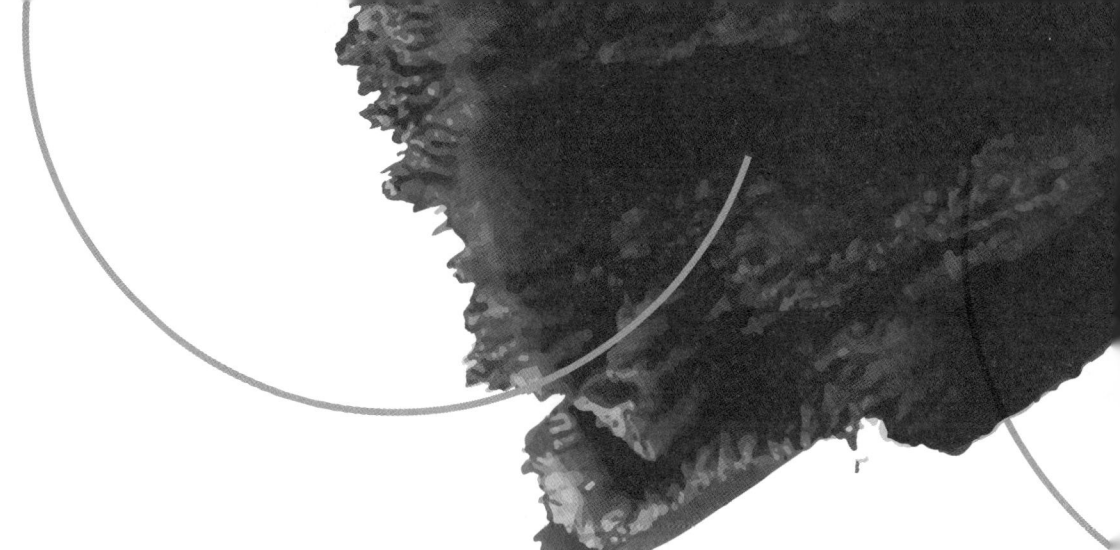

Chapter 9:
Interventions with Specific Populations of Children and Young People

> *While the central features of DDP remain constant, their various ways of being expressed are determined by the unique features of the child, family, and community context. (Hughes et al., 2019, p. 225)*

REFRESHER

In this chapter, we will explore the application of DDP interventions for different populations of children (Figure 9.1).

1. We explore how age and development can impact DDP, using the examples of work with preschool children and with older adolescents.

2. We consider how to adapt DDP interventions when developmental trauma interacts with other difficulties that children experience, such as learning disability or neurodevelopmental fragility.

3. Finally, we reflect on work with children who display risky behaviors through an exploration of children who engage in problematic sexual behavior and those who demonstrate violence toward their parents.

While this is not an exhaustive list, these examples provide an opportunity to reflect on how we can adapt and adjust DDP interventions depending on the context that the child and family brings.

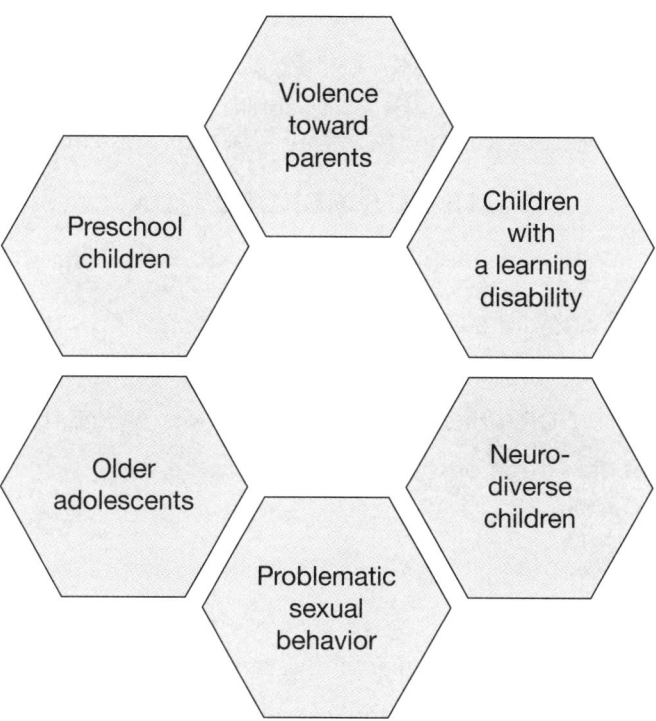

Figure 9.1 Range of Populations

ADAPTING DDP INTERVENTIONS FOR THE AGE AND DEVELOPMENTAL STAGE OF THE CHILDREN

In this section we will explore the way that DDP interventions can be adapted for children at two very different developmental stages. Whilst the DDP principles being used will be the same the application of these can look very different.

SUPPORTING PRESCHOOL CHILDREN

In this section we will reflect on providing DDP interventions for families caring for children in the preschool age group.

TIME FOR REFLECTION

Is this DDP?

Consider the following scenarios, and notice how the interventions draw on DDP principles.

How are DDP principles being adapted to suit the age and developmental stage of the children?

An 18-month-old girl is living with foster carers, following the traumatic experience of domestic violence and physical abuse. The foster carers describe her as very quiet, and often "zoned out." When they attempt to play with her, she may become animated with the toys but rarely looks at or interacts with the carers. If she starts to feel overwhelmed by the play, she typically will turn away from her carers. The DDP practitioner supports the foster carers to interact with the girl as if she is much younger. They do lots of interactional games, such as peek-a-boo and row the boat. They talk to her about what she is experiencing with lots of emphasis on their nonverbal communication. "Eh, you have had a big sleep. Here we go, time to get up. Oh-oh, time to get dressed. You really don't like this, do you? Here you go, nice and warm and safe." The practitioner helps them to develop a melodic rhythmic prosody including pauses, crescendos, and whispers to engage her attention. They learn to notice when she is feeling unsafe, triggered by past memories perhaps, and to provide cues of safety through voice, comfort, and their availability. Gradually, this child zones out less frequently. She appears more relaxed and ready to interact with them. They experience joy in her peals of laughter as she engages inter-subjectively with them. They start to introduce other toys, and she can now play in a way that feels more emotionally connected with them.

A three-and-a-half-year-old boy has been adopted after experiencing severe neglect in his birth home. He was often left in his cot, cold and wet. He now rejects his parents' attempts to cuddle and soothe him. He will remove his clothes, throw off his blankets, and resist any efforts to be nurtured by them. The DDP practitioner works with the child and parents together. They sit the child between his parents and place a blanket over him. As the child kicks the blanket away, the practitioner talks quietly and melodically about his current experience: "Oh, you have kicked the blanket off. And now you have taken off your jumper. Mummy, look how cold your son is. It's so hard for him to let you keep him warm." And now with animation, pauses, and suspense: "Oh my goodness . . . I am wondering . . . maybe, maybe. Let me think. I wonder. It could be. Yes, it could be. I wonder is this how your son felt when he was little. So cold, so alone. Could it be?" As the practitioner talks, the child cuddles closer to his mother. Gently, the practitioner picks up the blanket and places it around him. As mummy cuddles and warms him the practitioner plays some gentle music.

A four-and-a-half-year-old girl is living with her aunt, following the death of her birth mother. The child is quiet and withdrawn much of the time. When upset or tired, she calls for her birth mother and angrily *pushes her aunt away. A DDP practitioner works with the two of them. They try to engage the child with a range of toys, drawing materials, and puppets. The girl resists these overtures and hides under the table. She then picks up a blanket and hides under this. Remaining under the blanket she crawls toward the door. The practitioner talks slowly and quietly while picking the child up. They place the child in her aunt's lap. The practitioner sits close and continues talking to them both: "Aunty, your niece is having such a hard time. She has some big feelings, and it seems the only thing she can do is try to hide. It's so hard for her, so hard. I think she is missing her mummy." The child has visibly relaxed and is accepting her aunt's comfort. The practitioner continues, "I think she is trying to say to us: 'I don't know where my mummy has gone. I call her. Where is she? I miss her.'" The practitioner then guides the aunt to talk quietly to her niece, telling her that mummy was very ill and then she died. She describes what this means in simple language and in accordance with the family's religious beliefs. As the child sits up, signaling this is enough for now, the practitioner picks up a storybook suitable for the moment and reads it to the child and aunt. In the next session, the child uses the puppets to act out going into the hospital and seeing her mother for the last time. The aunt held her close as the practitioner put words to this poignant story.*

"Is this DDP?" is a question we are frequently asked. There is no simple formula. DDP is what it needs to be for each unique child and family. The principles will guide the practitioner as they adapt DDP to suit the circumstances, considering the age and experience of the child. In this way, DDP is an intervention that can be offered to preschool children, both through the support offered to the parents or carers and through direct work with the children.

As illustrated in the scenarios above, children of all ages, when feeling safe and comfortable, will engage with storytelling adapted to their stage of development. The verbal elements of the story are conveyed simply while the nonverbal elements convey safety and enhance the telling. Coregulation and cocreation are very evident within these interactions, with the practitioner using visual and verbal signals from the child about what they are experiencing to follow-lead-follow the child into their emotional world. In this way, affective–reflective conversations are developed both visually and verbally, and the child experiences their emotional life being held safely with PACE.

SUPPORTING OLDER ADOLESCENTS

When the DDP practitioner is engaged in therapy with a younger child, alongside the caregiver, the practitioner functions in part as a caregiver, parent substitute, or attachment figure. When the same DDP practitioner is providing therapy for an older adolescent, whether the caregiver is present or not, the practitioner may need to engage the adolescent more as a teacher, mentor, or coach.

The adolescent might be unwilling to rely on the practitioner for comfort and support but more willing to rely on them for information and guidance regarding the journey into adulthood. This is not to say that the practitioner is unavailable for providing comfort and support, but rather that such relational experiences need to be more in the background, more implicit than explicit.

The following are appropriate interventions and goals for the late adolescent:

1. While helping to reduce self-reliance as a personality trait, affirm the value and necessity of this skill. When self-reliance becomes a personality trait, it is the only way to be. We want to help the young person to develop self-reliance as part of a range of ways of managing difficult situations. The adolescent who experienced developmental trauma developed self-reliance because it was necessary for survival. Your willingness to assist them in using these skills more flexibly may be welcomed, as long as the adolescent does not believe that you are trying to make them dependent on you. Having you as a coach is likely to be less threatening than having you as a "parent."

2. Guide the development of these self-reliance skills by helping the adolescent to:
   - develop meaningful interests and habits to foster a sense of self-worth and contentment;
   - develop self-exploration through the integration of their life-story or autobiography as part of their identity as an emerging adult (the adolescent is likely to resist turning to the practitioner for comfort about their history; therefore, any support given by the practitioner will be implicit, not explicit); and
   - see that being alone may be the source of productive solitude rather than the means to avoid the experience of being rejected.

3. DDP involves both affective and reflective components. With the older adolescent, the practitioner might stress the reflective component to deemphasize any sense of developing dependency that might feel threatening. This may then enable the adolescent to choose to rely on the practitioner somewhat.

4. Having experienced betrayal or abandonment when they depended on another person, the older adolescent is likely to look forward to becoming an independent adult. They might anticipate a time when they won't need anyone. They are therefore unlikely to want to depend on someone else now. The practitioner might focus on helping them to have a reciprocal relationship that is characteristic of friendships. In such relationships, each person enjoys being with the other to share ideas, knowledge, or interests rather than seeking support.

5. The older adolescent might be more receptive to relationships in which they are a coach, teacher, or mentor, with others relying on them. This provides the adolescent with more control in the relationship than they would have if they were being taught or coached by another.

6. The older adolescent might be helped by learning that they do not have to choose between relying on themselves or relying on others. In some situations, relying on another might be in their best interest, while in other situations, relying on themselves might be best for them. Relying on someone for a specific reason does not make them a dependent person.

7. The older adolescent is likely to be more motivated to develop a relationship with a partner than to improve a relationship with a parent. This is understood and accepted. At the same time, the practitioner might suggest similarities in both relationships and notice that improving their relationship with their parent would be good practice for relating with a potential partner, leading to a stronger relationship. Examples include: communicating about emotional themes, resolving conflicts, engaging in relationship repair, cooperating about difficult issues, developing common goals, and sharing obligations.

8. The practitioner might go slowly in helping the older adolescent to rely on both the practitioner and the caregiver by suggesting that the adolescent turn to the other for information and practical matters first, and only later for emotional support.

9. The older adolescent might acknowledge that they have difficulty accurately understanding the motives of others and be quick to assume that others have a negative attitude toward them. The practitioner helps the adolescent to understand how this relates to their experiences of abuse or neglect with their parents. The adolescent might then understand how their parents' behaviors were due to their attachment histories and unresolved experiences of abuse and neglect. This reduces the adolescent's sense that what happened to them was their own fault.

10. The older adolescent might acknowledge that their relationship with their parent seems worse now, as they are thinking about leaving

home, than it did earlier. They can be helped to understand that viewing their parents more negatively can make leaving home easier.

All of us go through the important transition from adolescence to adulthood. During this time, we address anew how to balance our first way to manage distress—by relying on others in an attachment relationship—to managing distress through our gradually developing skills of self-reliance. The way we attain this balance can influence our manner of assisting others who are experiencing a similar transition.

When an adolescent has experienced developmental trauma, their transition is likely to be more difficult because their original developmental tendency to rely on others was compromised by being abused or neglected by those they relied on. Helping these individuals achieve a new balance may be especially difficult.

When we, as DDP practitioners, strive to help the youth who experienced developmental trauma to attain this balance, we use, in part, our own experiences with making this transition. If we achieved a balance that leaned toward relying on others more than self, we may well give priority to that strategy in guiding the adolescents in our care. If we formed a balance that gave priority to relying on our self, that is likely to be the perspective we take in our guidance.

TIME FOR REFLECTION

We invite you to reflect on your experience of transitioning from adolescence to adulthood.

- How did you manage distress? Did you predominantly rely on others, on yourself, or did you attain a dynamic balance between these two?

- Did your parents push you toward independence, hold you back by encouraging dependence, or attempt to support you to manage your confusing, often ambivalent strivings?
- Did your parents' psychological needs become interwoven with your own psychological needs to develop your autonomous journey into adulthood?
- Did you sometimes sense that what was best for you was being determined by what was best for your parents?
- Did the community and culture that you grew up in impact how you made the transition?
- Did your family composition—being an only child, being in a large sibling group, having a single parent, having separated parents, having same sex parents, losing a parent, or growing up away from birth parents—impact how your parents supported you?

If we are unclear how to resolve any differences between what seemed to be our parents' wishes for us and our own wishes, then we may be unclear as to where the adolescent client's best interests lie. If we have doubts about how well we transitioned into adulthood, then it seems wise to reflect on that aspect of our attachment history.

TIME FOR REFLECTION

Reflecting on these developmental themes in our own life is an important part of our clinical ability to understand and appropriately address our adolescent clients' best interests. We invite you to continue your reflections about your own experience:

- Were you aware of having ambivalence regarding independence and dependence that you had difficulty resolving?
- Did you experience guilt if your parents responded with distress to your wishes for independence or dependence?
- If, after leaving home, you felt a need to return home at times for support, did your parents encourage and support you? Or were they disappointed in you?
- When you thought about having your own family, did you hope that your family would be similar to or different from your family of origin?

When the DDP practitioner is providing therapy for the older adolescent, they are likely to emphasize different or additional issues when supporting the adolescents' caregivers.

These include:

- The older adolescent with developmental trauma is likely to want more independence than their caregivers believe they are ready for. They may well have given the adolescent many chances in the past, each one leading to failure. They may have little confidence that anything will be different now. And yet, if the adolescent is denied any chance to fail and (hopefully this time) learn from their mistakes, they will enter adulthood and actual independence ill-prepared to make some difficult decisions when on their own. The DDP practitioner holds empathy for the caregivers, while helping them to regulate their anxieties. Caregivers can then be supported to provide their adolescent with some choices even though these may well lead to mistakes. The focus is on allowing their adolescent to make choices in areas where the consequences will be manageable hoping that their adolescent will then accept limits on choice that would involve more serious consequences.

- The practitioner reminds the caregivers that if their adolescent is going to learn from their mistakes, the shame associated with failing needs to be regulated. Regulating shame reduces the adolescents' need to deny their mistake through lies, excuses, and blaming others. An empathic response will provide regulation; an attitude of "I told you so" will not. Better are comments such as "I know how much you wanted that to work out. It must have been so hard that it didn't." Or, "I can see that having made a mistake is very difficult for you. You're not alone in having that experience."

- The caregivers may need support to let go and recognize that they will no longer be able to control certain aspects of the adolescent's life. Making countless efforts to control their adolescent's behavior can lead the adolescent to experience themselves as a failure and a disappointment to their parents. If there are endless power struggles about things that the caregivers cannot control, then the repetitive focus on these issues may lead to a broken relationship, reducing the chance that their adolescent will be receptive to their perspective.

There always needs to be space for hope. One of us (Dan) was providing therapy for an older adolescent boy, Jason, and his adoptive family. Jason had been adopted eight years before and had been in therapy for the past year. His behavior was very oppositional. His parents were most concerned about his habitual drug use, including stealing from them to support his habit. When he turned 18, they told him that he must stop stealing from them or bringing drugs into their home. If he couldn't do this, he would not be allowed to continue to live with them. His behavior did not change and so they informed him that he had to move out within a month. They offered to help him to find a place to live, but the next day he left home without telling them where he was going.

Jason's parents didn't know where he was for the next seven years. When he was 25, he knocked on the door, accompanied by his wife and one-year-old son. They welcomed him in, and he told them his story. After leaving home, he was often homeless. He supported himself by selling drugs. He was eventually arrested and referred to a drug rehabilitation program where he lived for 18 months. During that time, he obtained a graduate equivalency diploma and managed to get and retain a stable job. He met his partner, they married, and a year later they had their son. They are renting a small home while they save to buy their own home.

Jason's parents asked him why he waited so long to contact them. He said that he wanted to show them that he had changed through his actions, not just his words. They then asked him how he had been able to change his life around so much. He replied, "Because you never gave up on me." They reminded him that they had told him he had to move out of their home. He answered, "But you did not want to do it!"

There is no way to determine if someone has the qualities that Jason had that enabled him to eventually take advantage of being loved by good parents. Some adolescents like Jason do not make it, while others do. We need to maintain our hope that the unique adolescent in front of us will succeed. When we communicate this hope and confidence intersubjectively, we may make it more likely to occur.

ADAPTING DDP INTERVENTIONS TO SUPPORT CHILDREN WITH LEARNING DISABILITIES AND/OR NEURODIVERGENCE

The interaction between environment, parenting, and intrinsic biological difficulties is complex (Figure 9.2). Questions about what demonstrates attachment difficulty and what is a result of biology are not easy to answer, as the two are so interlinked. We do know that traumatic experiences, inadequate social experiences (including nurture and parental availability), limited parenting because of parents own history, the child's biology, and inherited genetic differences

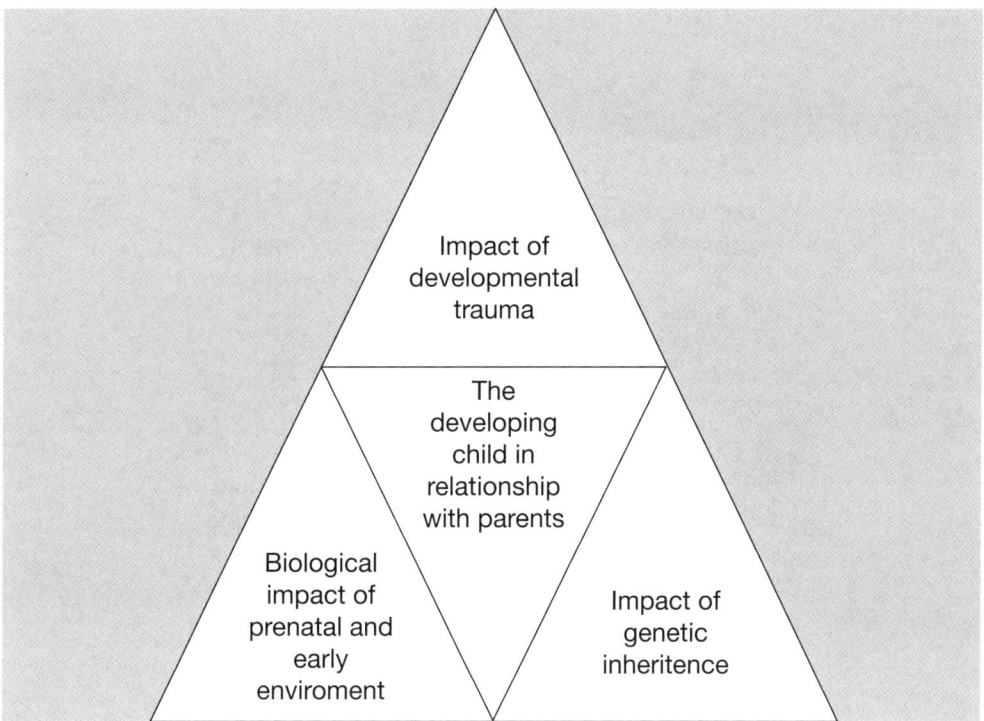

Figure 9.2 Interactions Between Environment, Parenting, and Biology

can all transact, leading to the child experiencing both trauma impacts and neurodevelopmental fragility.

As illustrated in Figure 9.3, children can inherit and/or acquire difficulties with sensory integration, emotional regulation, learning, and executive functions. All of these need to be considered when providing DDP interventions.

While maintaining a focus on the goals of DDP, including increasing attachment security, helping children to enter healthy intersubjective experiences, and processing and integrating traumatic experiences, we must also consider adapting DDP interventions to adjust for the additional needs that these children bring.

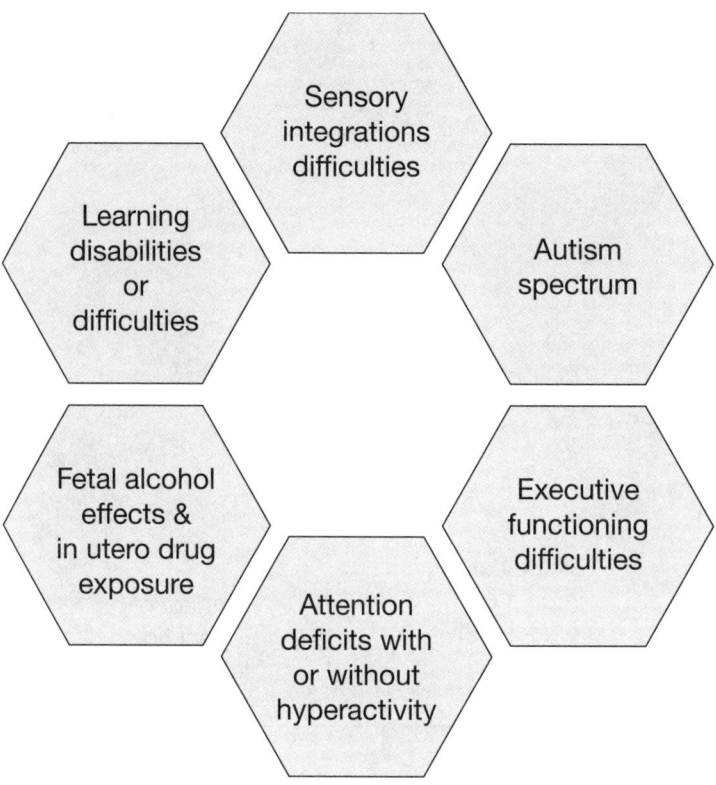

Figure 9.3 Examples of Children Who Are Likely to
Demonstrate Neurodivergence

This means

- combining DDP interventions with other interventions that can help
  the child with their neurodevelopmental functioning, for example:
  - interventions focused on sensory integration: the BUSS
    model understands difficulties within the context of trauma
    (Lloyd, 2020)
  - interventions that help attunement between parent and child:
    Theraplay complements DDP (Norris & Rodwell, 2017)

> – interventions that can adjust the environments that the child is living and being educated within: Marion Allen (n.d.), as part of the Family Futures team in London, U.K., has produced a helpful book for supporting children with executive functioning difficulties in school, with many ideas that could also be helpful for parents

- slowing down our interventions, and holding realistic expectations of what can be achieved

- increasing support for the parents, both to help them understand and have empathy for the child and the struggles that they encounter and to help them to adjust their expectations of what the child can manage (The box below provides an example of parenting a child on the autism spectrum.)

- helping the child to understand their own functioning and challenges; the child also needs support to help them with the impact of this on their sense of identity

SUPPORTING A CHILD ON THE AUTISTIC SPECTRUM WITH FAMILY EVENTS AND SPECIAL OCCASIONS

As I (Kim) am writing this in late December, the trials of Christmas for a person with autism are on my mind. This, of course, applies to any special family event or religious festival. Typically, these events cause alterations to routines and bring a need to manage experiences that are novel and unpredictable.

As a parent, it is so easy to become stressed and frustrated when trying to facilitate an enjoyable family event for everyone. Holding onto a DDP way of being, with its attitude of PACE, can be challenging.

As an autistic child, special occasions and family events signal a change in routine and can be extra stressful. Consider that these events often:

- increase demands on the child
- increase the need to be part of social gatherings
- increase visual and auditory stimulation
- increase novelty and surprises
- involve changes to the usual diet

When these events occur during a school holiday, the child will also have had to manage the school run-up to the holiday, with all the accompanying nonroutine events and activities. Many children will be masking to try and fit in and to meet the extra expectations on them, and consequently, anxiety increases. Emotional overwhelm builds, inevitably leading to dysregulation and meltdowns. Planned family events then become even harder to manage.

Helping parents to hold onto their playfulness, curiosity, acceptance, and empathy can make a big difference when riding the roller coaster of emotions that families experience when engaged in family events and special occasions. It is much easier when someone is holding PACE for the parents. With the emotional support provided by holding the attitude of PACE, the DDP practitioner can help the parents to understand their child's needs and to adjust their expectations.

Maintaining an attitude of PACE and enjoying the relationship with the child is easier when understanding replaces a defensive response to take things personally. Defensiveness in the child can feel very targeted! Instead of focusing on our disappointment and frustration at what can seem like ungrateful and selfish behaviors, we need to hold onto curiosity and to wonder what the child is finding especially difficult. With understanding comes empathy. The child really is trying their best to meet the expectations and demands upon them. They do not want to ruin the event and will be quick to experience shame, often blaming themselves when they cannot cope with the expectations on them.

As the parent is supported to maintain a PACEful attitude, they can step back and reflect on the needs of their child, adjusting routines and rituals to help the child. It will also help the parent to reduce their expectations of what their child can manage and on themselves of what they should be able to achieve in their parenting.

We invite you to explore an example, based on families we have known, where attachment difficulties and neurodevelopmental fragility intersect.

Esther was born to a young woman who had, herself, grown up in the care system. She drifted between homes and was a regular drug and alcohol user. Esther was taken into foster care when she was three months old. She continued to have erratic contact with her birth mother until she was adopted at 18 months. While Esther settled well into her adoptive family, she had to endure further trauma eight months into the adoption due to a prolonged bereavement in the family, during which her adoptive mom was away from the family home. Mom described her relationship with Esther as feeling different once she returned home. Esther's behavior became both controlling and rejecting.

Throughout her childhood, Esther excelled at music, enjoying playing the piano, but had limited play and imaginative skills. By early adolescence, Esther was demonstrating problems with anxiety, self-regulation, inattention, auditory sensory problems, and inflexible thinking. This all compounded her difficulties with learning, socializing, and regulating her mood and behavior. She also demonstrated features of a disorganized attachment pattern, leading to blocked trust with high levels of resistance to and rejection of adult support. She tried hard to avoid support in school and she actively and violently resisted support at home. Esther wanted and sought to be part of a social group, but this regularly ended in failure.

TIME FOR REFLECTION

Imagine meeting Esther and her family during Esther's adolescence.

- What do you need to understand to help you plan your DDP interventions?
- What do you think the relative impact of attachment and neurodevelopmental difficulties is on the challenges that Esther is experiencing?

Imagine meeting the family when Esther was younger.

- What difference might meeting Esther at this age make with regard to the interventions provided and to the progress you would expect to see by adolescence?

It is important to understand the neurodevelopmental and attachment profile presented by the young person and tailor DDP interventions to both. When planning interventions, the practitioner should also consider the developmental stage of the young person, as both attachment and neurodevelopmental challenges will manifest differently at different stages.

Understanding the parent's experience, in the context of their own attachment history and cultural expectations of their children, will also inform decisions you make about how to target DDP interventions.

It is also important to understand the transaction between all of these. For example, the child's attachment difficulties will affect the attunement between parent and child. The attunement can be further impacted by the parent's own history and cultural upbringing. This dynamic can, in turn, impact the child's level of stress, increasing their neurodevelopmental challenges. These challenges can create parental stress and frustration, as we saw in the box earlier exploring supporting a child on the autism spectrum, further impacting on the parent–child relationship. The child may end up feeling mad or bad, and the adults may view the child as willful and naughty.

REFLECTIVE EXERCISE: DEVELOPING ESTHER'S DDP JIGSAW INTERVENTION PLAN

- Consider what DDP intervention plan you would implement for working with Esther and her family.
- What modifications to these DDP interventions might you anticipate making to address the neurodevelopmental needs Esther presents?
- What network support would be helpful to build into your intervention plan?

In Worksheet 9.1 at the end of this chapter, there is an opportunity to explore what a jigsaw intervention plan might look like.

ADAPTING DDP INTERVENTIONS WHEN CHILDREN ARE DISPLAYING RISKY BEHAVIORS

In this section we will explore how DDP can be adapted to support children and their families where there is risk from the child. We have chosen to illustrate this with the examples of children who are violent towards parents and children who display sexually problematic behaviors.

CHILDREN WHO ARE VIOLENT TOWARD PARENTS

In families where there is violence directed from the child or adolescent toward the parent, the lack of safety for all members of the family is acutely apparent. Just as in the therapy session, the parent needs to experience their own safety before they can facilitate their child's safety. When not feeling safe, both parent and child are often defensive. Habitual defensiveness leads to a sense of failure and self-doubt. In order to address an acute problem successfully, the person needs to remain open and engaged with the problem, rather than responding defensively. Defensiveness is likely to be associated with fear and shame, which will impede the ability to learn from a mistake or solve a challenging problem.

> *Make the violence stop!*

More than most family problems, violence directed toward parents by children tends to mobilize everyone for action.

> *"We have to do something!"*

> *"What?"*

> *"I don't know! But we can't just do nothing! We have to try something!"*

DDP emphasizes that the best way to address a problem is to first know what it means and then reflect on how to approach it. Sometimes in a crisis we forget this. We must do something and do it now! DDP also stresses that we need to slow down to go faster. That remains true in situations where the child is violent toward a parent.

What are we doing when we are slowing down?

- We are understanding what the violence means.

- We are developing a story that contains the violence, while also describing its broader and deeper context.
- We are developing and exploring the story with PACE.

Our mind asks,

"What is the story?"

Followed by,

"Within this story, what does it mean?"

And only then,

"What do we do?"

Unless we slow down and reflect, we are likely to move too quickly through the story. There is a great deal of shame for both the parent and child involved in violence toward the parent. If we do not find a way to stop the violence, we can feel shame too. Reflection halts when we experience shame. We are likely to experience panic. We compulsively think that all that matters is that the behavior stops.

To develop the story needed to stop the behavior, we begin by anticipating that we will all feel a bit of shame. PACE must follow. The acceptance and empathy are likely to reduce the shame and open our minds to curiosity about the story that contains the violence. As we slow down and explore the story, we discover its features without evaluating them.

We begin this process by describing the family.

TELL ME ABOUT YOUR FAMILY

- Who are its members?
- What are your frequent activities, habits, and interests, both individual and joint?
- What are typical meals, games, and holidays you share?
- What are your favorite shared places and activities?
- Tell me about areas of differences and conflicts.
- How are differences resolved and relationships repaired?
- How is affection expressed and comfort given and received by each family member?
- What significant changes, losses, and events are approaching?

We then explore the violence.

TELL ME ABOUT THE VIOLENCE

- Who initiates and who receives the violence?
- Is the violence verbal, emotional, physical?
- Are there common themes, places, times of day?
- Are there associated stressors?
- Is it sudden or does it escalate slowly?
- What is the aggressor's initial expression?
- What does the recipient of the aggression then say or do?
- What impact, if any, does that have on the aggressor?
- Are other family members present and actively involved?
- Does their presence make it better or worse?
- What causes the aggression to decrease?
- How does the event end?
- Is the ending clear, or does the incident gradually fade away?

This leads to noticing how members of the family respond.

TELL ME ABOUT YOUR RESPONSES

- What is each person thinking and feeling during the incident?
- What does each person think the motives, thoughts, and feelings of the other person are?
- Do the individuals discuss the incident later?
- Do these discussions tend to lead to repair, do they make things worse, or do things stay the same?

It is crucial that, as we understand the violent events, we also understand the more varied, often satisfying, and enjoyable events that also occur among the members of the family. The acts of aggression don't define the family if they are understood and accepted as part of the larger context, both past and present. Knowing the events, along with their contexts, enables us to review them as problems to be addressed rather than as shameful aspects of each member of the family or the family itself.

As we discover and explore the family's story, it is crucial that they are able to accept their story. It is their story; it is not the total of who they are. They are engaged with us in an act of self-discovery, not self-evaluation.

SAFETY FOR ALL

The DDP practitioner assesses the degree to which the parent experiences safety in their home when their child is present. They explore the fear and anxiety the parent is likely to experience as they anticipate the child's return home, when they are about to set a limit that will make the child angry, or when the child raises their voice and makes threats in words or actions. Maybe their anxiety is so pervasive that it is present even when their child is cooperative.

Alongside this, the practitioner explores the parent's attachment history.

The child's anger might evoke anxiety associated with past relationships, for example, when their parents were angry with them. Where parents are coparenting, the way they handle disagreements will be explored along with whether the child's anger echoes how the parents show anger toward each other.

It is also important to assess whether the parent is in a state of blocked care, wherein they are habitually defensive.

The practitioner will help the parent to consider their coping and regulatory skills, to reflect on whether they are proactive or reactive in dealing with conflicts. Where two parents are coparenting the child, the parents will review the support they provide for each other. The parents will also consider which friends and relatives they can turn to for support. As they review this with the practitioner the parents might notice patterns that reduce the support they are getting. For example, they might have a tendency to hide their distress from other adults who would be willing and able to support them if asked.

Together, practitioner and parent consider how safe the child feels while also remembering the context of the child's experience of having been abused, neglected, or having lived in multiple homes.

REFLECTING TOGETHER

- Does the child habitually mistrust their parents and experience routine limits and corrections as being abusive or rejecting?
- When in distress, is the child able to turn to their parents for comfort and support?
- Is the child able to express sadness? Or is anger their only way of giving expression to their distress?
- Is the child sometimes able to demonstrate adequate coping and regulatory skills?
- Do certain times, limits, or expectations increase the likelihood that the child will become violent?

The practitioner next helps the parent to explore how they can engage the child in activities that generate safety and coregulation. The parent is helped to notice the practitioner's modeling of PACE and to consider relating to their child with PACE. They explore ways the parent can keep the need for connection with their child in mind, especially during conflicts. Keeping this need in mind will help them to consistently convey the attitude that their relationship with the child is more important than anger and conflict. Building security with their child is also helped when the parents engage in relationship repair fairly quickly rather than allowing long delays. Finally, the parent will be taught how to engage in deescalating behaviors and notice when they are reacting in ways that escalate the situation.

When there is violence in the home, safety needs to be supported and reestablished again and again. Parents need to continuously strive to see their child's worth and positive qualities, which exist in addition to their child's violence. Parents need to find and convey their positive experiences of their child as often and as soon as possible after times of conflict and violence.

THE NEED FOR LESS SHAME

When a child is aggressive toward a parent, both the child and the parent are likely to be mired in shame. The child's aggression is considered a bad, mean, and selfish act, all the more outrageous because of "all your parents have done for you." The child is likely to judge that their aggression toward their caregiver is proof that their original parents' abuse and neglect of them was justified. Each time they attack the parent, they become more convinced that they are unlovable and unwanted.

When parents experience aggression from their child, they often experience shame for failing to control their child as well. They may experience criticism from other adults for not being firm enough and not being able to prevent the child from being aggressive. They may feel that their child would stop being aggressive toward them if they were more capable parents. Additional shame will be felt when, pushed to their limit, they become aggressive toward their child in response to their child's aggression. They committed to parenting a child who has been hurt so much by others in the past; they now have the shame of having added to this hurt. They may have kept their aggressive acts secret, for fear of what others will say, which prevents them from asking for help. It will be a relief to talk about this with the DDP practitioner who meets the situation nonjudgmentally, with acceptance and empathy, and with a commitment to help these parents to find a better way to be with their child.

TIME FOR REFLECTION

Reflect on families you have worked with in which children have been violent. Notice the impact this work had on you.

- What anxieties or worries did you experience? How did this impact your work with the family?
- If there are any elements in your own relationship history that were echoed in this work, how did this affect you?
- Reflect on the attitudes toward violence within the family, communities, and culture that you grew up in. Did this impact how you related to the family?

Working with a family in distress, experiencing complex and severe problems that impact all members of the family, is hard. In the face of such violence, we can feel that we need to "do something, anything!" We may lose confidence in DDP and PACE.

We are aware that unsuccessful therapeutic interventions can lead to the breakup of the family. A breakup like this can feel like, and is often viewed as, a failure; although sometimes helping a child to move is the most helpful intervention. This might be the best way to preserve the relationship between the child and parents. Having the child spend time in foster care or a residential home can be very supportive for the family. It allows a break from the violence and creates time and space to provide the DDP interventions that will help the parent relate differently with the child so that the violence can decrease.

Before we react to the violence and despair, we need to reflect. And then:

1. Stay with PACE as a central way of being and engaging the members of the family.
2. Reflect on the historical roots of the violence for both the parents and the child.
3. Consider external sources of support for both the family members and yourself.
4. Develop compassion and empathy for all involved.
5. Help the parent to think about different ways of relating to their child, of providing regulation, and of communicating their unconditional acceptance of them, and explore ways to deescalate.
6. Violence of a child toward a parent presents a major challenge for the DDP practitioner, the family, and the child. The full range of DDP therapeutic interventions and child-rearing practices will be needed. Parents will need support more often than one hour a week and very likely will need support from trusted adults alongside the DDP practitioner. While the focus needs to be on the inner lives of the parent and the child, the behaviors of both also need to be addressed.

CHILDREN WHO ENGAGE IN PROBLEMATIC SEXUAL BEHAVIOR

Working with children and young people who engage in problematic sexual behavior is challenging. Talking about sexual abuse, including exposure to inappropriate sexual activity, is difficult and made harder when (often) so much is not known.

This work can also take place within a context that also includes making decisions about where children should live. For example, is it safe for siblings who have been engaged in sexual activity to remain together? There may be ongoing legal proceedings that further complicate the work.

Also, the current caregivers need support in how to care for and supervise the children and, sometimes, in how to manage uncomfortable sexualized behaviors directed toward the caregiver. Caregivers will have a range of experiences, from feeling a need to protect those they perceive most vulnerable to feeling anger and disappointment in those they view as instigating the behaviors. Holding PACE for all the children involved can be challenging for the caregivers..

We are going to consider an example where sexual activity among biological siblings has been reported within a foster family. Taylor, a 14-year-old boy, is suspected of instigating the sexual activity. Of the two younger girls, who are 11 and eight, the 11-year-old child is denying that anything has happened, whereas the eight-year-old has reported sexual abuse by her stepfather. The foster carers are upset with the social worker for placing these children with them. They had requested no children with a history of sexual abuse be placed with them. The male foster carer is also feeling uncomfortable by what he is experiencing as sexualized behavior from the girls toward him when he is trying to help with the bedtime routine.

TIME FOR REFLECTION

Imagine you have been asked to work with this foster family.

- Notice what comes up for you.
- Is there any immediate emotional impact on you that you need to be aware of?

There is a lot of discussion within the network about what should happen next. There is talk about moving Taylor into residential care, and there have been heated discussions about who is to blame within the sibling group. You are being asked to provide therapy but are warned not to get in the way of any future court case.

TIME FOR REFLECTION

Again, notice what is coming up for you.

- Where are your sympathies lying?
- Are you feeling irritated with parts of the network?

Consider the range of interventions that are likely to be needed to support these children.

- How can DDP interventions be helpful for the children, foster carers, and network?

Examples like this one demonstrate the complexity of the work when sexual abuse and sexualized activity are part of the emerging story. This work can be all-consuming, as interventions are needed within the network, with the caregivers, and with the children. Discussions can be heated, and the DDP practitioner can feel unpopular when they provide alternative viewpoints. For example, it is difficult when the eldest boy in a scenario, such as this one, is being viewed almost like an adult perpetrator, and you want to focus the network on remembering that he is also a child and likely to also have been a victim of sexual abuse. As a practitioner, you may also need to resist pressure to move too quickly into providing therapy for the children before a sense of safety has been established within the network and within the foster family.

Moving on, Taylor is now placed in a residential home at some distance from the foster home. He is allowed some limited, supervised contact with his siblings. Police investigations were carried out, and Taylor is now under a supervision order overseen by a youth worker. The sexual abuse allegation was investigated, but there was insufficient evidence to proceed. You are now working with Taylor and his key worker, Zoe, while a colleague is supporting the girls in their original foster home.

Some of us find talking about sexual abuse and sexual activity with a child as particularly challenging, especially when we have been brought up in a culture that discourages healthy discussions about sex. These conversations are, however, an important part of the work.

Let's explore one therapy session with Taylor and his therapist, Andie. They have been connecting and chatting for about 15 minutes, during which Taylor shared his enthusiasm for mountain biking.

Andie:	Well, Taylor, this is our third meeting, and I think I'm getting to know you—what you like to do, what you think and feel about things. Thanks for sharing with me your tales of mountain biking. It sounds cool.
Taylor:	No worries.
Andie:	(*to Taylor and Zoe*) And look at the two of you. Nice to see you getting on so well.
Taylor:	Zoe's alright.
Andie:	Are you settling into the home, do you think?
Taylor:	I like it. They're not on my back all the time.
Zoe:	We love having you, Taylor. (*to Andie*) He really makes us laugh, you know. A great sense of humor. (*Taylor smiles.*)

Andie: Yes, I have experienced Taylor's humor. (*laughing*)

Taylor: (*looking more subdued*) I wish it wasn't so far away though. I hardly get to see my sisters.

Andie: That's tough isn't it. You saw them this weekend, didn't you?

Taylor: Yes, but only for two hours, and we were watched all the time. I don't know what they thought we would do in the contact center!

(Taylor, feeling relaxed with Zoe and Andie, has perhaps said more than he meant to; he looks like he wishes he hadn't said this; his head goes down, and he turns away.)

Andie: Taylor, I can see how hard it is not seeing your sisters, not living with them anymore. I guess this is hard to talk about.

(Taylor's head remains down and he says nothing.)

Andie: (*to Zoe*) I think this is hard for Taylor to talk about. We were just talking about how Taylor is enjoying living with you and going mountain biking. I can see he is comfortable with you as his key worker. I think moving to the residential home has been a good move for him. Less intense than the foster home. As he says, no one's on his back all the time. But it's so far away, and Taylor really wants to see his sisters. The three of them coped with so much in their birth home. It has always been the three of them, and now it isn't.

(As Andie is talking, Taylor moves closer to Zoe, and she gently strokes his back.)

Taylor: They said I did stuff, but I didn't. I have always protected them. My mom always said I had to be a man, 'cause my dad wasn't.

Andie: Oh Taylor, I can see how much you are missing them, and not being able to protect them anymore . . . that is hard. And it sounds like your mom gave you some big responsibility. You were just a little boy. And now the adults are thinking that you and your sisters were engaging in sexual behaviors with each other in the foster home.

Taylor: (*more animated*) That's a bunch of crap.

Andie: (*increasing their animation to match*) This is so hard for you. It is feeling so unfair, and now I'm bringing it up too.

(*Taylor is feeling even more vulnerable; he draws back into defensiveness.*)

Taylor: I don't let it bother me.

Andie: And, to me that seems hard to do. After all that happened before, when you were living with your family and people thought that your stepfather had sexual behaviors with you and your sisters.

Taylor: That was crap too. He never did!

Andie: And people were so sure that it happened that the three of you were moved into foster care. Has it been hard being separated from your mom?

Taylor: What do you think?

Andie: I think it's been hard. All of it! And if your stepfather had done something, I'd understand why you'd not want to talk about it, or even admit it happened. And it's so unfair to you. I guess it gets mixed up with the fact that, at your age, you're becoming aware of the important place sex has in your life and in the lives of everyone. What people think happened with your stepfather, if he brought sex into his relationships with you and your sisters, would be so unfair to you three. Parents—and stepparents—should never do anything sexual with their kids. It makes something normal and natural for adults into something that is wrong, scary, and confusing.

Taylor: If he did do something like that—it's gross—why would me or my sisters do it too?

Andie: (*to help Taylor stay with this, Andie now talks with a degree of separation, so the topic is not directly about Taylor*) Great question. People like me, and social workers who get to know kids and teenagers who had a parent who had sex with them, wonder about that, because many of them did have sex with their siblings or peers too. It seems to me that they often were frightened and powerless to do anything about what had happened to them, and they somehow felt that if they were in control of the sexual behavior, it would not be so scary. They might have hoped that having sex together would help them to get over what happened to them. They would control it this time.

Taylor:	Well, it didn't happen to me.

Andie:	If something did, Taylor, and you don't trust me enough to tell me, I understand. I hope someday you do, because that would make it easier for you to let it go. You could then have regular thoughts about sex, where it's just part of your life, a special part, not a part with bad memories connected to it. And you'd know that what happened to you was not your fault. What you might have done because of what happened to you is connected to your trauma and is not a sign that you're a bad person.

(As Andie is talking, Taylor cuddles into Zoe and allows her to comfort him. For a while he looks vulnerable again as he allows Andie to talk. He then signals it is enough for today, but with vulnerability and not anger. This difficult work has begun.)

Taylor:	*(quietly and sadly)* Can we stop talking about this now?

Andie:	Yes, I think that is enough for today. Thank you for allowing me to think about this with you. Now, there are still a lot of things that I'd like to get to know about you and your life. You went to the cinema last week, didn't you? How was the film?

As Taylor starts to feel safe with Andie and Zoe, he is allowing a little thinking about the hard parts of his life. This is a good opportunity to help him reduce his shame and fear. This will give him a better chance to proceed with healthy development—emotionally, socially, cognitively, *and* sexually. This has been a good start. Andie needs to invite Taylor into exploring this traumatic part of his life carefully, sensitively, one bit at a time. Once this traumatic content has begun to be safely explored, questions that Taylor has about his sexuality in general will also be much easier to explore.

CONCLUSION

The DDP practitioner specializing in working with children who have experienced developmental trauma will encounter many different families representing many different populations of children.

DDP will look and feel different when working with a preschool child compared with an adolescent on the cusp of leaving home. Adjustments to our interventions will be critical if we are to meet the needs of children where developmental trauma interacts with learning difficulties and neurodiversity. Working with families where there is risk can be challenging. We have chosen to focus on children who are violent or demonstrating problematic sexual behaviors. These risky behaviors will require specialized DDP interventions, targeted at supporting the child, family, and network. These will have the usual goals of DDP interventions, building trust and security, increasing comfort in relationships, and processing and integrating trauma experiences. Additionally, attention will need to be given to reducing the behaviors that are so damaging to the child and to the family.

This is not an exhaustive list, but it provides a way to start to organize our thinking about how we provide DDP interventions and what adjustments we might make depending on the context.

Worksheet 9.1

 Reflective Exercise: Developing Esther's Jigsaw DDP Intervention Plan

This exercise imagines the intervention plan as a jigsaw puzzle of support for the child, family, and network. What pieces of a jigsaw would you put together, and what adjustments would be included within this jigsaw to additionally support the child with their neurodiverse challenges?

1. On each puzzle piece, write headings of different DDP interventions that could be helpful for Esther. Include headings for interventions which can meet Esther's neurodevelopmental needs.

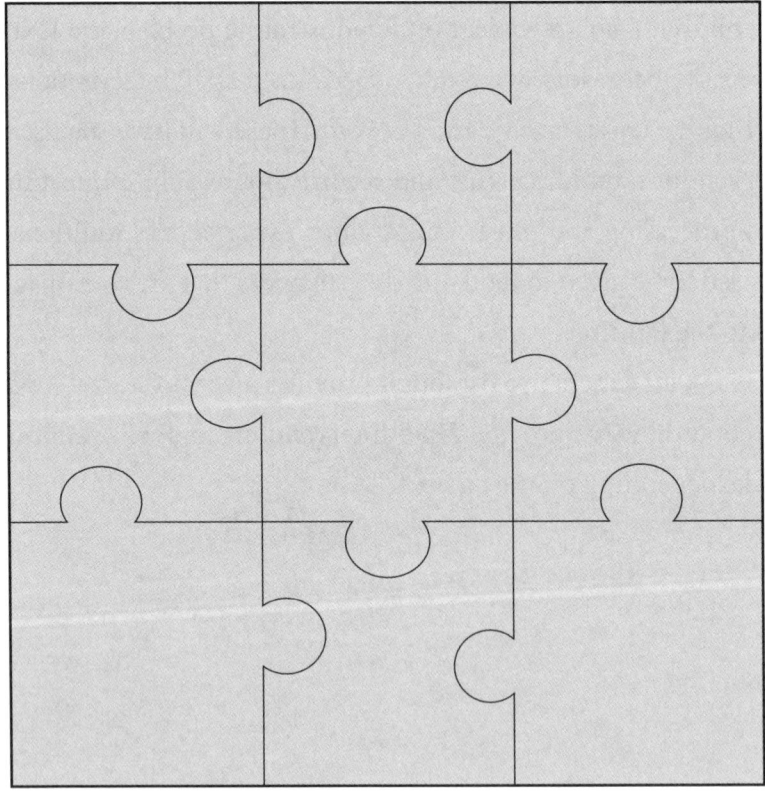

2. Make a note of what is needed under each heading.

Reflections on Worksheet 9.1:
Potential Response

A JIGSAW DDP INTERVENTION PLAN

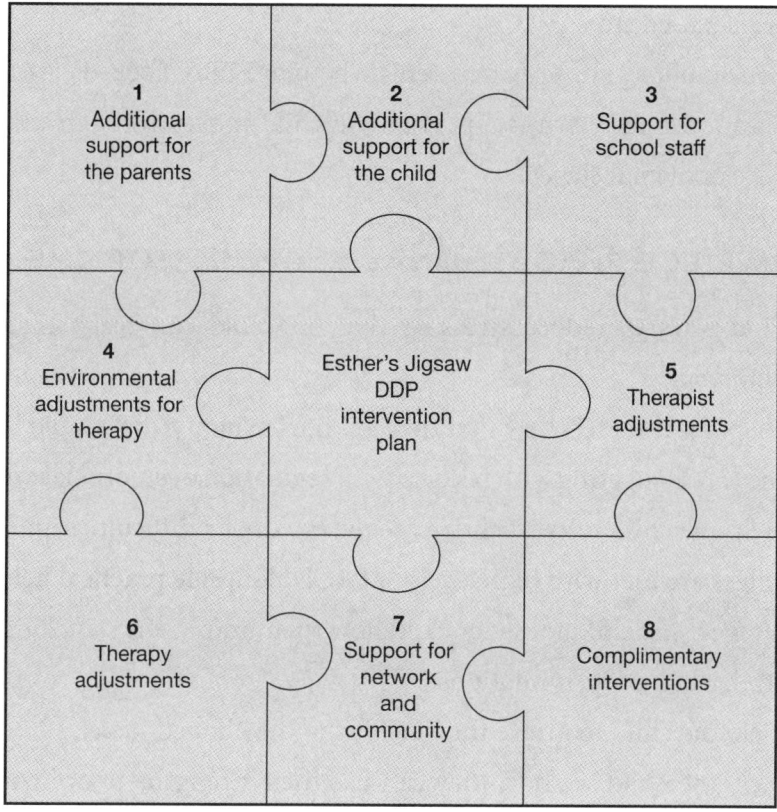

JIGSAW PIECE 1:
ADDITIONAL SUPPORT FOR THE PARENTS

- Help parents understand their child's difficulties.
- Support parents to adjust their expectations and to find ways to help the child with challenges.
- Provide emotional support for feelings of grief and disappointment as parents understand that the child's difficulties are greater than

initially expected. This also links to fears for the future as the parent wonders if their child will ever be independent of them.

- Notice progress. Celebrate moments of success and accomplishment for parents and for the child.
- Support more when progress appears to go backwards, often at times of increased stress.
- Look out for and support parents who move into blocked care.
- Plan for longer term support as the child moves through different developmental stages.

JIGSAW PIECE 2: ADDITIONAL SUPPORT FOR THE CHILD

- Find ways to reduce stress so that the child can reach their full potential.
- Help the child to know that they are not "naughty" or "stupid" when they are struggling with tasks or with regulation of emotional arousal.
- Help the child to trust their caregivers as their difficulties and challenges are met with high levels of PACE alongside practical help.
- Support the child to understand how their brain works, including its strengths and its limitations.
- Help the child to grieve the loss of who they hoped to be.
- Help the child see how they can use their strengths to overcome or surpass their limitations.
- Help the child communicate to teachers and parents what support they need.
- Help the child understand their own responsibilities alongside the responsibilities they expect of adults.

JIGSAW PIECE 3: SUPPORT FOR SCHOOL STAFF

- Help school staff understand the strengths and limitations the child is experiencing.
- Plan how the child will be supported coming to and leaving school.

- Identify the child's needs, and help the staff accommodate these. This includes environmental needs, such as reduced stimulation and where to sit in the classroom, as well as learning needs, such as additional support and scaffolding.

- Build in regulatory support, including tools for regulation, such as calm boxes and fidget toys. Provide additional regulatory breaks during the school day.

- Anticipate that the child will regress at times, that what is known one day might be lost the next. Notice how stress reduces progress, and find ways to reduce stress.

- Consider how to support the child when routines change, either planned or unexpected.

- Help the child manage unstructured as well as structured times, and increase support for managing peer relationships.

JIGSAW PIECE 4: ENVIRONMENTAL ADJUSTMENTS FOR THERAPY

- Plan the environment to match to the child's needs. Consider where the child is most comfortable, such as at the clinic or at home.

- Be aware of sensory challenges. Reduce auditory, visual, and tactile stimulation as needed.

- Provide additional aids to help child to stay regulated (e.g., objects to chew, hold, sit on, manipulate).

- Use visual as well as verbal cues to provide predictability and to signal safety.

JIGSAW PIECE 5: THERAPIST ADJUSTMENTS

- Ensure that signals of safety are very explicit.

- With a child experiencing very intense affect, stay regulated and animated rather than regulated and calm. This holds the child's attention and creates a meaningful intersubjective experience. Increasing animated, playful enjoyment of the child can build trust. Increasing animation with matched intensity and rhythm can help engage the child's interest.

- Match the affective expressions of the child to coregulate the cognitive, affective, and behavioral states, which may be agitated, disorganized, rigid, and inflexible. Help the child to calm and focus.
- Adjust therapist behaviors. For example, the therapist may need to reduce eye contact and touch for some children.
- Manage therapist expectations. anticipate and expect a bit less of the child cognitively, affectively, and behaviorally.
- Acknowledge and celebrate small successes.
- Accept and adjust for inflexibility and rigidity.
- Provide more repetition, increased structure, and lots of predictability to reduce stress.
- The therapist may need to do more leading to help focus the child's attention while also following the child's initiatives in response to this leading.

JIGSAW PIECE 6: THERAPY ADJUSTMENTS

- Transitions can be difficult, so plan and support the child entering and leaving the session.
- Go at the child's pace; expect slow progress. Don't move too quickly in helping the child reflect. Ensure good routines, structure, and regulatory support are established first.
- Anticipate emotional dysregulation, and provide regulatory activities and sensory breaks. Explore relational activities that help to soothe and regulate.
- Children may progress in bursts with longer periods of consolidation between. Adjust episodes of therapy to suit the child.
- Offer bits of challenge in very small steps—invite the child to try,

and accept resistance and failure without conveying frustration or disappointment. Support this with extra regulatory breaks.

- Anticipate that the child will enter states of shame more quickly. Provide a high level of acceptance and understanding to regulate these states.

- Be aware of attention difficulties and their impact on language, memory, planning, and initiating.

- Alternate talking with experiential interventions to reduce verbal demands on the child.

- Discover what helps the child to communicate: drawing, puppets, stories, etc.

- Work at getting into a nonverbal rhythm with the child wherever his attention is focused. Go slower, be simpler, and provide explanations of what is happening within the relationship.

- The child might produce fewer nonverbal cues, so check in with the child more often.

- Work toward the child engaging in reciprocal interactions; take slow steps, accommodating social communication difficulties.

- If the child monologues around a special interest, share attention and work to move into a dialogue. This involves slowing the child down, interrupting with curiosity, and increasing animation to convey interest.

- Develop storytelling as the child becomes used to the experience of being made sense of. Pay attention to tone of voice: Some children need to hear a more factual tone, others need a lighter, softer tone. Some children find indirect talking (talking about) more helpful; others will engage better with talking for. Ensure the storytelling tone of the DDP session is soothing and regulating.

JIGSAW PIECE 7: SUPPORT FOR NETWORK AND COMMUNITY

- Recognize the importance of network meetings to support DDP work.

- Ensure shared understanding and goals.

- Increase working together to support the family.

- Dispel myths about what therapy can fix.

- Advocate for the long-term needs of the family.

- Manage expectations about what we hope will change and what difficulties are likely to be ongoing.

- Work with the community and extended family. Recognize that culture and upbringing can affect how a community and a family respond to a child with disability and/or neurodiversity. Seek to understand as well as to inform.

JIGSAW PIECE 8: COMPLIMENTARY INTERVENTIONS

- Consider what additional therapeutic interventions could help the child with their neurodiverse needs. For example, DDP and Sensory Support; DDP and Theraplay.

- Plan to provide multiple interventions in a way that does not overwhelm the child nor the family. Interventions may be integrated or provided sequentially. If multiple therapists are involved, plan to work closely together.

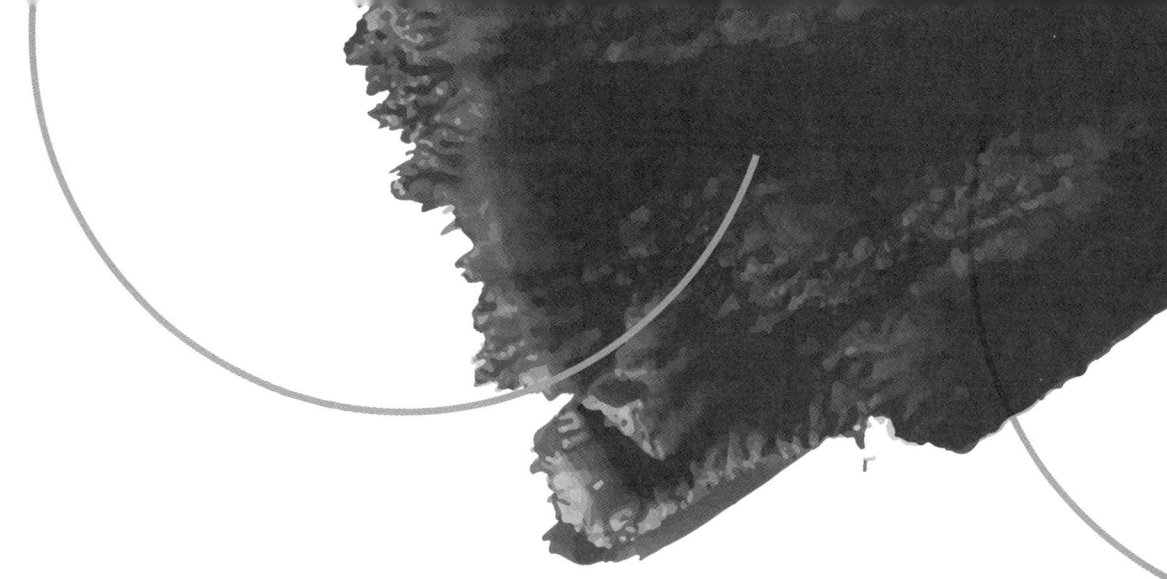

Chapter 10:
Interventions in Specific Situations

In all these quite differing situations, the principles and interventions of DDP provide the opportunity to develop a coherent narrative and safe relationships. (Hughes et al., 2019, p. 225)

REFRESHER

DDP interventions are applied in a range of situations. Safety is the starting point as the DDP practitioner adapts their interventions to the needs of the child and family. Wherever they are living, children with developmental trauma need a safe environment and help in developing confidence in that safety and in recovering trust in appropriate parental figures. This provides a foundation for healthy development.

In this chapter, we will explore several different situations (Figure 10.1).

GROWING UP IN FOSTER, KINSHIP, ADOPTIVE FAMILIES, OR RESIDENTIAL CARE

In this section, we invite you to reflect on providing DDP interventions for the range of families impacted by the care system. To inspire your reflections, we have chosen extracts from real stories (see stories described in the boxes below). Taken together, these illustrate how the DDP practitioner holds multiple stories in mind while helping the child and their current parents to discover their own story.

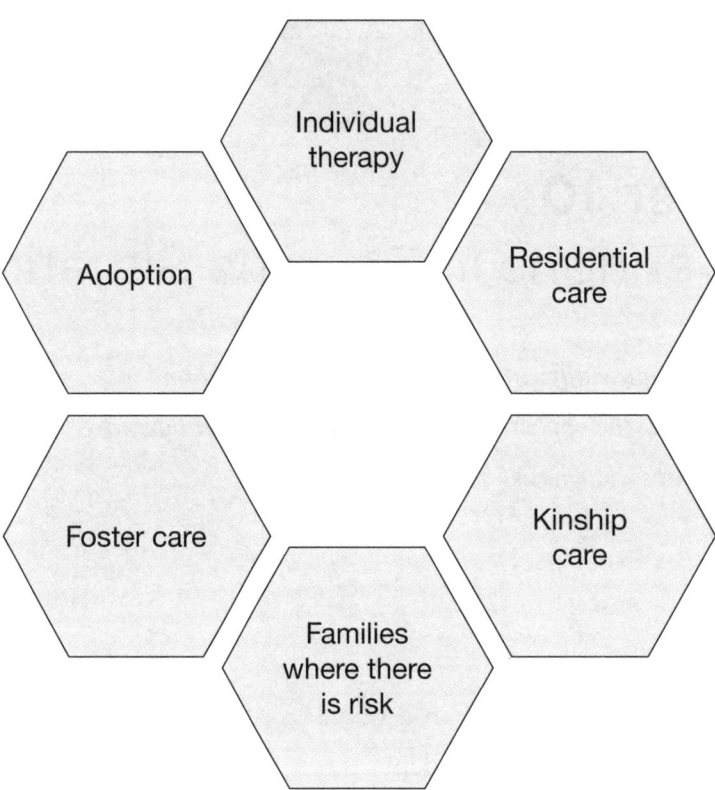

Figure 10.1 Range of Situations

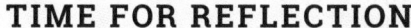

TIME FOR REFLECTION

Reflect on your experience of living within families. These reflections may be emotional. Give yourself time and space for this work. Take care of yourself and, use support.

- When you look in the mirror, how much of your biological family is reflected back?
- How do you feel connected to or disconnected from families you grew up in?
- How do you feel connected to the families' history and heritage?
- What gets in the way of feeling such connections?
- How did you gain a sense of belonging?
- What got in the way of feeling that you belonged?
- Did you imagine being in a different family while you were growing up?
- Did you experience any feelings of grief or loss when you imagined a different family?
- Think about your origin and life stories. Who shares these stories with you?

Do these reflections change your understanding of living in families?

How might this understanding impact on you as a DDP practitioner?

FOSTER AND KINSHIP CARE

Foster care involves disrupted relationships, as children move in and out of care and between placements. These moves lead to multiple losses, including families, pets, school, leisure activities, and social workers.

Fostering is complex:

- The carer is parent and professional, parenting under scrutiny and within the guidance imposed on them.
- Parenting is scrutinized by the network around the child.
- Support and supervision are often combined.
- Parenting a child with a difficult relationship history requires the carer reflect on their own, sometimes troubled, relationship history.

Many foster placements are planned to support the child into adulthood. However, placement breakdowns are not unusual, as the challenges being presented often overwhelm the foster carers' resources. Other foster placements are contracted for the short term. A foster carer has to love a child whom they will have to relinquish.

Children identify with birth and foster parents, complicating their sense of identity. This is challenged further when impacted by multiple moves. Contact with birth family is variable and complicated. Some birth parents will be supportive of their children's foster placements; however, they are living with their own loss, their role in this loss, and their resentment at the intrusion of the state in their lives. This experience can impact their relationship with their children. This can lead to a conflict of loyalty for the children. Their longing for their birth parents can be intense, as is illustrated in the box below. In the next box, a foster carer reflects on her experience of DDP.

A FOSTER CHILD'S STORY

Alexia grew up in foster care. As an adult she explores her complicated feelings about mothers, longing, and belonging.

I realized that it wasn't any unconditional mother that I

wanted, I wanted my own mother. I wanted her to uncon-ditionally love me. In accepting that it was not my fault that I had felt unlovable, I also had to accept that I could not make that better. No matter how "good" I became, I could not make her what I needed her to be. This wasn't in my control. All the controlling behaviors I had found were now to no avail. This turned my world upside down.

I needed to grieve the loss of the mother I had always believed could be there for me if only I could make myself good enough. I also needed to face the reality that all of the women I had sought as mother could also never truly be my Mom. I needed something from my birth mother that no one else could give me.

This piece of work also helped me to find my true place in my foster family, neither birth daughter nor outsider—an accepted part of the family. It led me to realize that no one could replace my Mom, and in accepting this, I could claim my foster mother. I no longer had to put her on a pedestal that she could never achieve. I had been completely reli-ant on my foster mother's opinions. I had tried to gauge this so I could be what she wanted, an attempt to find the "mother" I longed for. It was in vain, the mother I wanted was my birth mother. She could never be that, no matter how hard I worked to please her. Now I did not need her approval of me anymore. I no longer needed to control my relationship with her. This paved the way for us finding an authentic relationship together. (Golding & Jones, 2021, pp. 116–117)

A FOSTER CARER'S STORY

Liam grew up in foster care. Here his foster mother describes helping her foster son, supported by DDP.

The first day I met Liam, his foster carer left me with a comment: "He'll give you no trouble." She ruffled his hair and shoveled him in through the gate, and that was it. I mean, right there on the pathway was this little clown, a little entertainer, and (*to Liam*) living with you, I began to realize how much trouble you were in. I couldn't get close to you, at the beginning. You know that's not surprising, is it really? I mean things happen and you get put somewhere and that must be the most horrendously scary thing. Although I felt we were moving in the right direction, I still felt that you were very vulnerable, and I wanted to try and help with that. I tried lots of things, you know, tried and tested things, and you did respond to lots of those things. Loving you was the biggest thing and caring about you, actions speak louder than words; the things I did for you. I began to feel very concerned about you: When anything emotional happened, suddenly this little jack-in-the-box creature came out and entertained everyone. I could see it all going on, I just needed some help to deal with it. As soon as Kim started working with you and I'm watching her, I can begin to see how I can help you. Sometimes we adapt things, don't we? We adapt things and we go about it maybe a different way, but with Kim, she gives us the tools to work things out. (Golding, 2011, p. 153)

Living with relatives, in kinship placements, brings additional complexity. The children have a sense of belonging within their extended family. However, this involves additional losses. For example, when a grandparent becomes a parent, the child loses a grandparent. Contact with birth parents can be complicated by the extended family members' feelings toward their relative, including feelings of guilt and shame at not having prevented the harm to the child. All of this can create further conflict and confusion about the child's identity within the family. The DDP practitioner needs to take this context into account.

In foster and kinship care, there is more state involvement in the lives of the children. Consequently, DDP interventions may be more complex. Therapy for the child and support for the carer is insufficient. Interventions must also be put in place for the networks around the child.

TIME FOR REFLECTION

Reflect on the journeys that foster and kinship families make.

- What DDP interventions are needed?
- How might these be tailored to the needs of the child, to the foster carers, and to the network?

ADOPTION

Adoption is often seen as the fairy tale ending. The child has a permanent and legal family where they can grow up in a healthy environment, allowing them to develop to their full potential.

In reality, adoption is messy, with many conflicting stories of need, loss, and trauma. The adopted child needs a family, and the family needs a child, but these needs do not always align, and everyone may feel disappointed.

When the family created by an adoption does not turn out as expected, the parents—and the child—may experience grief. Feelings around the loss of an imagined family can be intense. When parents' and children's grief touch, the family may need additional support to navigate through this.

In the following box, we explore one person's adoption story.

AN ADOPTEE'S STORY

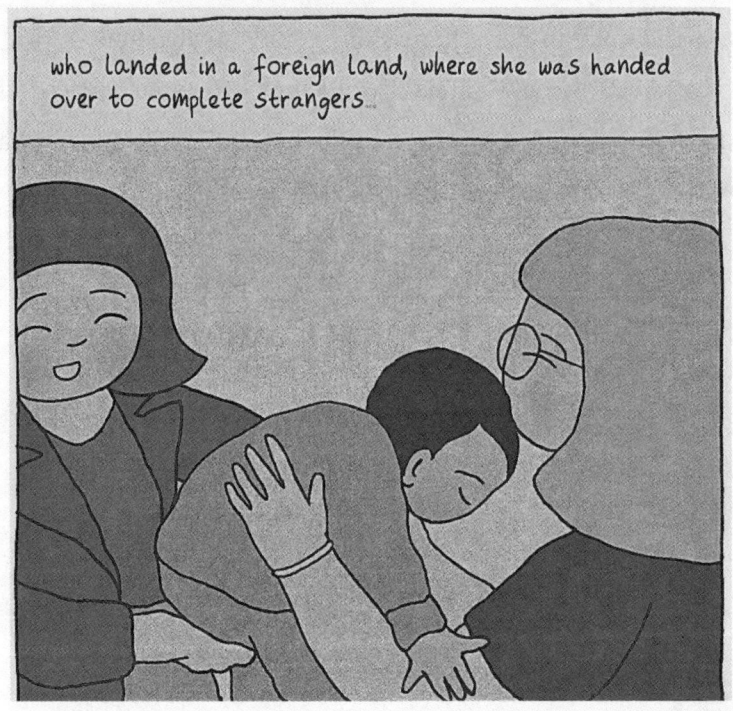

Source: From *Palimpsest.* Copyright Lisa Wool-Rim Sjöblojm. Used with permission from Drawn & Quarterly.

Lisa Wool-Rim Sjöblom was adopted in Sweden. Her graphic novel chronicles her search for her birth family and explores what happens to origin stories in adoption. The title, *Palimpsest*, is a metaphor for adoption and for having your origin story erased. "We become an empty vessel for other people to fill with their own story" (Sjöblom, 2019, p. 14).

Sjöblom (2019) shares:

> I'm a person who manifested out of thin air, a person without roots. Not born but still here (p. 11) . . . . Back then, when I embarked on my first search, I believed my adoption was proof that I was never supposed to exist. I'd grown up with the feeling that I was a mistake. Who gives up a wanted child? (p. 55)
>
> . . . To me being adopted didn't mean I was chosen, like others wanted me to believe. It meant I was rejected. (p. 28)

Giving birth to her own children brought back her own origin story in a very embodied way:

> Night after night, I watched over my newborn son, ready to pick him up if he woke up feeling lonely. Each cry tore me apart. I thought he sounded like an abandoned child. I was tormented by nightmare visions, in which I die, and Teddy is taken away to an orphanage . . . to later be adopted and taught to forget that I had ever been his mother. (Sjöblom, 2019, p. 16)

Making contact with her birth mother added another narrative to Lisa Wool-Rim's origin story. She also learned that her Korean name, Wool-Rim, had been mispronounced:

> I realize that I and everyone I know have been pronouncing it wrongly all my life. . . . I was always a bit embarrassed about it and thought it sounded harsh and ugly. But "Oolim"

is soft, and the pronunciation fits its poetic meaning: "forest echo." I have the most beautiful name in the world. (p. 73)

All my life I have fought to tell my own story. It's always been there, but it's gone through many edits before it finally felt authentic. (Sjöblom, 2019, postscript)

TIME FOR REFLECTION

Reflect on adoptive families that you have worked with or had personal contact with, including your own if this is your experience.

- Consider the themes that you have come across during your experiences.
- How does understanding these themes impact your interventions?
- How have your DDP interventions given a voice to adoptees and adopters?

Another, often silent, voice is that of the birth parents. Their presence will be felt in the stories told:

- The adoptive parent tells the child why they were adopted.
- The child tells themselves why they were rejected.
- The birth parents hold a story of why they lost their child.

Multiple stories impact the lives of all involved. The following box shares Carrie's story, giving a voice to the birth parent, so that they are not forgotten in our DDP interventions.

A BIRTH MOTHER'S STORY

Carrie is a birth mother with a traumatic history. Her children were removed from her care and then adopted. Carrie initially blames the social worker for removing her children, but during counseling, this narrative starts to change.

> Carrie starts to share her most painful feelings. She makes it clear that she hates herself; feeling completely to blame for her difficulties in being able to parent her children. Sometimes the intensity of the pain is too much, and she will rage to avoid her feelings of intense shame. Carrie feels to blame, and it is important for Jane to be alongside her in this process. Ultimately it is Carrie's truth, and she and Jane will need to find a way that Carrie can go on living with the knowledge that the children have been lost because of behaviors that she engaged in. Understanding that some of these behaviors might have stemmed out of the influence of her early abuse history will come later. For now, Carrie needs to experience Jane's compassion for her, even when her darkest feelings about herself are revealed. Carrie voices that it would be easier to die. How can she live with this level of self-blame and self-loathing? (Golding & Gould, 2019, p. 127)

The counselor supports Carrie with PACE while continuing to cocreate Carrie's story. As the counseling continues, the counselor writes: "She couldn't quite forgive herself for the loss of her children, but she was now compassionate towards herself and accepting of who she was and why she had made the choices that she had" (Golding & Gould, 2019, p. 130).

TIME FOR REFLECTION

When working with adoptive families:

• What thought have you given to the birth parents' stories?

• If you haven't given any, why do you think this is?

• How does holding these stories in mind impact the DDP interventions that you provide?

RESIDENTIAL CARE

There are many reasons why a child moves into a residential home, including the lack of an available, suitable family placement. Mostly, and more positively, a residential setting is an option for children who have not been able to live successfully within a family, especially when the child is putting themselves or others at physical risk. Residential care can provide them with the support they need but are unable to accept within a family. It can also help preserve relationships with family (birth, foster, or adoptive) in a way that cannot be achieved when they are living together.

Historically, residential care has kept children physically safe while paying little attention to emotional well-being. More recently, there is increased understanding about the importance of providing a therapeutic environment with some residential homes working hard to provide this. DDP practitioners can be helpful to residential staff groups who want to ensure that trauma-informed, attachment-based principles are built into their organization.

TIME FOR REFLECTION

We invite you to reflect on different ways that DDP practitioners can support children living in residential settings.

Additionally, what would help the staff embed DDP throughout the residential organization?

Here are a few of our thoughts, which illustrate our impression of the importance of DDP practitioners being therapist, support worker, trainer, and consultant for the organization. For a more comprehensive exploration, see Grant, Thompson, and Golding (in press).

- DDP as stand-alone therapy is unlikely to be sufficient. DDP principles need to be embedded in the daily milieu of home and school.

- Training helps the staff to understand the children and what they need.

- Ongoing support for staff helps them to absorb the impact of trauma on the young people, often displayed through their behavior. This includes helping the staff to understand their own relationship history and how challenges from their past can be triggered when caring for young people in the present.

- The staff will be at risk of experiencing blocked care and vicarious traumatization; they deserve good quality therapeutic support.

- DDP practitioners can help staff provide relationship-based discipline, such as providing regulatory and emotional support before behavioral support.

- The school needs support. Children placed in residential care benefit from a small, developmentally appropriate school that focuses on safety and emotional support before, and alongside, learning.

Residential care brings its own stories of loss, fear, and bravado, adding to the narratives from pre-residential experience. These stories impact the child's sense of self, their expectations of the future, and their relationship with past families, including their birth family. The following box explores one person's search for a narrative to help him understand who he is.

A RESIDENTIAL TEENAGER'S STORY

The BAFTA-nominated, award-winning, international writer, poet, and broadcaster Lemn Sissy tells the story of being taken into care against the wishes of his birth mother. Assigned to long-term foster carers as an infant and then moved to residential care as an early adolescent, his memoir tells the story of a life in care that should never have been.

> When I was tucked into bed the staff wrote their reports. They had the last word on everything. My teenage self could not deal with this at all. The report seemed only to document anything untoward. My wellbeing [*sic*] was defined by how many marks *against* my name were in that report. . . . I was three years away from leaving care. I started to ask questions about my origins. Who was my mother? Why was I in care in the first place? Where was I from? Why was I here? In realizing my foster parents didn't want me I wanted to know about my birth mother. The only person who could help me was my social worker.
>
> A fourteen-year-old boy should never have to ask the questions *Who is my mother?* and *Who are my family?* These were not easy questions to formulate in the mind or the

mouth because the question comes with others. . . . *What did I do to deserve this?* (Sissy, 2020, p. 104)

DDP interventions with foster, kinship, adopted, and residential families will be centered around many stories both historic and current. Like the stories shared here, the interventions will be personal, individual, and unique, while also touching on common themes. Understanding and exploring these stories will enhance DDP interventions, whether in therapy, parenting support, or consultation with schools and networks. When we hold common themes in mind, it needs to not be at the expense of the unique stories we are exploring. Rather holding the common themes and unique stories together will help us to be more vigilant to elements of the stories that need exploring. We can bring this understanding to our cocreation of stories with the family members we are working with. From our not-knowing-but-wondering stance, we can help deepen the awareness of themes that are impacting this family and explore how they influence the interventions that the family will find helpful.

TIME FOR REFLECTION

We invite you to reflect on the stories we have touched on in this section.

What stories have you discovered from your experience of supporting or knowing children living in families away from their birth parents?

FAMILIES WHERE THERE IS RISK

The foundation of DDP is safety. The theoretical foundations of DDP—attachment, intersubjectivity, and interpersonal neurobiology—all demonstrate the importance of safety for building relationships and healing trauma.

PACE is central in creating and maintaining safety. The acceptance of PACE means that all evaluations are restricted to behaviors, with none directed toward the inner life (thoughts, feelings, wishes) of the other. This allows members of the family to remain open and engaged rather than becoming defensive when behavioral challenges or differences are addressed. This enables them to address the behaviors while also protecting the relationship, repairing ruptures as needed. This method protects against shame, meaning that the person does not have to defend themselves by denying having engaged in the behaviors or by responding in anger.

A family at risk has an increased likelihood that behaviors harmful to some members of the family and to the relationships within the family will occur. The DDP practitioner is often able to contain the behaviors of children by attending to what they mean. This helps the child to communicate through a story rather than to express it through behaviors. With less need for challenging behaviors, the child will be more likely to rely on their parents for understanding and support.

When the source of risk is the parents' behaviors, these may have to be addressed more quickly and directly to ensure the safety of the children in the home. Here, the DDP practitioner needs to maintain the balance between addressing the behavior while maintaining the safety generated by the attitude of PACE. If there is too much focus on the need for behavior change without the support of PACE, the parents are at risk of withdrawing or becoming habitually defensive and not engaged in the therapeutic process of change. If there is too little focus on behavior change, risks to the child may fail to be addressed and may become more severe.

REFLECTIVE EXERCISE: BALANCING PACE AND ADDRESSING PARENTAL BEHAVIOR

In Worksheet 10.1 at the end of this chapter, there is an opportunity to explore the challenges of balancing the attitude of PACE with being clear about parental behaviors that seem to be harmful to the child and/or the parent–child relationship.

In DDP, the practitioner is encouraged to develop an intersubjective experience of the parents as: good people, who care about their child, doing the best they can. Once that experience is communicated to the parents—primarily nonverbally—the practitioner is more able to address the concerning behaviors. In addition, if they are experienced as good parents, they are more likely to remain open and engaged, rather than becoming defensive, to guidance regarding their behavior.

Here is an example of a practitioner creating an intersubjective relationship with a parent who has become critical of her son.

Practitioner: You're trying so hard; it must be very discouraging that Cam doesn't seem to be responding to your care.

Parent: I'm not discouraged. I'm angry that he seems to be so selfish no matter what I do for him!

Practitioner: And I hear that you're a bit angry with me too for commenting on how difficult it is trying to raise him right.

Parent: I don't want your pity!

Practitioner: I must be communicating poorly. I'm not sorry for you over how hard it is with your child. I'm trying to be with you in your challenges, to show you that you're not alone in your distress.

Parent: That doesn't make it any better!

Practitioner: Maybe you're annoyed with me because his behavior hasn't shown more improvement. If things don't seem to be getting better, I can understand why you would say my empathy for you isn't what you need.

Parent: I want him to be glad that I'm his parent!

Practitioner: Ah! That's it! You want to matter to him! He matters so much to you and you're not sure if you matter to him! That would be so painful!

Parent: Why can't he see how much he matters to me?

Practitioner: Ah! And I have to find a way to help him to see that! I see it! But he needs to see it! And if he doesn't see the place he has in your heart, I think there must be a lot of sadness under your anger.

The practitioner remains regulated and relates in an open and engaged manner with the parent, whether they are agreeing or disagreeing. The practitioner maintains an attitude of PACE throughout, which makes it possible to move on to addressing behaviors without causing the parent to become defensive.

SAFETY AND FAMILY PRESERVATION

When DDP is being used with families considered to be at risk, it is fair to say that one or more members of the family are not safe, physically and/or psychologically. While the goal of DDP is always to increase the safety of all members of the family, there is some danger that the DDP practitioner might overlook signs of risk out of a commitment to preserve the family. When this occurs, the results can be tragic.

TIME FOR REFLECTION

We invite you to reflect on some of the other reasons why DDP practitioners might overlook signs of risk to safety.

Here are some thoughts from us:

1. The DDP practitioner begins therapy by meeting and creating an alliance with the parents without the child present. The practitioner might underestimate the risk to the child as they develop empathy for the parents and all the challenges the parents are facing. The focus on discovering that the parents are good people, who love their child, doing the best that they might reduce the focus on the parents' behaviors and the possibility that they are hurting the child.

2. If the parents acknowledge their maltreatment of their child and show regret and a desire to change, the practitioner might too readily accept and have confidence in the parents' belief that they will not do it again.

3. The DDP practitioner might worry that if they address the parents' punitive behavior toward their child, the parents will no longer

trust them and will either withdraw from therapy or speak less openly about their behavior. As a result, the practitioner might wait too long before addressing any seemingly harsh treatment of the parents toward their child.

4. The DDP practitioner might hold unrealistic confidence that the therapeutic relationship will reduce the risk of maltreatment, even when the original maltreatment has not been addressed and/or the parents are in denial about what they have done.

5. The DDP practitioner might assume that they are in the best position to know what is best for the child and family and might conceal from other professionals details about the family, which might place the child at risk.

It is crucial that the DDP practitioner not focus on family preservation without keeping in mind whether safety is present.

When the DDP practitioner provides therapy to a family at risk, they should consider:

- meeting with the parents alone for additional sessions to address the behaviors that are creating risk
- meeting with the child alone for some sessions to ensure that they have an opportunity to express those experiences that they don't want to talk about in front of their parents
- having regular contact with social services and education (with permission) to obtain their perspective on the presence of risk

REFLECTIVE EXERCISE: RESPONDING TO INDICATIONS OF RISK

You can explore responding to indication of risks within conversations using Worksheet 10.2 at the end of this chapter.

We are going to imagine a scenario wherein you have been working with the parents for six months. The aim is for their son to return to their care from foster care. The child, now 10, entered foster care a year ago because of the parents' domestic violence and substance misuse. He had a previous period in foster care for the same reasons when he was seven years old. Both you and the social worker believe that this time, the progress is more substantial and that he will be able to safely return home. However, the child does not want to return home. He likes his foster parents and his life with them. It is the same foster home he had been in previously, and he believes that the same bad things will happen if he is returned home. He describes the marginal care he had when living with his parents before, and he does not believe they have changed. The social worker wonders if he also likes the middle-class life of his foster parents, something that his parents cannot provide for him.

TIME FOR REFLECTION

Consider some typical (non-DDP) ways that practitioners might try to help the family in this situation.

Reflect on difficulties that might arise from these suggestions.

Finally, reflect on how DDP interventions might prove more helpful.

Here are some examples of typical professional interventions to this scenario that we thought might not be helpful:

1. The professionals assure the child that this time will be different. They are confident that his parents will now take better care of him.
    - If the professionals are wrong, the child's trust and confidence in them will be undermined.
2. The professionals tell the child that adults know best what the source of the problems is and what to do about it.
    - While such comments are meant to reassure him, in that it is not his responsibility to resolve the problems, the child might instead experience such comments as suggesting that his thoughts and ideas are not important.
3. The professionals tell the child that when he is returned to his parents' care, the professional will be evaluating how things are going. If it is not working out, the professionals will ensure that the child is safe, including removing him if needed.
    - Such comments are likely to undermine the child's confidence that there will be significant change. He is likely to become more anxious, having less confidence in his parents and in the professionals.

Here are some possible DDP interventions that might have a greater chance of success.

1. The child is shown that his doubts are being taken seriously and are not being ignored. The professional relates with the child with PACE, demonstrating acceptance and understanding of the child's concerns. The child's concerns are not minimized, nor is the child given a "quick fix." The professional shows that they are now aware of the child's doubts, even though there might not be a simple way to make them go away.

2. The DDP practitioner and child meet separately from the parents. The practitioner focuses on understanding the child's doubts and exploring what, if anything, might help to reduce them.

3. The practitioner holds joint sessions with the child and parent. The practitioner supports the parents to acknowledge their parenting mistakes, accept responsibility, apologize, and express commitments to be different in the future. The practitioner also supports the child to tell his parents how he has been affected by his parents' behaviors and what worries he has, if any, about the future.

The DDP practitioner is conveying to both child and parents that the practitioner's goal is to support the relationship so that they all feel safe and valued. Challenges will be addressed while conveying that the relationships are more important than whatever conflicts they face. At the same time, the practitioner will ensure that the child's safety will not be forgotten.

INDIVIDUAL THERAPY

Generally, DDP involves the child, caregiver, and DDP practitioner. The practitioner builds a relationship with both the child and the caregiver to facilitate their relationship with each other. When the caregiver is not able to engage in DDP with the child, or the child will engage only in individual therapy, the practitioner may still engage the child in DDP. When this occurs, it is the relationship between the therapist and child that facilitates therapeutic change.

Individual DDP therapy may be indicated when there is no caregiver to become engaged in the therapy. The therapeutic relationship continues to manifest features of attachment, intersubjectivity, and integrative neurological functioning, characterized by safety. Within this relationship, the therapist engages in the coregulation of the child's affective states. This differs from some individual therapies, wherein the therapist presents the child with a neutral stance with the expectation that the child will autoregulate their affective state. Just as in dyadic interventions, the DDP therapist communicates their experience of the child in a way that contributes to the child's intersubjective experience of self and other. The difference is that they cannot facilitate the parent also communicating their experience of the child in this way. When, during the course of DDP therapy, the child struggles to develop a more integrative sense of self, the therapist assumes a more active role in the process of cocreating a coherent narrative.

In many forms of individual therapy, the child (or client of any age) is perceived as transferring features of other important relationships in their life onto the therapeutic relationship. Thus, if the child experienced habitual rejection or indifference in their relationship with their parents, they are likely to be highly sensitive to signs of possible rejection or indifference from their therapist. An important therapeutic goal becomes helping the child to begin to differentiate the therapist (and others) from the child's previous significant relationships.

In DDP with child and caregiver, the main therapeutic focus is to assist the child to differentiate their current relationships with caregivers from their prior significant relationships. The child is likely to have transferred aspects of their relationship with their biological parents onto their relationships with the foster or adoptive parents. The child who was abused by their biological parents may experience routine limits and discipline from foster carers as abusive. The child who was neglected might experience routine times when their adoptive parents are unavailable to interact with them as neglect. The DDP therapist focuses on helping the child become aware of the story they hold that they are using to interpret current interactions with the foster carers: *"They say 'no' to me because they do not like me"* or *"they are mean to me and think I'm bad."*

The therapist then helps the child to develop a new story about the foster carers' intentions: *"They do understand that I want that and am sad, but they are trying to teach me something important. They want to help to make it easier for me to understand that they say 'no' and still love me."*

By putting the focus on the foster or adoptive parents, the child is less apt to transfer their perceptions onto the DDP therapist. In fact, in DDP therapy, the child's relationship with their current caregivers becomes the source of the child's new learnings about self and other. The DDP therapist provides safety and the structure of affective–reflective dialogue with PACE to help this process. It is the child's new intersubjective experiences with their caregivers that are the most important sources of therapeutic change.

When the child is engaged in DDP in individual therapy, the relationship with the therapist becomes the key agent of change. In this relationship, the child experiences relational safety and discovers the positive effect they are having on the therapist. The child discovers that their birth parents' experiences of them are different from those of the therapist. They experience trust in the therapist rather than the mistrust that was present in their relationship with their parents.

TIME FOR REFLECTION

Below we present two different experiences of engaging children in individual therapy. As you read these, notice the ways that DDP has been adapted for there being no parents involved in the therapy.

Alisha is a 13-year-old girl who lived with her parents until she was seven. She experienced physical and verbal abuse, domestic violence, and emotional neglect from her parents, who habitually abused substances. Over the next five years, she lived in three foster homes, each time being asked to leave due to her oppositional–defiant behaviors. She is now living in a group home. The DDP therapist works with her individually because there is no primary caregiver in her life. Alisha shows little sign of trusting others and relates to the DDP therapist in a very belligerent manner. This interactive sequence occurs in the third session.

Therapist:	It's been a very hard week, Alisha. Though in some ways it hasn't been much different from most of your weeks here . . . or even most of your weeks everywhere you've been.

Alisha: Why don't you say it! I've brought it all on myself! I need an "attitude adjustment." Maybe I need to be taken apart, and you can put me back together so that I'm a good little girl.

Therapist: That would really wear you down, if you think something is wrong with you!

Alisha: I don't think that, but I know that you do! You say, "Poor Alisha," but you also think, "That bitch deserves whatever she gets."

Therapist: No wonder you don't trust me if that's what you think I'm saying to myself about you.

Alisha: I don't think it, I know it! And you'd say it if you wouldn't lose your job for it. You have to pretend you're interested in me and want to help me.

(The therapist tries to have a conversation with Alisha about her experience. The therapist accepts whatever Alisha says and then replies with alternating empathy and curiosity, each comment being determined by how Alisha responds to the previous comment.)

Therapist: So, to you, everything I say is fake. No wonder you're angry with me. Have you ever known someone who was interested in you and truly wanted to help you?

Alisha: Yeah, but it's not you!

Therapist: I'm glad you knew that someone was truly interested in you! What do you think that person saw in you?

Alisha: How do I know?

Therapist: Whatever it was, I hope you have some confidence that it does exist! There is something about you that the other person cared about . . . something about you.

Alisha: Hard to believe, isn't it?

Therapist: I wonder if it's hard for you to believe. If I'm truly interested in your life—in you—how would you know?

Alisha: Like that's going to happen.

Therapist: I worry that you would have trouble trusting your experience if you did think that I might care for you. It's so hard to believe that I really care about you, that you're not just a job to me.

Alisha: Why should I trust you?

Therapist: I hope you might a bit more each time I listen to you, feel sad with you about the hard times you've had to face for so long, and understand some of what you are saying to me.

Alisha: But you'll probably get bored just like everyone else has.

Therapist: I don't find you boring and it's hard to imagine that I will. You're alive! You're a fighter! You didn't choose the crazy world you were born into, and you haven't given up. No, I will not be bored by you.

Alisha: Suppose I decide that I never want to be good.

Therapist:	You'll have your reasons. Rather than thinking about whether you're good, I'll be thinking about whether you're finding the life that you want, that brings you some joy. No, I don't think I'll be bored if you let me get to know you as you go forward on your journey.
Alisha:	We'll see.
Therapist:	Thanks for suggesting it might be possible.

It is likely to take many conversations like this one before a child trusts that you are not like others who have violated their trust. These conversations are much more than words; they are expressions of your mind and heart that, hopefully, the child will gradually be able to experience. If Alisha had been in a residential program run based on attachment principles using a DDP framework, there would be a residential worker present in the sessions. This worker, from a stance of PACE, would be serving as an attachment figure for Alisha, and the practitioner would be facilitating Alisha's ability to trust that person. The frequency and variety of her interactions with that person would complement the features of her relationship with the practitioner.

Here is a conversation with another child, ten-year-old Jonah, who is also in individual therapy. His elderly foster parents are committed to providing ongoing care for Jonah but were clear that they did not want to be part of his therapy. As with Alisha, Jonah also needs to differentiate the relationship with the therapist from his relationship with his parents during his first few years. Jonah also experienced significant physical and verbal abuse and neglect. His defensive response is the opposite of Alisha's response. He compulsively tried to "be good" to avoid rejection and shame. Rather than using anger to distance himself from others, he tries to be liked to be close to others and to feel safer. Jonah tries to ensure that the therapist will like him through constant agreement, cooperation, denial of differences, and by vigilantly attending to the therapist for hints as to what might make him more likeable.

Here, the therapist would need to relate to Jonah with PACE in a manner both similar to and different from how they related to Alisha. The following represents typical examples of what the DDP therapist might say in this conversation.

- Jonah, I notice that we agree on most everything! What's that about, do you think?
- Jonah, when I asked you to tell me about the conflict that you had with your teacher, you did. I sensed that at least part of you would rather not tell me. Is that right? What do you think I would have said if you had expressed that part of you?
- Jonah, is it hard to disagree with someone that you like and who you want to like you? No? Could you give me an example of a disagreement that you had with someone you like?
- Jonah, what do you think would happen if you got annoyed with me during one of our meetings? Do you worry that I might not enjoy seeing you as much? Do you worry that I might even want to stop seeing you?
- Jonah, when do you think you started putting so much energy into being sure that people like you? Do you think, maybe, that you started doing that after your father hurt you, when he was annoyed with something you did?

If Jonah's caregiver was engaged in the DDP therapy, the practitioner would be discussing events at home involving similar themes with the caregiver. The daily events occurring in the home would provide many more opportunities for Jonah to begin to create a new story about his relationship with his attachment figure. With the help of the practitioner, Jonah would be able to reflect on his differences and conflicts with his caregiver without experiencing pervasive shame or a fear of abandonment.

CONCLUSION

DDP practitioners will find themselves working with children who have experienced developmental trauma and who are now living in a wide range of situations. Where they are living is the context in which their development is facilitated or hindered, experienced, and expressed. It is the practitioner's responsibility to strive to understand these living situations so they may understand the impact the situations are having on the child. These contexts may provide protective features that enhance the child's ability to resolve their traumatic past. They may also provide risk features that make it difficult to achieve resolution of trauma. As the DDP practitioner assists the child on their developmental journey, they need to get to know the context within which the child is trying to move forward. If the practitioner can have an impact on this context, the journey is more likely to increase the child's sense of safety, resilience, and capacity to thrive.

Worksheet 10.1

 Reflective Exercise: Balancing PACE
and Addressing Parental Behavior

Reflect on the following scenarios. Explore how the practitioner might respond in a way that addresses parental behaviors while maintaining an attitude of PACE.

1. **Parent:** I do become angry with them when they get annoyed at my decisions. It is completely disrespectful.

2. **Parent:** You're blaming me for this!

3. **Parent:** Don't feel sorry for them! They need to be held accountable for their behavior!

_____

_____

_____

_____

4. **Parent:** My kid needs to accept my rules! You seem to encourage him to question my authority.

_____

_____

_____

_____

5. **Parent:** I don't care what it means! I want the behavior to stop, and I want you to tell me what to do to make it stop!

_____

_____

_____

_____

6. **Parent:** Are you saying I don't love Danny? Are you agreeing with him when he said that I don't love him because I wouldn't let him do what he wanted? I'm his parent! My job is not to please him all the time, I have to do what is best for him even if he doesn't like it!

_____

_____

_____

7. **Parent:** I know I'm raising my kid the way my parents raised me! And I'm proud of that! They did a good job raising me.

_____

_____

_____

Reflections on Worksheet 10.1: Possible Responses

1. **Parent:** I do become angry with them when they get annoyed at my decisions. It is completely disrespectful.

   Therapist: I agree with you on the importance of respect within family relationships. I worry that any time your child seems annoyed with something you've done, you consider that to be disrespectful. Is there room in your relationship for your child to express annoyance with something you've decided and it to not be considered disrespectful? Is it ever allowable for your child to raise their voice and show their annoyance in their facial expressions, which are the most clear and direct expressions of annoyance?

2. **Parent:** You're blaming me for this!

   Therapist: I'm sorry I said that in a way that feels like I'm blaming you. I wanted to get us thinking about another way to address their behavior that did not generate such anger on their part. If they could more easily accept your correction, your relationship would remain closer despite your differences.

3. **Parent:** Don't feel sorry for them! They need to be held accountable for their behavior!

   Therapist: I think we might disagree on the place of empathy in your relationship with your child. Could we explore it again? Because I didn't intend to convey that I am sorry for them over how strict you are, nor am I suggesting that you are too strict. Rather I simply want them to know that I understand how hard this is for them.

4. **Parent:** My kid needs to accept my rules! You seem to encourage him to question my authority.

   Therapist: Either we disagree about this, or I gave my recommendation poorly. I was suggesting that you restrict your rules to your child's behaviors, without limiting the value of your child being able to develop his own unique thoughts and feelings about things. You're more likely to have a child who becomes habitually rebellious or submissive—not just with you but with others too—if your child isn't able to have thoughts and feelings that disagree with yours.

5. **Parent:** I don't care what it means! I want the behavior to stop, and I want you to tell me what to do to make it stop!

   Therapist: I would if I could, but if I don't know what the behavior means, I'm likely to give you poor recommendations. I think you're telling me that his behavior is really, really hard for you and that you are desperate to get it changed as soon as possible. I promise to give you a suggestion as soon as I possibly can. To do that, I need to know what the behavior means. I'm sorry it is so hard for you just now, and I am asking you to wait.

6. **Parent:** Are you saying I don't love Danny? Are you agreeing with him when he said that I don't love him because I wouldn't let him do what he wanted? I'm his parent! My job is not to please him all the time, I have to do what is best for him even if he doesn't like it!

   Therapist: Your love for him is obvious to me and I regret if I haven't been clear about that! I'm saying that the conflicts you two have are so frequent and so intense that he may not feel loved at times. His brain may know you love him, but his heart may not feel it! I want to help you find ways to give him the guidance and limits that he needs without creating any doubts in his heart about your love. I'm not asking you to love him— that's not in doubt! I'm asking you to work with me in finding ways to show your love for him—so he feels it even when you are saying no to him!

7. **Parent:** I know I'm raising my kid the way my parents raised me! And I'm proud of that! They did a good job raising me.

   Therapist: I am sorry if you feel that I'm being critical of your parents' relationship with you. My sense is that you respected your parents and took advantage of their guidance. I also think you were not emotionally close to them. You didn't share your hopes and dreams, doubts, fears, anger, or sadness with them. Seems that you and your parents believe that you cannot have that emotional closeness and at the same time respect and rely on your parents' authority. I'm saying that I disagree. Would you explore with me what having both of these would look like, and then decide if you want to learn how to make it happen?

IN CONVERSATION FIVE

Kim met with Shani Sephton to talk with her about her experience as a Black British practitioner attending DDP Level One and Two trainings. Shani is Black British-Caribbean and has had a career as a social worker and is currently training as a clinical psychologist. Kim was the trainer for both Shani's DDP Level One and Two trainings. Between these two trainings, Kim participated in racial equity training.

Following this conversation, Kim asked Ahoora Baranian and Swati Uniyal to read her conversation with Shani and reflect on their own experiences of attending DDP Level One training. Ahoora is a psychotherapeutic counselor trainee. He is Iranian, born in Iran, and has lived in England since he was 15 years old. Swati is a psychotherapist trainee. She was born in India and moved to the U.K. 18 years ago.

KIM AND SHANI

Kim: Shani, I'm really interested to hear about your experiences of DDP training.

Shani: Even at the point of signing up for DDP Level One, I was thinking, "What's this going to be like? I'm probably going to be the only Black person in the room." Attending the training, I had to take a deep breath, put a layer of skin on, as I anticipated microaggressions. I expected to feel singled out and alone. I expected that I would not see any videos that included people that represented or looked like me. I guess it feels like being an elephant in the room, because I am the only Black person, but, strangely, you also feel invisible as the only Black person, if that makes sense. This isn't just with DDP Level One, this is what I feel quite often when I go to any professional training.

Kim: I remember, there was only a little cultural diversity within your Level One group.

Shani: Yes, everyone was really lovely and welcoming, at my table particularly, but it was very much a white space. I remember looking at the training material; it felt very white, Eurocentric. I had to think, "OK, how do I apply this to my situation, my life, or people that look like me?" I really liked much of what I was hearing, but I didn't feel that it fully related to me. I had to think, "How can I tweak that? How can I adapt that so that it applies to people that look like me?" One of the recordings made me feel really uncomfortable, the comment directed at Black people; that felt really overt.

Kim: I didn't look at it through your eyes. That is one of the things the work I have done has helped me to be more mindful of; who is in the room and how might they receive this.

Shani: The difficulty is, even within the Black community, there are varying levels of racism and internalized racism. What might be offensive to one Black or BIPOC person might be acceptable to another. So, I was trying to suss out the room, and I think that probably contributed to me feeling slightly anxious. So, then I was in limbo, thinking, "Right, how do I honor the trainer, this person I respect, but equally highlight some of my concerns?" And then I sort of plucked up the courage to highlight my concerns. I was met with so much openness from you. You were open to understand and learn a bit more and that is when you suggested that there might be some opportunities for me to help shape things within the DDP community.

Kim: When I think back to that Level One, I feel I didn't give much thought about how to make the training applicable to a diverse group. I was very open to whomever came to the training. I wanted them to feel welcomed and included, but I didn't go that extra step of, for example, noticing you as a black woman. I wasn't curious about what this would be like for you. You were extremely welcome. I would consider myself someone who would welcome anyone into the training space, whatever their race, sexuality, gender, disability. I was open to anybody, but I was blind as well. My idea of welcoming was to not see color, to not see difference. This led to mistakes, as you experienced. I was welcoming to you, but it wasn't with careful thought.

Shani: Why do you think it's important, realizing how being color-blind wasn't inclusive?

Kim: Because I didn't know that you would come in with all that anxiety. It wasn't in my consciousness that you'd be worrying that you would be the only Black person in the group and that you were not going to see yourself represented. My idea of being open and welcoming to the group was to not notice difference. That's what I was socialized to do. I thought I was being open and welcoming to you by not noticing you were a black woman. That's where I had to shift my perspective. This shift happened between your Level One and Two, and so I am wondering how Level Two was for you.

Shani: I didn't go into Level Two with the same level of anxiety that I went into Level One with. I felt more comfortable and confident because of our conversations, because of the work we had been doing. I anticipated a safe environment, or at least a safer environment. This meant that I could learn and connect better, right from the start. Then you brought race, culture, and difference into the room seamlessly. It felt comfortable.

Kim: That's lovely to hear, because at times I have been clumsy; in trying to include and welcome people, I have made them uncomfortable. I don't want to ignore difference anymore; but in noticing it, I have caused discomfort too. DDP values the importance of repairing relationships. That has been so important for me to hold onto. Go to them, and repair it, and then, if they are ready, move on.

Shani: It sounds like you didn't purposely try to offend. In racism, it is often true that the person did not purposely offend. Intentions might be well-meaning however the impact is important. How did that land with the person? The good thing is, you felt comfortable and confident to repair and then move on. Whereas if you had not addressed it, then that person may have felt anxious for the rest of the training. Myself, as a Black woman, I respect people who are able to reflect and think: "Ooh, that didn't quite come out right. I'm sorry, but this is what I meant. I wonder how I could rephrase it." It's a new language in terms of the things that you're saying and talking about. It's about how you bring all these words, sentences, and phrases together so that it makes sense and also is respectful and honors the person that you're in conversation with.

Kim: In training, it's really hard to know how to be inclusive in a way that is helpful for everyone. That's where I'm struggling.

Everyone's different, and everyone wants something different. At the beginning of a training, when you don't know people, it's really hard to get it right.

Shani: Yes, maybe notice that there is diversity in the room, mentioning intersectionality, but without singling anyone out. It gives people a sense that you are open to these conversations, and then they can choose how much they want to share.

Kim: OK, comment that I want us to think about how DDP interventions can be sensitive to diversity and the intersectionality between race, sexuality, gender, disability, class, and religion. Invite reflections on this as we move through the training. And maybe, if it is a nondiverse group, I could say, for example, "I notice our training space is predominantly white, and I want us to think about diversity in a way that feels safe."

Shani: Yes. I think there is always going to be a degree of discomfort when a person of color is inhabiting a predominantly white space. It's going to feel visually uncomfortable. You look beside you and think: "I'd better not laugh too hard. I've got to mind the way that I say something because someone might tone-police me. What microaggressions might I expect?" There's always going to be a layer of uncomfortableness.

Kim: And this is likely to be similar for other trainees from marginalized groups. Someone who is gay, for example, or has a visible or invisible disability. They will be wondering what they should share and how they will be received by the rest of the group.

Shani: Yes, the way you model talking about diversity will open up avenues for further conversation in line with what people are comfortable sharing.

Kim: This is making me think about the opening introduction, when I ask people to talk about themselves. By providing that general acknowledgement of the diversity or lack of obvious diversity in the room, it might help people to feel safer sharing.

Shani: Doing the general acknowledgement provides a signal for people within the group; for example, people with hidden disabilities, people from a Black Asian race, someone who's not heteronormative. It will help them to see that you are open to these conversations. Then when you do go into the introductions, people might feel more comfortable to say, "This is my identity."

Kim: I'm thinking, as we are talking, that it's also important to remind people to only share what they feel comfortable to share. Take a moment to think: "Do I want to share this?" It's all about establishing safety, safety to share and safety not to share. This sets the tone for the rest of the training. The opening part of a training is such an important time, isn't it?

Shani: First impressions last.

Kim: Yes, and I have found that when you do this, conversations emerge quite naturally during the rest of the training. I notice opportunities to reflect, or someone in the group makes a reflection and we have a conversation about supporting people with diverse identities and diverse needs within our DDP interventions.

Shani: Yes, that felt really comfortable. It didn't feel tokenistic, like, "Here's the script. I've got to remember to say that word. If I don't say that word, then I'm not hitting all my diversity markers." It didn't feel like that at all. It felt like a conversation, a comfortable conversation, throughout the whole training.

Kim: Thank you so much Shani, for spending this time with me. It has been really helpful talking about this with you.

Kim and Ahoora

Kim: Hello Ahoora, I am interested in your reflections of experiencing a DDP training.

Ahoora: Introductions feel important. I've noticed that when I introduce myself, I'm aware of my skin color. I always start with a joke. I say: "I'm Ahoora Baranian, it's a typical Yorkshire name," just to break that barrier down. I think it's for my protection. People may hear my Yorkshire accent, too, and realize I've lived in that part of the country, and although I am not white, I have some Britishness in me. This may help to establish some credibility and that I have roots in this country.

Kim: That feels important for you to do, in a way that I don't feel the need to. That is a tough part of being in a minority within the community you are living and working. Shani and I were thinking about how I, as a DDP trainer, can help people from marginalized groups feel welcome in the training space. What are your thoughts about this?

Ahoora: I think vocalizing it is important. It's the wording of it that is hard. Naming the difference feels important to me but I think it's tricky when meeting for the first time. That might be more uncomfortable. Naming the difficulty could work. Discussing the difficulty will help people to relax. Right at the beginning, it can be very uncomfortable. Over the training I started to feel more comfortable.

Kim: What do you think helped you to feel comfortable?

Ahoora: I liked the way you shared about yourself. It was very congruent, in the way you said it and your body language. You were approachable. You invited us to share. You said, "Please interrupt me if you would like to." I would have liked to see more people from around the world in the training materials. The recordings were all white people. Looking for people who are similar to me is something I've become aware of. When I looked for a therapist, for example, I wanted an Iranian therapist.

Kim: Yes, that is something we are aware of and need to address. It will take time to build more representation of all kinds within DDP, therapists, consultants, and trainers. This would then be reflected in the training materials. It's work we need to do.

Ahoora: Maybe just state that at the start. Say that this profession is white, middle class, and heterosexual dominant and we would like to change that. If I had heard you saying that, it would have made me feel more comfortable.

Kim: I see what you mean. It's important to acknowledge that we are not representing everyone in the room within the training materials. I would also add that I welcome your contributions, if you feel comfortable to share, so that our discussions can represent everyone's views and experiences. Thank you so much, Ahoora, it has been lovely talking with you.

Kim and Swati

Kim: Swati, I am interested in hearing about your experiences of DDP training.

Swati: I think I have been using invisibility and silence as my defense to feel safe. So, when we started discussing diversity, I felt this discomfort. Perhaps, it heightened the awareness of being "seen" by you and my peers. But your compassionate approach made me feel safe enough to share my feelings and experience as a person of the minority. Since I developed an internalized racism from a young age, perhaps this feeling "Am I worthy of taking space?" or "who will be interested in what I have to say anyway?" meant the use of disengagement as my coping strategy, which I used very often in the class. And perhaps that's why, even though you created an inviting space, initially, I felt resistance. However, it was my choice not to speak up, and that in itself felt empowering. I finally spoke, even though it took a lot out of me to speak up and share how I felt about it in the group. Also, I noticed that once I said it out loud, my discomfort was replaced by anger. Perhaps it was underneath the defenses all this while. I didn't realize the level of intensity until you presented me with this opportunity where I came in contact with my vulnerable feelings about it. It has been an eye-opening experience. Gradually, I am noticing my patterns. For instance, when some of my white peers are unhappy or would like to make suggestions to improve in certain areas related to the course, they would raise it and generally seem more comfortable in putting their suggestions forward. However, I would usually tend to focus on the positive experiences and try to stay compliant. Perhaps, I don't feel entitled. I am wondering if my cultural values and how we view authorities has a role to play here too.

Kim: What advice would you give to me, as a DDP trainer, to help people from marginalized groups feel welcome in the training space?

Swati: I think your tentative approach regarding your understanding of marginalized groups and the thoughtful manner with which you shared it made me feel welcome. For me, it created a room for addressing power imbalance, which might have stayed invisible otherwise. I have felt this hidden pressure as a person of color, and by naming it and talking about it during our DDP training, it is slowly helping me to take some of that pressure away. However, in general, and of course in my experience so far, I feel that although we acknowledge diversity, we are not really addressing it. I would like to see more videos and case studies of people of color and the challenges a DDP practitioner might face while working with different ethnicities. Also, I wonder how we can integrate culture-centered theoretical approaches in our training programs. I have also noticed that we talk about working with diversity as something we would need to consider in the context of our future clients. It makes me wonder if we are overlooking the racial diversity or lack of it here and now in the classroom. This is because there is a lot of emotion and a lot of suppressed hurt in the room, and if we are not being attentive to that, then this will only further deepen the invisibility and silence and disempower the trainee psychotherapists of different heritage. I feel if our training courses become more inclusive, it will help minority trainees to navigate their identity better and to understand their defenses and develop skills rather than feeling preoccupied [by trying] to blend in.

Kim: Thank you so much for your thoughts and advice, Swati. Your insights are so helpful to increase my learning.

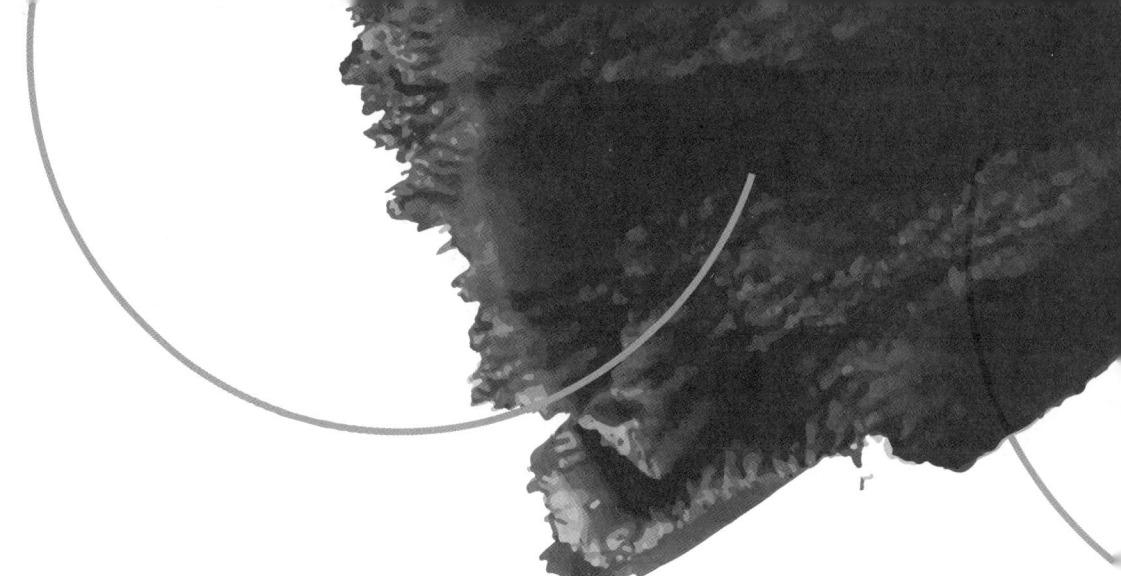

Chapter 11:
Training and Supervision the DDP way

. . . *through DDP-informed supervision [and training], the practitioner is provided with the same safe relational engagement and discoveries that they are attempting to provide for the children they are trying to help.*
(Hughes et al., 2019, p. 278)

REFRESHER

In this chapter, we are going to explore how DDP principles can be used to support practitioners of DDP as well as the parents. We will consider providing supervision and the application to training.

As we will explore, any training in or supervision of a relational model will benefit from a relational approach. The DDP principles adopted by the trainer or supervisor can help to achieve this aim. This relational approach also lends itself to promoting inclusion within supervision and training.

Many practitioners and parents have their own relational trauma history. To some extent, this is what has drawn them to a relational model. Additional support might be needed to help these individuals access the training or supervision.

Trainers and supervisors also need to be aware of and be committed to understanding social justice and the impacts of trauma and discrimination whether because of race, sexuality, gender, class, religious beliefs, neurodiversity, or disability. In this chapter, we will also explore how to make trainings and supervision inclusive, so that everyone feels welcome, providing a richer experience for all.

BRINGING A DDP-INFORMED APPROACH TO TRAINING

TIME FOR REFLECTION

Reflect on training that you have experienced. What engaged you? What did you bring to the training, and was there space for this?

Training focused on the DDP model needs to do more than just provide instruction on the model. If the practitioners and parents attending the training are going to embed DDP principles into their practice, then the model must also be experienced. DDP is a relational model, and its training needs this same focus. This requires a move away from a didactic teaching style so that those attending (i.e., the trainees) can get an experiential feel for DDP. The content, while important, must be provided in a way that embeds it within the relationships facilitated by the trainer. If the trainees get an embodied sense of DDP alongside cognitive understanding, they will be learning about the model from the inside out.

REFLECTIVE EXERCISE: DDP PRINCIPLES IN TRAINING

Worksheet 11.1, at the end of the chapter, provides an opportunity to explore bringing DDP principles into a training.

BRINGING DDP PRINCIPLES INTO ALL STAGES OF TRAINING PROVISION

In this section, we explore how a trainer uses the DDP principles throughout the different stages of training (Figure 11.2). The relationships between trainer and trainees, and within the whole group, will be an important focus. These relationships rely on everyone feeling safe and welcome.

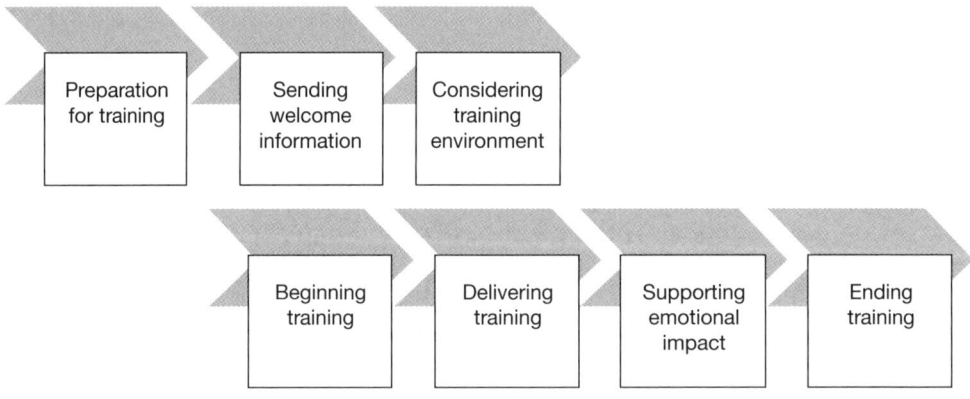

Figure 11.1 Stages of Training

1. Preparation for training:

Slowing down is an essential part of DDP interventions. It encourages reflection, beginning with self and extending to others. It stops precipitous action, ensuring that action follows understanding. Slowing down is as necessary in training as it is in other DDP interventions.

Starting with self, the trainer has a responsibility to know what they, personally, bring to the training: the values, beliefs, and biases that they might hold. The trainer reflects on their own experiences, including their attachment history and any trauma experiences that they have lived through. The trainer considers how these might be similar or different from the trainees experiences and how this could enhance or impede their training. The trainer must be especially attentive to areas of anxiety and shame and how these could be, unhelpfully, evoked while they are training. A simple example would be if a trainer who parented their own children quite behaviorally is now advocating a very different parenting approach. A sense of "if I knew then what I know now" could impact their ability to train if they have not yet worked through this in supervision.

Next, the trainer is curious about the trainees who have signed up for the training. While the trainer is likely to have limited information at this stage, they should be aware that the trainees will bring their own attachment, and sometimes trauma, histories to the training. The trainer reflects on potential clues that these histories are impacting the trainee. They will consider what support the trainees might need should the training content or process evoke emotions such as anxiety or shame.

In addition, the trainer will get a sense of the group in terms of the preliminary information provided: job role, employer, gender when indicated, even names can provide clues as to the mix of the group. During preparation, the trainer will:

- Consider the mix of trainees who will be attending.
- Reflect on what coming into the training space will be like for the trainees.

- Consider which voices might dominate the discussions.
- Explore what voice they will bring and how this might influence participation.
- Wonder how they can ensure that quieter voices are heard.

PROVIDING AN INCLUSIVE TRAINING SPACE

As part of the pretraining reflection, the DDP trainer will wonder who is likely to occupy the training space. Consider how will it feel for attendees:

- who are white, Black, or brown
- from the range of sexualities and genders
- who are impacted by physical difficulties
- who have been impacted by life experiences and/or mental health difficulties
- with neurodiverse challenges

The trainer considers how the trainees might be the same or different from themselves.

Using this reflective process, the trainer can stay mindful of the additional challenges that might be present for trainees as well as for themselves.

The trainer also reflects on the content that they are sharing in words, pictures, examples, and recordings.

- Consider how welcoming each element will be to the range of people who are attending the training.
- Are handouts designed with those with dyslexia in mind?
- Do video and audio recordings reflect the diversity among the trainees?

Kim has grown up in a heteronormative family. This led to an unconscious bias in the way she talked about and depicted families in her trainings. Consciously considering this, she reviewed her training materials to contemplate how welcoming her materials would be for people with different experiences. A simple example of a modification to increase welcoming is changing the images. All the images of families included in her slides and handouts included a father and a mother. There were also no images of people with a physical disability. With some conscious thought, this was easy to change.

2.   Sending welcome information:

All DDP interventions begin with safety and return to safety whenever it is lost. Until trainees feel safe, learning will not happen and they will not benefit from immersion in the model.

Welcome information is often sent out to trainees in advance of the training and can be written in a way that signals that the safety needs of the trainees are important to the trainer. While respecting peoples' wishes not to disclose, trainees can be invited to privately share information about themselves with the trainer.

> *Do contact me if you would like to share anything about yourself prior to the training. This includes if you have any needs to improve accessibility. I am happy to think solutions through with you and make any adjustments that are possible.*

Possible responses to this welcome:

- I have a trauma history that might be triggered by the topic of the training. I might leave the room to look after myself if this happens.
- I am likely to be quiet and don't want to be encouraged to talk.

- I am starting back at work after a bereavement and will need to pace myself during the training.
- I am neurodiverse and find processing a lot of information difficult. I might need more time, adapted handouts, and more sensory breaks.
- I am deaf and will need interpreters with me.
- I will need a prayer room at specific times during the day.

These early contacts provide an opportunity to model PACE. The trainer will listen attentively, be curious about the needs of the trainee, and meet these needs with acceptance and empathy as well as by suggesting adjustments. The trainer offers a regulating presence, helping the trainee to relax and feel confident that the training will be adjusted to their needs as far as possible.

3.   **Consider the training environment:**
Safety and comfort can also be created with attention to the training environment.

- Is the room welcoming, with access to natural light and sufficient space for the trainees to sit comfortably?
- We generally provide some refreshments upon arrival. Are these reflective of the needs of all in the group?
- Does the space accommodate trainees with disabilities?
- Are there quiet spaces for those who need them?
- If there are aspects of the room that might cause discomfort—harsh artificial lighting, noisy heating/air conditioning unit—the trainer can consider how to mitigate these difficulties. What lighting can be turned off? Are there alternative heaters or units that can be used? Will there need to be more breaks to compensate for these difficulties?

When Kim was unhappy with the room that had been provided for a DDP training because it was airless with little natural lighting, she built in some group work that could be done outside. This gave trainees a break from the room. Fortunately, the weather was suitable!

PROVIDING AN INCLUSIVE TRAINING

The trainer will consider ways to make the training environment inclusive.

How will trainees who are observing Ramadan be accommodated? Is there space for prayer so that trainees can observe their religious practices? Where might an autistic trainee go if they experience sensory overload? Do sight or hearing-impaired trainees need to sit where they can see the trainer or use any sort of sight or sound enhancing device?

TIME FOR REFLECTION

We invite you to reflect on involving interpreters in a training.

Imagine that you have learned that a deaf trainee will be attending your training and will be bringing two interpreters with them.

- What do you need to do to prepare for this training?
- What adjustments can you make to increase the accessibility of the training?
- How will you welcome this trainee?

We give ideas from our own experience in Worksheet 11.2 at the end of the chapter.

This reflective exercise is one example of meeting the needs of trainees during training. Trainers will have different experiences within different training groups. Knowledge can be shared among trainers, to help all trainers to be prepared for the range of people who might arrive in the training space.

4. Beginning training—welcome and introductions:

The beginning of training is an important time for the trainer to establish a safe environment. The aim will be to help everyone to feel safe, be able to connect with each other, and be ready for learning. This is a time for encouraging connect-and-chat; just as at the beginning of DDP therapy sessions, this can help people to settle down, to feel comfortable with each other, and to begin the process of relating intersubjectively.

- If it is a small group, each person might be invited to introduce themselves. This generally consists of first name and area of work. Can we extend this to respectfully demonstrate deeper interest in them? For example, questions about names, where they live, and where they were born might invite personal as well as professional reflections, signaling that we are open to conversations based on lived as well as professional experience.

- Hold sensitivity when asking questions of the trainees. For example, on one occasion when Kim asked trainees to tell the group something about their names, she later found out that a trans trainee was uncomfortable. Talking about his name might have disclosed his trans status before he was ready for this to be known. Providing choice about what to talk about (e.g., "Tell us something about your name or the name of the place where you live.") and helping people to pass if they don't want to participate can avoid such discomfort.

How can we bring this same perspective to large groups when there isn't time for individual introductions?

- Can we ask questions of the whole group that encourage getting to know each other?
- Could we invite people to volunteer thoughts about what they would like to get from the training personally as well as professionally?

PROVIDING AN INCLUSIVE TRAINING

- An inclusive training begins with a welcome that acknowledges and honors the range of differences and diversity within the group and the intersectionality of race, culture, sexuality, and range of abilities represented by the participants.

- If comfortable doing so, the trainer may disclose something about themselves relating to their own heritage, sexuality, or disability.

- Be aware of expectations and assumptions. For example, there may be trainees who have anticipated being in the minority, and this will impact their level of engagement, trust, and readiness to begin. If their minority status is obvious—a physical disability, Black or brown skin color—they may be preparing themselves for experiences based on past trainings. They may anticipate others' curiosity, microaggressions, or their needs and experience being dismissed. If their minority status is not evident, they may be anticipating not being seen and the training being less applicable for them. A gay trainee may be anticipating heteronormative content; a person of mixed heritage who passes as white might anticipate incorrect assumptions being made about their heritage; a person with dyslexia may worry about being asked to read. These trainees may come into a training with hypervigilance to how they are treated. They may have a level of anxiety that is not conducive to learning. They may also be reluctant to challenge, provide feedback, or simply raise questions because of past experience.

- The trainer needs to work hard to ensure that negative expectations and assumptions are not met within their training.

**5.	Delivering the training:**

Within all training contexts, the DDP practitioner balances content with process (Figure 11.2). Clearly, there is content that needs to be delivered. However, it is the process of delivering the content that facilitates affective–reflective learning. The trainee will both learn and experience. For example, trainees will discover PACE as a way of being while also learning about how the attitude helps people to feel more secure and confident to emotionally connect.

While there is a training plan, the execution of it is flexible, allowing the training process to unfold in a way that moves between content and experience. The trainer introduces content and then encourages AR discussion. Lectures are kept to a minimum, while a storytelling style maintains engagement and immersion in the DDP model. As trainees engage with the content of the training, they will be reflecting on its relevance to their lives, both personally and professionally. This is the power of affective–reflective discussions. Trainees engage emotionally with the content as well as learning from it.

There is space for relationships within this training, as intersubjective sharing of the experience of the training is encouraged. The trainer provides coregulation and facilitates the cocreation of narratives. In this way, trainees are introduced to the model cognitively and experientially.

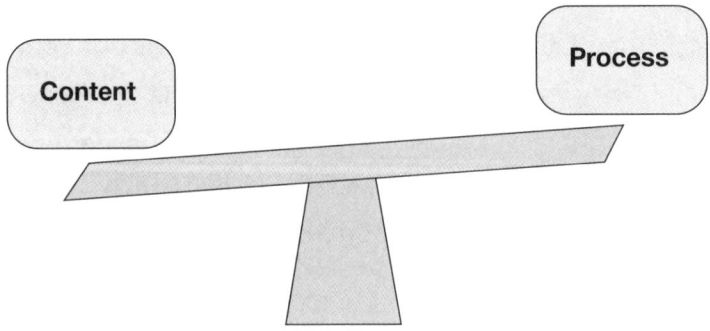

Figure 11.2 Balancing Content and Process

Individual experience becomes a seamless part of the learning, arising from the value placed on curiosity and the sharing of stories. In this way, trainings are collaborative, learning from the expertise of the trainer as well as the expertise of the different trainees. This sharing of expertise provides a richer training experience for everyone, including the trainer. The training becomes a conversation, or series of conversations, guided by the trainer and within the parameters of the training content.

PROVIDING AN INCLUSIVE TRAINING

For some trainees the training will have another layer of complexity. For example:

- A deaf person will be wondering how DDP interventions could be provided meaningfully within the deaf community. For example, how might signing convey the subtlety of a PACE response?
- Someone working with communities whose first language is not English may wonder how the intervention can be provided through interpreters.
- Trainees whose heritage is non-European—African, Latinx, or Asian, for example—will be reflecting on how to make a model that is grounded in Eurocentric theory relevant within their culture.

Discussing differences in experience and making the training relevant to all means that tokenism can be avoided and there is a more natural flow to conversations, allowing each participant to feel that their perspective and expertise are valued.

Sensitivity is necessary. For example, it would be uncomfortable to be put on the spot because of your color or sexuality.

There will be times when the trainer makes a mistake and realizes that they have been insensitive. It is important to acknowledge the mistake and offer a repair before moving on. This can be brief and still honor the insensitivity.

Example: A trainer realizes an example they have given to a wheelchair user assumed full mobility. Acknowledging this assumption and rephrasing the example provides a brief and respectful repair. At other times a private repair might be more appropriate. Kim remembers a time when she drew attention to a Black member of the group in a way that made him feel singled out. She didn't attend to this within the group, as this would have caused further discomfort. Instead, she talked to the trainee during a break. She noticed what had happened and apologized. The apology was accepted, and they went on to have an interesting discussion about a theme introduced in the previous session.

The DDP model provides a way of being that can aid trainers in embracing individual identity within their training groups. This relational approach encourages an interest in the trainees. As this interest broadens into curiosity about their lived experience and their professional thinking, we can all become richer from the process. A model that sits within Western psychology can broaden and grow to encompass many different perspectives when it accepts influence from non-Western ways of being. In addition, an interest in the individual will encourage thinking about the way that differences in race, gender, sexuality, ability, social class, religion, and the vast array of experiences within each of these broad terms can influence our thinking about how to help children with developmental trauma. This will build on and extend beyond the theories that have guided us thus far.

6.   Supporting trainees with the emotional impact of the training:

As we have been exploring, training with a DDP lens means that the trainees will get an affective–reflective training experience. Immersion in the model, alongside training about the model, will impact the trainees emotionally as well as cognitively. The trainer needs to keep this in mind. This way, they may anticipate some of the multitude of feelings that trainees might experience, including anxiety, sadness, worries, and sometimes shame.

Trainees who have their own trauma history are likely to be especially impacted by a relational training with a focus on understanding parenting and supporting children with trauma histories. A trainee's experiences can be triggered through the exploration of a child's trauma. The trainer needs to be aware of, sensitive to, and able to engage with these trainees.

In DDP Level Two training, as well as within the group work programs, *Nurturing Attachments* and *Foundations for Attachment*, (see list of resources), we explicitly ask trainees to engage with their own attachment histories. This can be a very emotional experience, and those with traumatic attachment histories may need additional support from the trainer or cofacilitators.

It is our experience that trainees will respond to these invitations for self-reflection in different ways, some sharing a little, others using the opportunities to reflect more deeply. While generally trainees will share only what they are comfortable sharing, it is also important to acknowledge that when a group is feeling safe and supported, trainees might share more than they were initially intending to. They can be surprised by the emotional depth of this. Ensuring that there is sufficient support and time for returning to emotional equilibrium will be important. Moving into a break following self-reflection can be a helpful part of this support.

TIME FOR REFLECTION

Kim remembers attending a training when she felt very anxious. It was hard to concentrate or focus. The trainer seemed to be going very fast. There was no time to take in one point before the trainer moved on to another. This created a sense of panic in her. When the trainer posed a question, Kim could not make sense of the question, never mind think of an answer. This added to Kim's anxiety as she worried that she would appear disinterested in the training.

- Reflect on times when you have been emotionally impacted within a training.
- Reflect on how you made sense of this impact.
- What got in the way of engaging with the training?
- What helped you to settle and re-engage?

The degree of support a trainer can give to trainees will depend on how much the trainee makes the trainer aware of their need. In larger groups, it may be less obvious that people are impacted. Thus the trainer needs to allow space in the program for sitting with the experiences and having quiet reflection time. Moving into small groups might provide an opportunity for sharing these experiences and getting support from colleagues.

With small groups, emotional impact will be more obvious. The trainer, in supporting the trainee, will also model DDP in action. This will include taking an open and engaged stance that avoids trying to reassure or fix, sitting with discomfort for longer than feels comfortable, and responding with an attitude of PACE. Some trainees will want to share a little of what they are experiencing, supported by the trainer's regulating presence. Some cocreation of the trainee's story can then occur, allowing the trainee's experience and their reflections about it to be witnessed. This can be a powerful experience both for the individual and the whole group.

Kim was in the middle of a DDP training with a small group who were highly engaged and supportive of each other. After showing a recording of a DDP session, one member of the group was visibly impacted. She felt safe enough to share that she recognized herself in the stories being shared in the recording. She told a little of her own story, supported by Kim's PACEful response and the sensitive witnessing of the group. These types of experiences can be life changing for the individuals involved, giving them new insight about themselves and strengthening themselves as a practitioner and/or parent.

This individual chose to share her story openly within the group. Other trainees might approach the trainer more privately. The trainer needs to find time within or after the training to hear and witness trainees' stories. Others might have shared their trauma experiences with the trainer ahead of the training, alerting them that they are anticipating the impact the training might have. Knowing this, the trainer can seek an opportunity to quietly check in with the trainee during the training and can support them to take a break if needed.

The most powerful demonstration of the DDP approach being applied in training is within group work with parents, including foster carers, adopters, and kinship carers. These groups meet over a longer time, creating safe spaces for sharing. Emotional experience can be intense as the group laughs and cries together. As well as learning more about themselves, the parents are understanding more deeply the impact of trauma on their children while learning about different approaches to parenting. This can lead to many feelings, such as sadness, regret at not knowing this sooner, and hope that the program will offer a way forward. There can also be some shame in discovering that one's well-intentioned parenting might have added to the child's insecurity and in reflecting on the parenting they did with previous children, who may now be struggling as adults. The trainer is advised to provide coregulation and cocreation of these experiences, aided by a strong attitude of PACE. Alongside this, the trainer looks for opportunities to link back to the content, increasing learning and understanding.

Perhaps one of the hardest parts of managing the training process is when trainees move into shame and become defensive. Shame may be expressed as anger, frustration, humor, or criticism. The trainer needs to avoid being pulled into defense themselves, responding PACEfully to the individual and maintaining safety for the group.

When the trainer notices a trainee moving into shame, they first reflect on what has been happening within the group that might have caused this response. If the trainer suspects that something they said or did has unwittingly caused shame, they will ensure that they seek the individual out and repair the relationship. If it was an interaction within the group, the trainer needs to sensitively notice the difficulty and mediate understanding between all those involved. When a trainee moves into defensive behaviors on more than one occasion, it can be helpful to take the person aside and wonder PACEfully about the trainee's experiences, including their sense of safety. The trainer would enquire if there is anything the trainee wants to share with them alone or with the group. This will help the trainer become alert to potential triggers during the remainder of the training, so that they can try to maintain the safety of the trainee. The trainee, themselves, might have ideas for what would be helpful for them, such as being warned when triggering material is going to be discussed and having a safe way to leave the training for a while if necessary.

7.   Ending trainings:

DDP-informed trainings can be an emotionally intense experience, especially in small groups. The trainer will allow space and time for the ending that includes opportunities for reflection on the experience and recognizing the importance of goodbyes. If certificates are being provided, handing them out also allows a moment of celebration of the time spent together.

TRAINING THAT EMBRACES DIVERSITY

Kim recalls a time during a Level One training when she was facilitating a discussion about providing DDP interventions in a way that is inclusive. It started with reflections about working with individuals from different racial backgrounds before widening to thoughts about differences of gender, sexuality, and disability:

I was aware of one British member of the group who was of Asian heritage. She remained silent throughout the discussion. I noticed myself becoming anxious. I perceived her as being upset with me. Had I said something wrong? Was she unhappy with the way I was facilitating this discussion? When I met her at the break, she told me that she had enjoyed the discussion. She volunteered that staying silent was the way she kept herself safe when race was being discussed in groups that were predominantly white. I realized that, feeling anxious, I had perceived her silence through my own lens of needing approval, rooted in my unmet needs from childhood.

TIME FOR REFLECTION

Reflect on trainings that you have provided.

- Think about how the person you are and the lived experiences you have had influence the way that you deliver trainings.
- Notice how experiences can enrich your trainings and ways in which your experiences might limit them.
- How do you embrace diversity, and what are the ways that you could extend and develop this?

To be effective, it is important that training be relevant to the diverse groups who are interested in it. We need to be aware of DDP's interconnection with race, gender, sexuality, and disability. Social class and religious background will also impact the experience of training. Some attendees will have their own trauma history, and there will be trainees who have grown up in care environments outside of their birth family. The trainer will also sit within this diversity. Reflecting on self and how it might impact training is an important part of engaging the trainees. The trainer has a responsibility to make the training safe and applicable to each person in attendance.

As part of embracing diversity, it is important to acknowledge that DDP has its roots in mainstream Western psychology and to think about the implications of this for all who are impacted by the DDP approach. For example, research informing psychological models and theories is based on data generated from Western, middle-class participants. As explored in Chapter 2, Henrich et al. (2010) coined the term WEIRD to describe Western psychology (Western, educated, industrialized, rich, and democratic). This describes less than 12% of the world population (Arnett, 2008,). While DDP has developed from this narrow demographic, within training and DDP practice, we are working toward being open to ideas and practices rooted in non-Western cultures. It is interesting to note the oral tradition of using stories to share social knowledge within many Indigenous cultures, and how much DDP interventions, which are grounded in storytelling, could learn from this Indigenous wisdom (Pitama, 1997, as cited in Haenga-Collins & Gibbs, 2015).

DDP will develop and grow through the influence of DDP recipients, practitioners, and trainers who bring their unique and precious family, cultural, racial, sexual, gendered, physical, and socio–economic stories to the global community. The more DDP trainings can provide a learning culture rooted in curiosity and in shared storytelling within intersubjective relationships, the more trainers and trainees will learn together from a powerful blend of their own life experiences, integrated with the theory, practice, and research evidence.

TIME FOR REFLECTION

Think about social justice and inclusivity within DDP.

1. What does social justice mean to you?
2. What does practicing within an inclusive DDP model look like?
3. What barriers to inclusivity can you foresee within DDP interventions?

Reflections from practitioners attending DDP Level Two trainings are included in Worksheet 11.3 at the end of the chapter.

TRAINING: AN EXAMPLE

TIME FOR REFLECTION

We are now going to imagine a training scenario.

Reflect on this example and consider how the DDP principles are being and could be used by the trainer to provide a richer learning experience for the whole group, including themselves.

The trainer is introducing DDP principles to a group of social workers interested in applying the DDP model when supporting adopted families. As the trainer reflects on the importance of curiosity, stories of individual experiences of family are shared. This prompts a member of the group to share his experience of transracial adoption.

Magnus was born to a white European mother and Māori father. He was removed into foster care at birth and then adopted by a white European family in what is known as a closed stranger adoption (Haenga-Collins & Gibbs, 2015[7]). He shares that he never felt that his parents, or those supporting them, ever took the time to understand his story. While he knew of his Māori heritage, he was not encouraged to be curious about it, and elements of his story were therefore lost to him. He gave an example of visiting New Zealand and feeling like a stranger in the country he was born in. He had little knowledge of his native Māori language, and this felt deeply painful. Visiting and witnessing Māori culture led him to wonder about the person he would have been had he grown up within this society. The trainer, with the trainee's permission, chooses to follow this story.

The trainer thanks the participant for sharing and reflects on a sense of sadness at hearing this story. They invite affective–reflective responses from the group, while modeling an attitude of PACE toward the responses.

One participant, Lisa, then wonders if it would be better to discourage an interest in heritage other than the white-European heritage the child is adopted into. Wouldn't this help them to feel a greater sense of belonging in their adopted family?

The trainer, with acceptance and empathy for Lisa, moves the focus away from the personal story that has been shared by Magnus by noticing the positive motive to help adopted children feel a sense of belonging in their adopted families. The trainer is then curious about the narrative that belonging will arise out of an avoidance of birth heritage and wonders if there is an alternative narrative that might sit alongside this.

The group, helped by the anecdotes of Magnus, who continues to feel safe to share, then has a rich discussion about how to provide adopted children with a sense of belonging. They start by thinking about how hard it is to hold and feel a sense of belonging in two very different cultures. One trainee, reflecting on a family they are working with, notices how the young person's sense of identity

---

7   We would like to acknowledge the paper by Haenga-Collins & Gibbs (2015) that provided the inspiration for this fictional example.

has arisen from their knowledge of both their heritage as well as the culture they have grown up in.

Magnus tells the group of the Māori tradition called *whakapapa*, which recognizes identity as being formed from an understanding of personal genealogy and a connection to ancestors. This leads to a thoughtful response from Lisa, who reflects on her previous comment and the child she was thinking about when she made it. She observes that this child was not protected from racism, despite immersion in the adopted family's culture. She now wonders if some affiliation with people from the child's birth family's heritage might have been supportive for her. Magnus remembered how finding out about Māori culture was like finding a part of himself. It did not take away his identity within his adopted family but rather gave him a dual identity, enriched by learning about Māori language, culture, tribal affiliation, and spiritual practice. He regretted that his adoptive parents were not encouraged to take an interest in this while he was growing up.

The trainer now encourages the group to think in pairs about the ways they did or did not feel a sense of belonging while growing up. This leads to a discussion about the importance of understanding a child's sense of difference, their feelings of loss and grief, and possible feelings of rejection within their adopted culture. Children can be encouraged not to notice their difference at home, while this is all that seems to be noticed in the community, often in discriminatory ways.

The trainer then extends the discussion to reflect on same-culture adoptions. A trainee reflects on her own experience of being adopted and invites the group to imagine looking at adoptive parents and not seeing their own physical features mirrored back. The group notice how differences of socio-economic status, religious beliefs, ability/disability, gender, and sexuality can also challenge sense of belonging. The discussion rounds off by the group developing a set of principles to help adopted children feel they belong:

- Help a child understand and feel connected to both their birth and their adopted family, including the parents and child exploring life story information together.

- Talk about feelings of loss from the separation from birth and foster families and helping the child to grieve these losses.

- Help adoptive parents to understand, and help their child to understand, the culture, subculture, and heritage of their adopted child.

- Notice and talk about differences between the child and their adopted family and between the birth and the adopted family.

- Support adoptive parents to help their child engage with cultural and other appropriate activities related to their birth family.

- If safe and practical, help the child to visit their place of birth and, if appropriate, meet with family or birth community members.

- As the child matures, help them to integrate a sense of who they might have been, as well as who they have become, as the complexity of their identity is embraced.

At the end of this discussion, the trainer thanks everyone for sharing and acknowledges both Magnus and Lisa for initiating the discussion about belonging and adoption support. They then circle back to the DDP principles, noticing how they have been used within this discussion.

DDP-INFORMED SUPERVISION

Supervision informed by DDP principles follows a similar process to DDP work with families. Safety and relationship building is a prerequisite to any successful supervision. This recognizes the importance of slowing down, discovering stories together, and emotional coregulation. Ensuring safety and privileging the relationship allows a deeper experience, with both consultant and supervisee feeling safe to be vulnerable. This supervision feels less task focused. Opportunities are provided to explore the emotional impact of the work. The supervisee explores connections with aspects of their own life alongside reflections of the work and how to move forward. The supervision helps the supervisees to develop their DDP skills through modeling, reflection, and instruction.

DDP-informed supervision takes several forms:

- individual or group case supervision
- working with networks and systems
- practicum supervision (This type of supervision was explored in Chapter 10, Healing Relational Trauma [Hughes et al., 2019]. DDP consultants also provide supervision for consultant practicums and DDP trainers for the trainer practicum.)
- Organizational supervision (DDP consultants and experienced practitioners work with organizations to embed the DDP principles into their ways of working.)

TIME FOR REFLECTION

Think about key themes that can arise within DDP-informed supervision. How are DDP principles used to address these themes?

- How can DDP supervisors model the DDP principles within their supervision?
- How can DDP-informed supervision intersect with the exploration of racial equity and social justice?
- What space is given within supervision to consider race, sexuality, gender, religious beliefs, class, neurodiversity, and disability?

One of the central themes that you probably identified is the need to slow down. In the following example, we will explore slowing down during some case supervision. This is a fictional supervision session inspired by a newspaper article that Kim read (Amelia Hill, *The Guardian*, February 3, 2022).

TIME FOR REFLECTION

As you read through this example, reflect on what themes you might have followed if you were the supervisor.

Christy is a clinician working on a team that supports families who are on the edge of having their children removed from their care. Christy has engaged in DDP Level One and Level Two training and is keen to bring those principles into her work with these families. She has sought supervision from a DDP consultant, Lev, to help her with this aim. Here, we reflect on part of an initial supervision session between Christy and Lev. They begin with some getting to know each other. Lev describes his current work as a gay clinician with a particular interest in supporting same sex adoption. Christy talks about working with families who are often oppressed and marginalized. She is excited about how a DDP-informed approach could help her support these families. They then begin to explore Christy's work with one of the families.

Christy: I'm working with a single mother of three young children. I've been asked to help with basic parenting, helping her with routines, boundaries, you know the sort of thing; but am feeling a bit stuck. She seems to get it when we are talking together, but it doesn't seem to have an impact on her parenting. She's very isolated, and I have the sense that her childhood was difficult, but she's reluctant to talk about it. I don't think she's feeling particularly safe with me yet. I want to slow down and get to know her better but I'm not sure how to do this.

Lev: That does sound tricky. Tell me a bit more about the mother.

Christy: Well, Honor is 26 years old, unmarried, and looking after three children under the age of six. She has recently separated from her boyfriend and is working hard to move away from the drug lifestyle he introduced her to. I feel I'm developing a relationship with her, but she's very distrusting, which is not surprising, really, given her experience of services. She feels judged by everyone. She has very real fears that the children could be removed into foster care if she doesn't make some progress.

Lev: That feels like a lot of pressure, on both of you.

Christy: Yes, my manager is keen for me to demonstrate improvements. She wants me to focus on Honor's parenting, but I'm not so sure. She doesn't feel safe with me, and I need to build a relationship with her. I want to know more about her and her background. It's going to take time though. She isn't going to talk openly until she can start to trust me.

Lev: So, it sounds like you're trying to go slowly, build some safety and trust, get to know her better, just as DDP would recommend. However, you are under pressure to make some progress on her parenting. That sounds tough.

Christy: It is tough! Our team is under pressure to get results. We have to prove we're worth the funding investment. I

	can see the stress my manager is under, but it sometimes feels like I'm not trusted. She's very directive about what I should be doing.
Lev:	Some parallel issues about trust here then. It must be hard for you to take the time you need to build trust with Honor when you're also trying to earn trust with the manager. I'm wondering what that's like for you.
Christy:	To be honest, this feels a bit uncomfortable. I want help with the family, and you're asking about me. I guess that is the DDP way, but I'm not used to it. And as I'm saying this, I'm thinking maybe that's how Honor feels, wondering why I'm interested in her and her experiences instead of telling her what to do with the children.
Lev:	That's an interesting reflection. And discomfort can easily reinforce distrust if it's not talked about, so thank you for being honest with me. I am sorry that I'm making you feel uncomfortable. I guess in our own ways we're both trying to take a step back and understand the whole picture. Are you OK to continue?
Christy:	It's helpful, in a way, to understand Honor's experience. I always feel uncomfortable having the focus on me. I'm not the most socially confident. I think Honor is a bit the same. I can feel her anxiety whenever I visit: I get all these feelings, a bit sick, heart beating, tension. I know she's anxious, I'm just not sure how to help her with it.
Lev:	Wow, that is impressive. You're really attuned to her then.

Christy: Well, yes. I can attune to people easily. It's like I vicariously experience other people's emotional and physical sensations. It helps me understand their difficulties, and I have an instant resonance with them.

Lev: I've heard of people who can do this, a kind of synesthesia. How do your clients find it, being understood so quickly?

Christy: I think it can be helpful. I can get people at a deep level, and they feel felt by me, if you see what I mean. That's why DDP is so important to me. As long as I respond PACEfully and they don't experience any judgment from me, I think it helps. Some of the teenagers can find it a bit freaky, but I can be playful with them.

Lev: It sounds like you have a real skill, Christy. It will be good to explore how you develop your use of DDP alongside this sensitivity to others.

Christy: I'm glad you think that. Some of my team think I'm too sensitive, that I get over involved. They question my boundaries; it can be quite hurtful.

Lev: That sounds really hard, feeling unsupported within your team while working with families where there are a lot of challenges. I'm concerned about how you're managing. The emotional toll it's taking. I don't want to intrude, but how do you feel about us thinking about this? I think it might help me to support you with your families.

Christy: Actually, it's a relief to be talking about this with someone who doesn't leap to judge me. I think I need to tell you something that I don't usually share professionally.

Lev: Of course, I'm happy for you to share anything that feels important. We're just getting to know each other, so make sure it feels comfortable for you.

Christy: You might have figured it out. I know I don't always follow all the social rules. I find them tricky. You see, I'm autistic. I was diagnosed in my late teens. I think it helps me in my work, but not everyone agrees.

Lev: Christy, thank you so much for sharing this with me. You are a remarkable woman, and I can see already what sensitivity you bring to your work. Does any of your team know?

Christy: Well, I'm not sure about remarkable, but I think autism is a superpower. Not everyone agrees. I haven't told anyone at work. I have met so much negativity in previous jobs that it can feel like professional suicide to disclose this about myself. I decided to keep quiet this time. It's hard work, making sure I get social interactions right, you know, remembering to make eye contact, have I understood what they have asked me, that sort of thing.

Lev: That sounds like very hard work. I feel so sad for you having to hide such an important part of your identity.

Christy: (*smiling*) Yes, I can experience your sadness! I have a choked feeling in my throat.

Lev: Superpower indeed! As you know, I've had times in my life when I have had to hide parts of myself from others. It's exhausting as well as invalidating.

Christy: Yes, I can see some similarities, your identity as a gay man and mine as an autistic woman. It's exhausting, but just as you are using your experience to work with the adoptive parents, I believe I can use my abilities, linked to my autism, to understand and help the families I'm working with.

Lev: I can see how the parents you work with feel held by you. You can get under the anger and frustration; the defenses they have in place and find the person who is hurting. We talk about follow-lead-follow within DDP; you will remember it from your training. I think your following and leading will be so well attuned to your clients. I really am looking forward to helping you bring the DDP principles into your work.

Christy: I'm excited about that as well. I can't tell you how relieved I am that I have told you. It feels like I can be authentic with you and that you understand me.

Lev: Well, I can't pretend that I know how you feel, being autistic in a nonautistic world, but I do know about my experience of hiding in plain sight. Not disclosing that I was gay was quite a strain. It's so much easier now that I can be myself at work. I'm not saying it's always smooth sailing. I'm not experiencing discrimination like I used to, but all the little moments add up. The looks I sometimes get or the embarrassment when someone mentions sex, that sort of thing. I think I can understand some of the strain you are under. All the masking and camouflaging; having to hide or minimize your autistic traits so that you can fit in with the neurotypical world, it must take its toll.

Christy: Oh, I have plenty of meltdowns when I get home! Luckily, I have a supportive partner. There is something called "autistic burnout," well, I know what that feels like. My manager is kind, but I think we also think differently about things. that's why I've been reluctant to tell her.

Lev: I do get that. It's huge, not knowing how such a central part of yourself will be received. I know I've been more at peace with myself since I've been open about who I am, the whole of me. It has to be your decision, but I'm happy to think more about it with you.

Christy: I would like that, but for now can we return to this family? I want to check out the way I'm trying to be PACEful. Am I getting it right? And how can I balance this with making sure she makes the changes she needs to make if she isn't going to lose her children?

Lev: Sure, let's focus on the family now.

TIME FOR REFLECTION

We invite you to reflect on this example.

- In what ways does the supervisor slow this supervision down?
- What would it be like being this supervisor supporting Christy?
- Now, imagine being the supervisee and what it would be like to experience this supervision.
- Notice the way the DDP principles are brought into this supervision session.
- How do you think the supervision will help Christy in her work with the family she is discussing and also in her work beyond this case?

CONCLUSION

In this chapter, we have explored how to bring a DDP approach into training for practitioners and parents and how to add a relational, affective layer to our supervision of others.

The DDP model incorporates a set of principles that guide therapy, consultation, and network support. These same principles can guide training and supervision, providing trainees and supervisees with an experience that is both educational and immersed in the model.

Worksheet 11.1

 Reflective Exercise:
DDP Principles in Training

For each of the DDP principles in the table below consider how these can be
applied when training.

DDP Principle	Application in Training
Creating a sense of safety	
Intersubjective relationships	
Attitude of PACE	
Co-regulation of affect	
Affective–Reflective	
Follow-lead-follow	
Cocreation of narrative with storytelling style	
Attending to verbal and non-verbal	
Rupture and repair	

Reflections on Worksheet 11.1: Possible Responses

DDP Principle	Application in Training
Creating a sense of safety	Take opportunities to help the trainees settle into the training space, including time for relaxed "connect and chat." The trainer attends to the trainees with the attitude of PACE. They are open and engaged, playful, responsive, and caring. The model is being modelled all the time.
Intersubjective relationships	While it is difficult to connect intersubjectively with everyone in the room, a general feeling of intersubjective connection is sought. This attends to all three components of intersubjectivity: shared attention, complimentary intention, and matched affect. If attention isn't being shared, the trainer will switch focus to what the trainees are attending to before leading the trainees back to the content. This means that the intention of the trainer can switch between talking and providing content and listening and sharing reflections. In this way intention remains complimentary.

Attitude of PACE	Throughout the training the attitude of PACE is modeled. The trainer remains attentive to the trainees with acceptance, curiosity, and empathy. There is also room for a healthy dose of playfulness as the trainer enjoys being with the trainees.
Co-regulation of affect	The trainer monitors the affective mood of the group, matching the affect being expressed and using this to further discussion and reflection. In matching the trainees' affect, the trainer needs to be sensitive to whether the trainee's affective state is becoming dysregulated, providing co-regulation when needed. The trainer also needs to reflect on their own affect to ensure that it remains regulated.
Affective–Reflective	The training experience is affective-reflective. This manages the content while allowing time for discussion, sharing, and storytelling.
Follow-lead-follow	The trainer leads the training, follows the response of the trainees, and then leads again.

Cocreation of narrative with storytelling style	The trainees' experience is engaged through storytelling rather than lecturing. Understanding is cocreated with the trainer drawing on their expertise alongside the expertise of the trainees.
Attending to verbal and non-verbal	Both verbal and non-verbal communications are noticed and attended to. If they are not congruent, the trainer may address that with the trainee.
Rupture and repair	If relationship ruptures occur the trainer makes efforts to repair. This relies on the trainer accepting their role in the rupture without shame.

Worksheet 11.2

 Reflections on Including Deaf
Trainees in Trainings

- Discuss with the trainee their needs ahead of the training. Don't generalize from previous experience with a deaf trainee. Remember, each person is unique and will have their own needs and preferred adjustments.

- Make sure the space can accommodate two interpreters who can be seen by the trainee.

- Ensure that there is quiet space for the trainee to engage in group work.

- Talk to the interpreters beforehand, provide them with training notes and go over any technical terms they may need to sign. This is also an opportunity to alert them to any emotional content within the training so they can look after themselves.

- Discuss with the trainee their level of hearing, ability to lip read, and preferred ways of engaging. For example, will they want to rely on interpreters or lip reading when working within a small group?

- Review recordings and add subtitles where possible. Provide a description of any recordings that do not have subtitles. Provide opportunities for the trainee to watch these before the training, if that is what they prefer.

- Provide the trainee with the training materials ahead of time so they have chance to review them.

- Help the trainee feel welcome in the training space. The trainer might learn to sign a simple welcome at the beginning of the training. Watching appropriate recordings without sound can allow the whole group to share the experience of the deaf trainee.

- Help the trainee to be involved in group discussions. This might involve the trainer managing the discussion in a way that brings in observations and questions that the trainee mentioned to them privately.

- Be aware that attending to interpreters and the trainer can be exhausting. Ensure that there are sufficient breaks. Agree with the trainee that they can take unscheduled breaks if needed and find ways to help them to catch up. It can be helpful to go through the program and identify what is most important they be present for and what could be missed and caught up on later.
- Check in with the trainee and interpreters during the training so that ongoing adjustments can be made.

Worksheet 11.3

Reflections on Cocreation and Inclusivity Within DDP

Kim has reflected with her DDP Level Two training groups on how to ensure that DDP interventions are socially just and inclusive. She includes here a summary of these reflections from five trainings.

"PACE is a direction, not a strategy. If we are truly PACEful, inclusivity (of difference of any kind) is authentically held in mind."

—Agnieszka Anna Pytlowana, discussion during DDP Level Two training, 2022

1. What does social justice mean to you?

work in progress
empowerment
progress
removing barriers   valuing   championing
fairness   authenic
compassion   listening
equality
kindness
advocacy   belonging
nonjudgmental   challenging norms
opening your eyes
inclusivity
sit with discomfort

2. Themes that emerged when asked: "What does practicing within an inclusive DDP model look like?"

    A way of being

    - Being open, accepting, and curious about similarities and differences and not shying away from talking about them
    - Being curious with the uncomfortable while regulating own discomfort
    - An environment for holding someone's emotions with empathy while accepting their individual experience
    - Treating and accepting others as you would wish to be treated and accepted

    Collaborative

    - Cocreation and not being the expert
    - Remembering you can never fully understand another's experience
    - Following the person's lead and working at their pace without judgment

    Self-reflective

    - Paying attention to your own prejudice, assumptions, and bias as you explore the identity and experience of the client
    - A reflective, responsive culture
    - Self-reflection about the inclusiveness of your own practice
    - Understanding yourself so you can hold genuine interest and understanding of the person in front of you
    - Being open to and actively seeking feedback
    - Willingness to be challenged and to be uncomfortable

    Diverse and inclusive

    - Diversity in action—reflected in therapy, support, training, research, and resources
    - Increasing access to DDP interventions and training
    - Increasing choice by increasing diversity

- Acknowledging and valuing difference while minimizing barriers
- Recognizing, hearing, and valuing individuality and differences
- Assertive engagement of parents of all sexualities, genders, classes, religions, abilities/disabilities, cultures, and backgrounds.

3. What barriers to inclusivity can you foresee within DDP interventions?

lack of self reflection

lack of self awareness   power imbalances

defensive organizations   prejudice   lack of resources

class expectations   values

confidence   no repair   cultural expectations

white privilege

cultural norms   fear   unconscious bias

heteronormative bias   western dominated

expectations   inaccessible buildings

fear of making mistakes

nondiverse practitioners

communication barriers

"I think the DDP principle of storytelling has been really helpful for me, as it has reminded me that everyone's story is very much their own, and it is important for me to hold that in mind (and never make assumptions). Formulation expects the therapist to 'make sense' of the information a client brings, which can mean differences of diversity are missed. Storytelling invites the therapist to listen and empower the individual to make sense of their own story thus, allowing for cultural influences or difference to come through in the narrative. This has been powerful for me."

—Lucy Rymer, Feedback on DDP Level Two training, 2022

IN CONVERSATION SIX

Kim met with Sherell Calame, a clinical psychologist working in the U.K., where she is supported by a white British DDP consultant. Sherell is Black British and has a Caribbean heritage. In this conversation, we chat about Sherell's experience of DDP-informed supervision and how this can support her with a Black family she is currently working with.

Kim:	Sherell, thank you so much for chatting with me. I'm interested in hearing about your experience of DDP.
Sherell:	I've known about DDP for a while. I've done my Level Two training and have been trying to put it into practice. It's been the experience of supervision that has had the most impact on me. Being supported by someone who is really curious about me and empathizes with my experiences of racial discrimination and racial trauma and how this impacts my work with families. In other supervisory experiences, with other models, we might have touched on this, but not to the depth that I experienced within DDP supervision. I think there is something inherent in the DDP model because we're trying to connect with people's experiences and to understand them on that deeper level, that means that this is brought into supervision.
Kim:	That's interesting. DDP is very much about curiosity, empathy, and acceptance. I have been guilty of not attending enough to these principles in my supervision of people of color. I am trying to take more notice of the individual I am supporting and their unique identity, how this intersects with their work that we are discussing.

Sherell: I came to DDP and the supervisory relationship with my own expectations. I anticipated that race might be touched upon but didn't expect to really go there. Maybe I've built up some defenses, not opening up so much about my experiences and my differences. It feels like a really vulnerable place.

Kim: Colleagues have said to me that, being Black, you put your armor on when you're going out and interacting with white people because you don't know what's going to come back at you. That's been the reality you've lived with that I haven't been noticing.

Sherell: The armor describes it quite well. I put on what I think is a professional self, based on observing other psychologists who have generally been white and middle-class. I feel that when I step out of that, I'm not being professional. Within DDP, I am encouraged to be my genuine self, to truly connect with people. This means opening up to feelings. It can be difficult to feel safe enough to talk about these things in supervision.

Kim: I would imagine it takes a huge jump in vulnerability, because you don't know what's going to come back at you. I'm guessing it's not the overt racism but more the microaggressions that you get bathed in?

Sherell: I'd agree with that. The microaggressions and having experiences dismissed or minimized when issues related to race or discrimination come up. When I've attempted to talk about things previously in supervision, it's kind of, "are you sure that's what they meant?" or they wonder if that really happened. I haven't felt safe enough to explore things, or I've felt that it's not appropriate to. On the other hand, my experience with a DDP supervisor gave me confidence to openly talk about differences in relation to both the family I was talking about and in relation to me. It was safe to explore some important feelings that were coming up in relation to the family. Without this, it would have been hard to understand the family when so much of my feelings were caught up in their experience as well.

Kim: So in a way, you were taken care of and therefore you could take care of the family at a deeper level.

Sherell: Yes, exactly that.

Kim: And I'm thinking we're not going to be looking after you very well if we're not comfortable with having these conversations. I'm thinking of white people worrying about saying the wrong thing. We're worried about being unconsciously racist and how this can shut down the conversations. If we're too preoccupied with "am I getting this right?" how can we be truly listening? That's why we have to do our own work so we can stay present.

Sherell: I guess that's the DDP way, isn't it? Curiosity, not being certain or knowing but being willing to explore. I think that approach just fits so well in raising these conversations and exploring experience. I think it's hard because you just described a supervisor second guessing themselves. Also me as a supervisee, I'm second guessing myself too. I'm not sure whether I feel OK to share these things. I'm not sure, even though it's something important that I need to share because it's going to have an impact on my work. There's a part of me that might be holding back because I'm nervous about how it might feel for you in talking about it. I'm nervous about whether a supervisor can handle talking about these difficult things or whether it might be really uncomfortable for them.

Kim: So, you end up taking care of them and not being able to get what you need from the time and space?

Sherell: At times, yes. That's really profound, isn't it? My families might not always get what they need because I'm not being adequately supported in the supervisory relationship and getting what I need.

Kim: As I'm listening to you, I'm thinking about the intergenerational racial trauma that you're holding and how that might get played out within those supervisory sessions, and potentially within your work with families. You're holding all that, you're trying to take care of the other person, and you're trying to protect yourself from what might come back at you. It's a really complicated existence, isn't it?

Sherell: When you said that, I just thought of being exhausted! There's the constant feeling of being different. There's the constant awareness of not feeling like you fit professionally. There's constant looking out for how people perceive or understand you, and there's the constant effort to put on this professional persona. If I'm not talking about these issues when they arise, because I'm not feeling that there are adequate spaces to share or to feel understood, I won't get what I need from supervision. I think all of this can be very draining.

Kim: I'm also thinking about the families with a white practitioner advising them, focusing on issues in adoption or fostering but the intersection with race left unspoken. I'm thinking about your experience, and I'm guessing the families would feel the same.

Sherell: That really was my experience with this family. When certain values came up, they were seen as not engaging. They were misunderstood. Then, meeting me, they could visibly see that I have some similarities and hoped that our shared experience would mean a deeper level of understanding and the possibility that I could help. For me there's a pressure that comes along with that.

Kim: A lot of weight of expectations?

Sherell: Yes, expectations that because I am a Black clinician, I will be able to relate and help them in a way that others haven't been able to. And there's the impact of the shared trauma as well.

Kim: And that can start to get played out in an unhealthy way.

Sherell: I think so, if there isn't a supportive supervisory relationship. How difficult it would then be to do the work, to be open and engaged with the family, to be my authentic self. I suppress some of the trauma that's potentially being triggered for me and then within the work with the family because of my fear that it may not be understood in the supervisory relationships, if that makes sense.

Kim: That totally makes sense, because how can you be confident in what you do with a family if you don't feel your supervisor is confident talking about this with you? How can you be freed up to do the work that really needs doing if they haven't got your back?

Sherell: Definitely, I need that to help me to maintain my curiosity with the family. With this family, for example, they are all Black, but they're from different cultures, and I'm from a different culture again. Assumptions were made that we'd have the same, or very similar, experiences. We have some similar experiences in society, but we also have very different ones. It's a reminder for me that even when I do meet a family that is similar to me, it's really important to maintain my curiosity. I don't have all the answers around race and discrimination. I have my personal experiences. There might be clients who have similar experiences, and we can relate in some ways, but it doesn't mean that I'm an expert in all issues of race or in what the clients experienced. The curiosity, the not-knowing element, and the willingness to be interested is important for my work with a family and, I guess, for my relationship with a supervisor.

Kim: Absolutely. It's so easy for me to see a Black person and assume all Black people are the same.

Sherell: I have experience of that. You know, "we've got this family and they're from this specific part of Africa. Could you work with them? They're looking for someone who's really experienced in that culture," and I'm thinking, but I'm not experienced in that culture. It's the assumptions that are made. It's difficult sometimes.

Kim: I can imagine that.

Sherell: It's making me think, in the supervisory relationship, how much both of us might be holding from our own experiences. You might find it hard to have the conversation. I find it equally hard with a white supervisor because I'm holding so much and expecting I won't feel safe or they won't feel confident. Then I don't feel confident in raising it. If I can't talk about myself and the impact on me, how can I relate to the family about their experience? How can I do that well without being able to have the difficult conversations in supervision? It was a very contrasting experience to have a supervisor say: "What does this mean to you? What's your experience of this been like?" It was things that I was thinking about, how racial trauma and discrimination might be impacting the family. How they might have been misunderstood. I was thinking about their experience, and being able to explore this with a supervisor was really helpful.

Kim: And knowing yourself as well, so that you understand your blind spots.

Sherell: Yes, someone being curious, encouraging me to reflect on myself and my own experiences. I haven't had that in other models of supervision.

Kim: Whereas DDP encourages that.

Sherell: Absolutely. This goes back to the beginning of our conversation. The use of self that DDP encourages: take off the professional persona and be human. That's it, Kim, that's the difference. In the training, we'd go through our attachment histories. It's an opportunity to think about other experiences as well. Things that have influenced you. How you respond to others and how you understand yourself. Feeling safe enough to bring this into supervision, from both sides.

Kim: Definitely. That makes me feel hopeful. Within DDP, we've got these principles and we can apply them to working with diversity and difference. We've just got to wake up and start doing it.

Sherell: It's really great to even be having this conversation and to know it's being thought about.

Kim: Thank you so much for talking with me, Sherell. I am so appreciative of your insights.

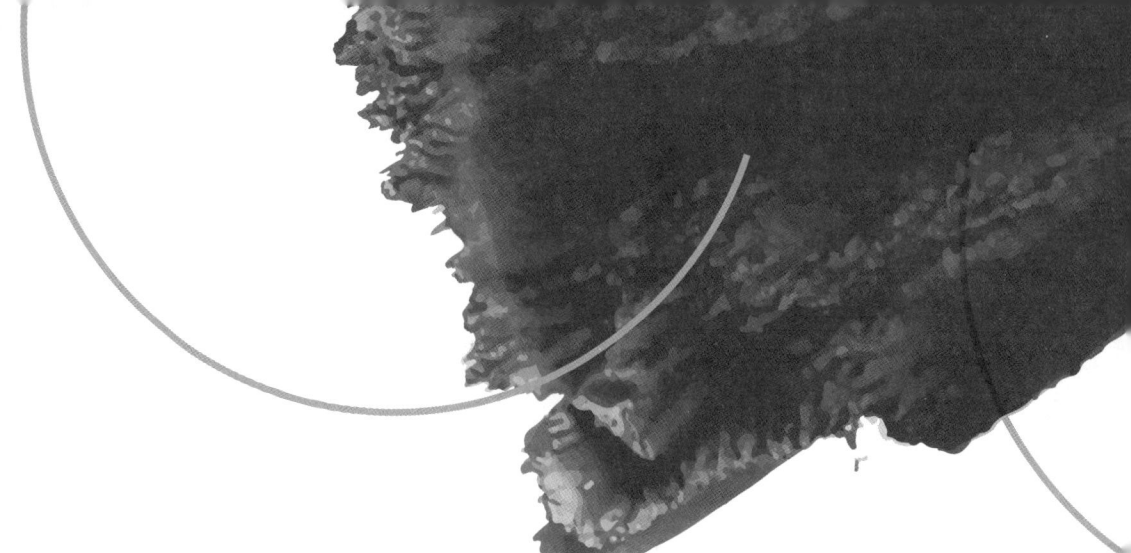

● Chapter 12:
Research and Evidence Base

Developing an evidence base for the efficacy of dyadic developmental psychotherapy, practice, and parenting will require a wide range of evidence using a range of research designs. (Hughes et al., 2019, p. 302)

REFRESHER

Developing an evidence base for DDP is complex because it is both a therapy and a practice model. We need to establish the efficacy of DDP as a psychotherapy and as a support for parents, schools, and networks.

DDP has established face validity because it is:

- grounded in psychological theory with supporting research,
- described in a large body of published work,
- supported by a website (https://ddpnetwork.org), and
- supported by robust processes for training, certification and supervision of therapists and practitioners overviewed by the DDP organization.

In addition, DDP is:

- research based—supported by qualitative and quantitative research through small scale projects and single case studies, including therapy, application to parenting support, and application to school support
- supported by a full randomized control trial (at the time of writing, Phase one and two have been completed and the full trial in phase three is ongoing)

(For more detail about the developing evidence base for DDP, the reader is directed to Chapter 11 of *Healing Relational Trauma* [Hughes et al., 2019].)

In this current chapter, we explore ways that our evidence base can continue to develop, supported by practitioners and the families at the center of DDP interventions.

THE RIGHT (RELATIONSHIPS IN GOOD HANDS TRIAL)

The U.K. medical research council provides a framework for developing and evaluating complex interventions, such as those commonly used in health and social care services (Skivington et al., 2021). The RIGHT methodology was informed by guidance on evaluating complex interventions that was updated by this new framework.

This trial is being run in the U.K., led by Professor Helen Minnis, University of Glasgow. It explores the clinical efficacy and cost effectiveness of dyadic developmental psychotherapy as an intervention to improve the mental health of children who have experienced abuse and neglect and are living in or who have been adopted from foster, kinship, or residential care. This is explored within three contrasting service contexts: National Health Service, social care, and private practice. The trial takes place across three phases (Figure 12.1).

The trial is being run with adoptive or permanent foster parents with children aged 5–12 years with symptoms of maltreatment-associated psychiatric problems (MAPP).

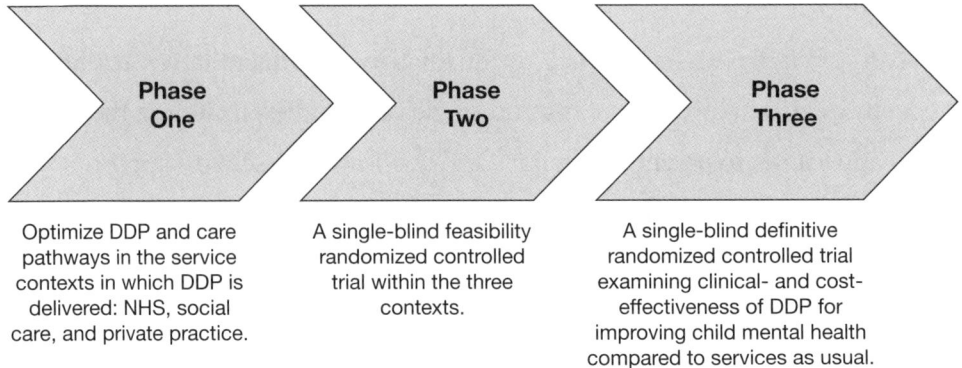

Phase One
Optimize DDP and care pathways in the service contexts in which DDP is delivered: NHS, social care, and private practice.

Phase Two
A single-blind feasibility randomized controlled trial within the three contexts.

Phase Three
A single-blind definitive randomized controlled trial examining clinical- and cost-effectiveness of DDP for improving child mental health compared to services as usual.

Figure 12.1 Phases of the RIGHT Trial

This trial explores three research questions:

1. What are the features (including barriers and facilitators) of safe and effective service delivery [whether DDP or service as usual (SAU)] for abused and neglected children with MAPP?
2. How clinically effective is DDP when compared with SAU?
3. What are the costs and consequences of DDP, and is it cost-effective when compared with SAU?

More detailed information about RIGHT can be found on the DDP website at the following link: https://ddpnetwork.org/research/research-announcements/ and on the University of Glasgow website: https://www.gla.ac.uk/research institutes/healthwellbeing/research/mentalhealth/research/projects/right/.

DEVELOPING DDP

DDP is spreading globally, providing more opportunities for growth and development. Though it was developed as a model of psychotherapy in the U.S., work is happening in Australia, China, and Singapore as well as other Eastern and Western European countries. A model that has roots in Western psychological theory and U.S.-based practice can both influence and be open to influence within the different countries it expands into—a truly intersubjective experience of learning. Change begins at home; this includes interacting with and learning from the multicultural societies within the U.S., Canada, and U.K., the foundation countries for the development of DDP.

TIME FOR REFLECTION

Since you became interested in DDP, what change and what growth have you witnessed as it has developed?

- What do you think are the main influences on this growth and development?
- What are the advantages and/or disadvantages of this growth?
- Have you noticed any missed opportunities as this development has happened?
- What would you like to see as DDP develops in the future?
- How might you influence some of this development?

The biggest development of DDP has been in its expansion outside of the therapy room. This includes:

- dyadic developmental parenting and practice, informing social care and educational practices
- the application of DDP to birth families (for example, counseling parents who have lost their children to adoption [Alper, 2019])
- working in specialized areas (for example, adult therapy [Golding & Jones, 2021])

Theoretically, DDP has grown influenced by the growing body of knowledge in neuroscience. This has led to more attention being given to blocked trust and blocked care, work led by Dan in partnership with Jon Baylin (Hughes & Baylin, 2012; Baylin & Hughes, 2016), and exploration of processes such as Nim Tottenham's research into social buffering (Gee et al., 2014).

Innovative developments, informed by the reflections of the practitioner and of the family, are an important way of developing DDP.

A practitioner might try a novel approach with a family or may explore blending DDP with another compatible model. They might explore whether a routine piece of work is improved by bringing in a DDP-informed approach. For example, how might life story exploration with a child be received when the practitioner is using DDP principles?

Practitioners who have received DDP training might move into a different service, perinatal care for example, and explore embedding DDP into this care.

At the time of writing, work is happening to increase DDP's relevance to a broader population, including being more inclusive of those from oppressed and marginalized groups. DDP will benefit when DDP practitioners bring their own lived experience to their practice. For example:

- An adoptive DDP practitioner might work in a different and helpful way when supporting an adoptive parent.
- A Black African DDP therapist, who is connected to their African cultural roots, might explore blending DDP with healing practices from within their African traditions.
- A transgender support worker might help parents of a transgender child.

The intersection of gender, sexuality, and race offers a wealth of lived experience that can enrich DDP interventions. DDP interventions will similarly be extended by increasing the number of DDP practitioners who live with disabilities and those who can contribute their unique talents stemming from neurodiversity. Experiences based on class, language, and religious beliefs will all increase the depth of DDP practice.

Disseminating the experience of this innovative practice will encourage other practitioners to innovate, thus building up a range of experience that can inform the development of DDP. With an ever-growing DDP community, we have burgeoning resources to advance this development.

EXPLORING THE POTENTIAL DEVELOPMENT OF DDP THROUGH CONTACT WITH NON-WESTERN COUNTRIES AND/OR POPULATIONS

As DDP expands to an increasing number of countries, there will be opportunities for the growth of DDP to be influenced by cultures, knowledge, and ways of healing from around the world.

Western psychology is dominated by cognitive models and a focus on the mind (Kinouani, 2021). Even with the expanded scope of psychological theory provided by attachment theory, intersubjectivity, and neuroscience, psychology is still underpinned by a largely Western world view. Though informed by Western psychology, DDP embraces emotional experience, engages in affective-reflective conversations, and privileges story. Could it go further through learning from non-Western practitioners and researchers?

Traditional healing practices have much to offer in enhancing DDP interventions. This includes the Indigenous populations of the Americas (including South America and Canada), Africa, Australia, and New Zealand. For example:

- Kinouani (2021) discusses how African cultures have a greater understanding of the body and the impact of movement.
- Atkinson (2022) explores the use of healing circles and the development of communities to support the healing of aborigi-

nal peoples transgenerationally traumatized by colonization and state interventions.

- There are also Eastern traditions that attend to well-being via the body. Yoga, for example, has gained much popularity in Western well-being practice.
- Similarly, Buddhist practices and their influence on mindfulness interventions and compassion-focused approaches (Gilbert, 2009) have encouraged DDP practitioners to consider how these interventions can be incorporated into DDP.

Within DDP, we focus on healing through relationships, something we share with the Indigenous peoples of Canada, the U.S., Australia, and New Zealand. Can we go further by also learning from these peoples' cultural activities and connectedness to country and to the land?

Can we learn more from the healing stories that these Indigenous peoples practice (Atkinson, 2002)? Within DDP, the importance of understanding, witnessing, and retelling stories of experience is an integral part of helping the child to heal. How much can we learn, then, from the depth of experience Indigenous people have in the use of story?

The Australian Aboriginal ceremonial process of *Dadirri* aids deep listening.

> When Dadirri is used within a circle, the circle holds the vulnerability of the person who has suffered the loss in sacred trust; it provides the space for them to be open and revealing of the depth of their pain. This provides the means by which loss can begin to heal as others support them in their grieving. (Atkinson, 2002, p. 203)

Through this process, cultural safety is created and communities are strengthened.

Here is one Aboriginal woman talking about her healing when she participated in a workshop providing such a circle:

> The word healing—it means to me [that] I need to look at all my pain. Feel the pain and release it. Work with it, talk about it and let it go, rather than holding on to it, locking it up inside myself. I need to have a safe place where I can talk about my pain, all the pain that I have had in my life, my drinking in my marriage, my childhood, to be able to sit and feel free enough to talk about it and get it out of me. (Lorna, in Atkinson, 2002, p. 142)

The Western process of DDP could be enhanced by learning from this Aboriginal use of connections and storytelling both with families and with the professional communities supporting the families. As I (Kim) read about *Dadirri*, I reflect on how little I currently extend DDP interventions into communities. Our focus is more on the child, family, and professional network. How much could be gained by also working with the communities within which these families live! For example, foster children live within two communities: that of their foster family and that of their birth family. What scope is there for working with these communities together, reducing the child's experience of confusion and conflict from being caught, as they are, between two worlds and enhancing the ability of the community to support and heal the child?

CONTRIBUTING TO THE DEVELOPMENT OF DDP

We would like to spend some time thinking with you about how we can all contribute to the development of DDP. First some self-reflection to get you thinking.

REFLECTIONS FROM KIM

Kim is white British, descended from many generations of Yorkshire people on her mother's side and from Eastern European Jewish people on her father's side. Kim has a love of story and storytelling, which she suspects has roots in her father's ancestry. She has memories of being told stories by her grandmother and her father. Kim imagines what it was like for her great-grandparents, having to leave their home in Russia to escape persecution, traveling to England, young themselves and with a small child. Did they tell stories to keep the child entertained? Or did fear and worry suppress stories? Kim knows that no stories from this time have come down through the family; an indication perhaps of the power of trauma to disrupt connections built through stories. Perhaps this is one of the things that drew Kim to DDP, the opportunity to help children experience their trauma stories being understood and witnessed so that healing from the trauma could begin. Perhaps this is also why Kim has explored the use of metaphorical story within her practice of DDP both with children and with adults (Golding, 2014; Golding & Jones, 2021).

REFLECTIONS FROM DAN

Dan descended from many generations of Irish on his mother's side and from a mix of Irish, Welsh, and German heritages on his father's side. His mother's mother spoke fondly of the "Irish gift of the gab," which she demonstrated quite regularly. Dan's father was a workman (welder) who worked long hours supporting his large family (seven children). One of his greatest influences on Dan's development was his storytelling. Beginning when Dan was two years old, until he had to work in the evenings, he would make up a story for Dan and his older brother, Jim, every night at bedtime, an activity that made going to bed enjoyable. Dan recalls often falling asleep imagining the events of that night's story.

TIME FOR REFLECTION

We invite you to consider what you can bring to the development of DDP.

1. Reflect on who you are and the intuition, knowledge, and skills that you bring that is linked to your ancestors. In what ways might this influence the way you practice DDP?
2. Consider how we can improve our understanding of how DDP can be applicable to the needs of different populations by learning from each other. How can the richness of DDP be enhanced because of what we all bring?
3. Reflect on how we can learn from each other about the needs of people with disabilities, people across the range

of sexuality and gender, people from different racial groups, people within different age groups and across class and religious backgrounds. Think too about the intersection of these groups and the impact of this extra complexity.

- What experience can we offer about adopting and being adopted, fostering and being fostered, living in and caring for those in residential care?
- How does this intersect with transracial adoption and fostering, same sex parenting and being parented, transgender parenting and being parented, caring for and being cared for when disabled?
- How can all this knowledge impact on the practice of DDP?

4. Consider how this learning can be disseminated.

- How do we tell the stories of what we have learned?
- How do we encourage each other to contribute to reflective articles, books, peer reviewed journals, conferences, podcasts, blogs, and in other ways we haven't yet thought about?

BUILDING AN EVIDENCE BASE

DDP is a complex intervention, as defined by the U.K. guidance for developing and evaluating complex interventions (Skivington et al., 2021).

DEFINITION OF A COMPLEX INTERVENTION

An intervention might be considered complex because of properties of the intervention itself, such as the number of components involved; the range of behaviors targeted; expertise and skills required by those delivering and receiving the intervention; the number of groups, settings, or levels targeted; or the permitted level of flexibility of the intervention or its components (Skivington et al., 2021, p. 2).

The authors suggest that researching the efficacy of such interventions needs to consider the complexity of both the intervention's components and its interaction with the context within which the intervention is being provided. This means an evidence base is not just about the efficacy of the intervention and requires a range of research methods, both qualitative and quantitative.

For intervention research in healthcare and public health settings to take on more challenging evaluation questions, greater priority should be given to mixed method, theory based, or systems evaluations that are sensitive to complexity and that emphasize implementation, context, and system fit (Skivington et al., 2021, p. 5).

An additional challenge for researchers arises because of the difficulties in standardizing DDP as a therapy. Describing a uniform therapy which can be replicated by therapists and researchers is not possible when providing a relational therapy, with every new therapy session emerging out of the relationship between therapist and child/parent.

> The renowned psychotherapist and psychiatrist Irvin Yalom describes that the "very act of standardization renders the therapy less real and less effective" (Yalom, 2002, p. 33). He goes on to describe that: ". . . therapy is spontaneous, the relationship is dynamic and ever evolving, and there is a continuous sequence of experiencing and then examining the process" (Yalom, 2022, p. 34).

Therefore, researchers must apply their research methods to a process within which fidelity is measured against a set of DDP principles, as described in this workbook, and applied by the therapists, within the context of the unique needs of the child and family they are working with.

Developing an evidence base for DDP thus requires:

- understanding the efficacy and effectiveness of the interventions currently used based on the application of the DDP principles to a variety of therapy and nontherapy situations
- exploring how interventions impact the child, family, and the systems that DDP also tries to influence, including schools, social care, health networks, residential organizations, youth support, and youth justice systems

This evidence base is a living, breathing body of work, influencing and being influenced by the continuing practice of DDP and the innovative, imaginative practice that the DDP community of practitioners and families contribute.

To develop an evidence base for DDP, we need research that is imaginative drawing from research methods embedded in Western and non-Western practice. For an example of a non-Western practice, see Judy Atkinson's culturally appropriate research with Indigenous people in Australia, referred to above (Atkinson, 2002).

There are several facets to the work ahead of us:

- We must draw upon both quantitative and qualitative research, relying not only on randomized control trial data but also encompassing smaller scale projects.
    - We must carry out quantitative research that can help us know what is effective.
    - We must develop qualitative studies to enrich our understanding of why.

> Qualitative studies make most use of one of human beings' unique attributes—the use of language (Banister et al., 1997). We can draw on self-reflection, researcher and participant conversations, and group discussions to better understand what works for whom. "It [qualitative research] may be the voice that carries through the sense of the phenomena under investigation, while the quantitative research component circumscribes the scope and extent of the topic" (Banister et al., 1997, p. 15).

- We must include a range of research encompassing outcome studies, service evaluations and audits, single case studies, focus groups, reflections, testimonials, and storytelling. This will allow us to ask a broad range of questions moving beyond "is DDP effective?" to consider how DDP works for whom, how it interacts within the context in which it is implemented, what its impact is at the child, family, and systems level, what its cost effectiveness is, and how best decisions can be made on the interventions needed (Skivington, 2021).

- We must understand what package of DDP interventions are needed for children in the context of their age, family context, identity, and placement stability or instability. Family context includes residential care, and families include birth, kinship, adoption, foster, and respite parents. Family context also includes the racial identity, sexuality, gender, religious affiliation, ability or disability, age, and class of the parent(s). Many children and families are at risk from systems of oppression and thus the intersection of gender, sexuality, race, class, religion, and disability also needs to be considered in understanding how DDP interventions can be most effective.

- We must explore optimum length of interventions, and consider the ratio between parent/child and parent work that is needed. We need to understand what benefits can come from a school supporting the DDP interventions and how a DDP approach can help network members to work together most effectively.

- We must extend beyond DDP as a single intervention to explore how it can be part of a package of interventions to support the family. These might include sensory interventions, relationship focused approaches (such as Theraplay), narrative approaches, parent approaches to manage extreme difficulties (such as nonviolent resistance [NVR] for managing child to parent violence) and adult therapy approaches (such as compassion focused and attachment focused interventions).

Developing an evidence base is a job for all of us. Evaluating DDP interventions on the ground, in real world settings, with user involvement is as important as carefully constructed and resourced research programs.

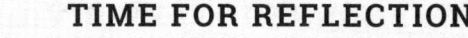

TIME FOR REFLECTION

We invite you to reflect on the DDP interventions you provide for the organizations you work within or for.

1. How can you routinely build in evaluation?
2. What client feedback are you collecting, and how is it used to improve services? How can this be expanded and used to inform the evidence base and to contribute to the continuing development of DDP?
3. How can you extend this to also encompass small scale research projects?
4. Consider how this can influence research methodology. How can you contribute to the development of quantitative and qualitative research methods? What stories can be told? What questions can be asked? What experience can be explored?

DDP AS A CULTURALLY SENSITIVE INTERVENTION

Culturally adapted interventions involve "the systematic modification of evidence-based treatment or intervention protocol to consider language, culture and context in such a way that it is compatible with the client's cultural patterns, meanings and values" (Bernal et al., 2009, p. 362). In the ecological validity model (Bernal et al., 1995), eight dimensions of intervention are suggested: language, persons, metaphors, content, concepts, goals, methods, contexts. These can guide the development of culturally sensitive interventions in collaboration with the community.

WAYS TO ENSURE INTERVENTIONS
ARE CULTURALLY SENSITIVE

- Integrate cultural context into all areas of psychological practice.
- Ensure congruence with client's cultural experience.
- Specifically include cultural values and concepts in the intervention.
- Personalize interventions to needs and context of the individual.
- Match race or ethnicity between client and therapist.
- Use client's preferred language.
- Incorporate cultural world view and values into sessions.
- Agree on intervention goals that the family values.
- Provide cultural sensitivity training.

(after Rathod et al., 2018 and Bernal et al., 2009)

DDP practice needs to be relevant to the cultural, class, and religious backgrounds and the different identities of the diverse populations DDP practitioners work with. We therefore need an evidence base exploring:

- how DDP interventions can be culturally responsive, appropriate, and effective (Rathod et al., 2018)
- how DDP practitioners can be sensitive to difference in terms of sexuality and gender, including the additional struggles that this identity can bring to those who are already impacted by developmental trauma
- the impact of living with neurodiverse talents and disability in a neurotypical and nondisabled world and the intersection of these with trauma

When evidence-based practice relies too much on systematization of intervention protocols, culturally competent practice can be reduced (Bernal et al., 2009).

DDP, a flexible and individualized model of intervention, is well suited to cultural and contextual adaptation. The DDP practitioner has the flexibility to adapt their practice to the needs of the children and families they are working with.

WAYS DDP PRACTITIONERS CAN ADAPT THEIR PRACTICE TO MEET THE NEEDS OF THE FAMILIES FROM NON-WESTERN CULTURES

- In some non-Western cultures, professionals are expected to be directive and prescriptive. For example, being direct with Chinese clients increases the strength of the therapeutic alliance (Guo & Hanley, 2015, cited in Golker & Cioffi, 2021). Perhaps, in DDP interventions, a lead-follow-lead approach might be more helpful than follow-lead-follow.

- Explain interventions using culture-specific language, metaphors, and stories (Hinton & Patel, 2017, cited in Golker & Cioffi, 2021). DDP's storytelling approach helps the practitioner to talk with the families based on an understanding of the families' culture and worldview. This includes adopting cultural and religious ideas to develop cultural common ground with the family (Guo & Hanley, 2015, cited in Golker & Cioffi, 2021).

- DDP already works with family members to support the work with the child. When working with sociocentric cultures, the DDP practitioner might also draw on the families' community as a resource to facilitate therapeutic change (Guo & Hanley, 2015, cited in Golker & Cioffi, 2021).

- Religious diversity can be overlooked in Western cultures dominated by Christianity (Schlosser et al., 2009, cited in Golker & Cioffi, 2021). As the DDP practitioner builds a relationship with the family, understanding religious beliefs will be an important part of establishing safety.

OUTCOME MEASURES

Quantitative research involves collecting and analyzing numerical data through statistical analysis. This relies on outcome measures that can be collected before, during, and after an intervention. More sophisticated studies will also include a follow-up in which the outcome measure is repeated at an interval after the intervention is ended. Comparison groups can help us to have confidence that any changes we see are related to the intervention. For example, a waiting list control group can complete the same outcome measures at two intervals while waiting for a service. The randomized control trial, as reflected in the RIGHT trial, is the most rigorous and expensive method of collecting quantitative data.

There are a range of outcome measures that clinicians can use in their services. Some of these lend themselves to routine evaluation with all families, while others are more likely to be incorporated within a research project. This represents a greater burden on families who are being asked to complete the measures, and therefore clinicians have an ethical responsibility to inform and support the families with this process.

Further discussion about potential outcome measures can be found in the article "Measurement in DDP guidance and recommended measures," available on the DDP website (see https://ddpnetwork.org/backend/wp-content/uploads/2017/05/Measurement-in-DDP-Guidance-and-recommended-measures-April-2017.pdf).

TIME FOR REFLECTION

We invite you to reflect on the many ways you are and could be increasing your understanding of what works for whom and within which contexts where DDP interventions are being provided.

Reflect on ways that this developing awareness can be disseminated within the DDP community.

CONCLUSION

An enriched evidence base keeps a model alive and developing. There are many ways that DDP practitioners can contribute to the evidence base, even with little research experience. The combination of research projects, large and small, with practitioner and family experiences of DDP interventions will bring a much-needed depth to the evidence base for the complex intervention that is DDP.

LIST OF RESOURCES

EDUCATION

Bomber, L. M., & Hughes, D. A. (2013). *Settling to learn: Settling troubled pupils to learn: why relationships matter in school.* Worth Publishing Ltd.

Golding, K. S., Phillips, S., & Bombèr, L. M. (2021). *Working with relational trauma in schools: An educator's guide to using dyadic developmental practice.* Jessica Kingsley Publishers.

Phillips S., Melim, D., & Hughes, D. A. (2020). *Belonging: A dyadic developmental practice framework for trauma-informed education.* Rowman & Littlefield.

Trauma informed education website: https://traumainformededucation.org.uk/

PARENTING

Elliott, A. (2013). *Why can't my child behave? Empathic parenting strategies that work for adoptive and foster families.* Jessica Kingsley Publishers.

Elliott, A. (2021). *Superparenting! Boost your therapeutic parenting through ten transformative steps.* Jessica Kingsley Publishers.

Golding, K. S. (2014). *Nurturing attachments training resource running parenting groups for adoptive parents and foster or kinship carers.* Jessica Kingsley Publishers.

Golding, K. S. (2017). *Everyday parenting with security and love: Using PACE to provide Foundations for Attachment.* Jessica Kingsley Publishers.

Golding, K. S. (2017). *Foundations for attachment training resource: The six-session programme for parents of traumatized children.* Jessica Kingsley Publishers.

Golding, K. S., & Hughes, D. A. (2012). *Creating loving attachments.* Jessica Kingsley Publishers.

Hughes, D. A. (2009). Attachment-focused parenting. W. W. Norton & Company.

Page, D., & Swann R. (2021). *Therapeutic parenting with PACE: An attachment, trauma and DDP informed group programme and training resource.* Pavilion Publishing and Media Ltd.

RESIDENTIAL CARE

Grant, E., Thompson, G., & Golding, K. S. (in press). *Working with relational trauma in children's residential care: A guide to using dyadic developmental.* Jessica Kingsley Publishers.

SOCIAL CARE

Keith, A., & Lister., A. (in press). *Working with relational trauma in children's social care: a guide to using dyadic developmental practice.* Jessica Kingsley Publishers.

TRAUMA-INFORMED ORGANIZATIONS

Treisman, K. (2021). A treasure box for creating trauma-informed organizations, Vols. 1 & 2. Jessica Kingsley Publishers.

REFERENCES

Allen, M. (n.d.) Retrieved April 26, 2023, from https://www.familyfutures.co.uk/product/attachment-developmental-trauma-and-executive-functioning-difficulties-in-the-school-setting-handbook/

Alper, J. (Ed). (2019). *Supporting birth parents whose children have been adopted.* Jessica Kingsley Publishers.

Arnett, J. J. (2008). The neglected 95%: Why American psychology needs to become less American. *American Psychologist, 63,* 602–614.

Atkinson, J. (2002). *Trauma trails, recreating song lines: The transgenerational effects of trauma in indigenous Australia.* Spinifex Press.

Banister, P., Burman, E., Parker, I., Taylor, M., & Tindall, C. (1997). *Qualitative methods in psychology: A research guide.* Open University Press.

Baylin, J., & Hughes, D. A. (2016). *The neurobiology of attachment-focused therapy: Enhancing connection and trust in the treatment of children and adolescents.* W. W. Norton & Company.

Bernal, G. Bonilla, J., & Bellido, C. (1995). Ecological validity and cultural sensitivity for outcome research: issues for the cultural adaptation and development of psychosocial treatments with Hispanics. *Journal of Abnormal Child Psychology 23,* 67–82.

Bernal, G., Jiménez-Chafey, M. I., & Domenech Rodriguez, M. M. (2009). Cultural adaptation of treatments: A resource for considering culture in evidence-based practice. *Professional Psychology: Research and Practice, 40*(4), 361–168.

Dana, D. (2018). *The Polyvagal Theory in Therapy: Engaging the rhythm of regulation.* Norton.

Dent, H. R., & Golding, K. S. (2006). Engaging the Network. Consultation for looked after and adopted children. In K. S. Golding, H. R. Dent, R. Nissim, & E. Stott (Eds.), *Thinking psychologically about children who are looked after and adopted: Space for reflection* (3rd ed., Vol. 47, pp. 265–284). John Wiley & Sons Ltd.

Downs, A. (2012). *The velvet rage: Overcoming the pain of growing up gay in a straight man's world.* Go Hachette Books.

Gee, D. G., Gabard-Durnam, L., Telzer, E. H., Humphreys, L., Goff, B., Shapiro, M., Flannery, J.; Lumian, D. S.; Fareri, D.S.; Caldera, C.; & Tottenham, N. (2014). Maternal buffering of human amygdala-prefrontal circuitry during childhood but not during adolescence. *Psychological Sciences, 25*(11), 2067–2078.

Gilbert, P. (2009). *The compassionate mind.* Constable.

Golding, K. S. (2011). Exploration and integration: When present and past meet. In A. Becker-Weidman (Ed), *The dyadic developmental psychotherapy casebook* (3rd ed., Vol. 47, pp. 265–284). Jason Aronson Inc.

Golding, K. S. (2014). *Using stories to build bridges with traumatized children: Creative ideas for therapy, life story work, direct work, and parenting.* Jessica Kingsley Publishers.

Golding, K. S., & Gould, J. (2019). "No quick fix": The benefits of longer-term counselling for birth parents with complex histories of trauma and abuse. Carrie's story. In J. Alper (Ed.) *Supporting birth parents whose children have been adopted* (3rd ed., Vol. 47, pp. 265–284). Jessica Kingsley Publishers.

Golding, K. S., & Jones A. (2021). *A tiny spark of hope: Healing childhood trauma in adulthood.* Jessica Kingsley Publishers.

Golker, C., & Cioffi, M. (2021). Cultural adaptations of cognitive behaviour therapy for the Orthodox Jewish community: a qualitative study of therapists' perspectives. *The Cognitive Behaviour Therapist, 14*, E3. https://doi.org/10.1017/S1754470X20000616

Haenga-Collins, M., & Gibbs, A. (2015). "Walking between worlds": The experience of New Zealand Māori cross-cultural adoptees. *Adoption & Fostering, 39*(1), 62–75.

Harwood, R. L., Miller, J. G., & Irizarry, N. L. (1995). *Culture and attachment: Perceptions of the child in context.* The Guilford Press.

Henrich, J., Heine, S. J., & Norenzayan, A. (2010). Most people are not WEIRD. *Nature, 466*(7302), 29.

Henrich, J. (2021). *The weirdest people in the world: How the West became psychologically peculiar and particularly prosperous.* Penguin Random House.

Hughes, D. A., & Baylin, J. (2012). *Brain-based parenting.* Norton.

Hughes, D. A., Golding, K. S., & Hudson, J. (2019). *Healing relational trauma with attachment-focused interventions.* Norton.

Keller, H. (2017). Culture and development: A systematic relationship. *Perspective on Psychological Science, 12*(5), 833–840.

Keller, H. (2022). *The myth of attachment theory: A critical understanding for multicultural societies.* Routledge.

Kinouani, G. (2021). *Living while Black: The essential guide to overcoming racial trauma.* Penguin Random House.

Lancy, D. F. (2017). *Raising children: Surprising insights from other cultures.* Cambridge University Press.

Lloyd, S. (2020). *Building sensorimotor systems in children with developmental trauma: A model for practice.* Jessica Kingsley Publishers.

Norris, V., & Rodwell, H. (2017). *Parenting with Theraplay®: Understanding attachment and how to nurture a closer relationship with your child.* Jessica Kingsley Publishers.

Menakem, R. (2021). *My grandmother's hands: Racialized trauma and the pathway to mending our hearts and bodies* (U.K. edition). Penguin Random House (first published in USA by Central Recovery Press 2017).

Norcross J. C., & Wampold, B. E. (2011). Evidence-based therapy relationships: Research conclusions and clinical practices. *Psychotherapy, 48*(1), 98–102.

Nouwen, H. J. M. (2017). *You are the beloved.* Hodder & Stoughton.

Porges, S. (2011). *The polyvagal theory.* Norton.

Porges, S. W. (2017). *The pocket guide to the polyvagal theory: The transformative power of feeling safe.* Norton.

Rathod, S., Gega, L., Degnan, A., Pikard, J., Khan, T., Husain, N.. Munshi, T., & Naeem, F. (2018). The current status of culturally adapted mental health interventions: a practice-focused review of meta-analyses. *Neuropsychiatric Disease and Treatment, 14,* 165–178.

Ryan, F. (2011). Kanyininpa (Holding): A way of nurturing children in aboriginal Australia. Australian Social Work: Vol 64, No 2 (tandfonline.com).

Siegel, D. J. (2020). *The developing mind* (3rd ed). The Guilford Press.

Siegel, D., & Hartzell, M. (2003). Parenting from the inside out: How a deeper self-understanding can help you raise children who thrive.

Sissy, L. (2020). *My name is why.* Canongate books.

Sjöblom, L. W-R. (2019). *Palimpsest: Documents from a Korean adoption.* Drawn & Quarterly.

Skivington, K., Matthews, L., Simpson, S. A., Craig, P., Baird, J., Blazeby, J. M.; Boyd, K. A.; Craig, N.; French, D. P.; McIntosh, E.; Petticrew, M.; Rycroft-Malone, J.; White, M.; & Moore, L. (2021). A new framework for developing and evaluating complex interventions: Update of Medical Research Council guidance. *British Medical Journal,* 374. http://dx.doi.org/10.1136/bmj.n2061

Sprince, J. (2002). Developing containment. Psychoanalytic consultancy to a therapeutic community for traumatised children. *Journal of Child Psychotherapy, 28*(2), 147–161.

Sprince, J. (2005, Mar 1). *Towards an integrated network. A psychoanalytic perspective on consultation* [Paper presentation]. 7th Annual Fostering & Adoption Conference, Bristol, U.K.

Van der Kolk, B. (2005). Developmental trauma disorder: Toward a rational diagnosis for children with complex trauma histories. *Psychiatric Annals, 35*(5), 401–408.

Yalom, I. D. (2002). *The gift of therapy: An open letter to a new generation of therapists and their patients.* Piatkus Books Ltd.

INDEX

Note: Italicized page locators refer to figures; tables are noted with *t*.

ABOUT THE AUTHORS

Daniel A. Hughes, PhD, is a clinical psychologist who founded and developed dyadic developmental psychotherapy (DDP). For over 20 years, he has conducted seminars and workshops, and has spoken at conferences throughout the U.S., Europe, Canada, and Australia. He is also the founder of DDPI, a training institute responsible for the certification of professionals in DDP, engaging in extensive training and supervision of therapists being certified in his treatment model, in addition to conducting ongoing consultations with various agencies and professionals. Dan is the author and coauthor of many books and articles including *Building the Bonds of Attachment,* 3rd ed. (2017), *Brain-Based Parenting* (2012), *The Neurobiology of Attachment-Focused Therapy* (2016), *Healing Relational Trauma with Attachment-Focused Interventions* (2019) and *The Little Book of Attachment* (2020). Dan can be found online at www.danielhughes.org.

Kim S. Golding, PhD, is a clinical psychologist living in the U.K. Kim has always been interested in collaborating with parents and carers to develop their parenting skills tailored to the particular needs of the children and young people they are caring for. She is a consultant and trainer in DDP and provides training, consultation, and supervision to a range of individuals and teams. Kim is the author of several books written for parents, educational staff, and practitioners supporting children and families with experience of developmental trauma. In 2020, Kim was honored with a CBE for her work.